MANUAL OF SCLEROTHERAPY

MANUAL OF SCLEROTHERAPY

Neil S. Sadick, M.D.
Associate Clinical Professor
New York University Hospital
Cornell University
New York, New York

LIPPINCOTT WILLIAMS & WILKINS
A **Wolters Kluwer** Company
Philadelphia • Baltimore • New York • London
Buenos Aires • Hong Kong • Sydney • Tokyo

Acquisitions Editor: Beth Barry
Developmental Editors: Glenda Insua and Carol Field
Production Editor: Jonathan Geffner
Manufacturing Manager: Tim Reynolds
Cover Designer: Mark Lerner
Compositor: Maryland Composition

227 East Washington Square
Philadelphia, PA 19106-3780 USA
LWW.com

Printed and bound in China

Library of Congress Cataloging-in-Publication Data

Sadick, Neil S.
Manual of sclerotherapy/Neil S. Sadick.
p. cm.
Includes bibliographical references and index.
ISBN 0-397-51742-4
1. Varicose veins—Treatment Handbooks, manuals, etc.
2. Injections, Sclerosing Handbooks, manuals, etc. I. Title.
[DNLM: 1. Varicose Veins—therapy. 2. Sclerosing Solutions.
3. Sclerotherapy—methods. 4 Telangiectasis—therapy. WG 620
S125m 2000]
RC695.S14 2000
616. 1′4306—dc21
DNLM/DLC
for Library of Congress 99-16112
CIP

---

10 9 8 7 6 5 4 3 2 1

CONTENTS

PREFACE

Varicose veins have existed ever since human beings assumed an upright posture—that is, when gravity took on the role of inhibiting venous return from the extremities. The oldest record of venous disease was found on a religious tablet dedicated to the gods by a citizen of ancient Greece in the hope of healing a case of disabling varices.

Until the end of the eighteenth century, varicose veins were considered a local disease and were cauterized. Their relationship with the circulatory system was only suspected.

After the Second World War, the stripper invented by Babcock in 1907 was formally introduced on a large scale and surgery for varicose veins reached a new impetus. Heated debates over surgical and medical interventions reached maximal intensity over the next two decades, with a more generally accepted consensus on therapeutic principles emerging over the past decade.

Important historical leaders in the field of phlebology have included the following:

- *Fabricus of Aquapendente.* Circa 1584, Fabricius discovered the venous valves, recognized their critical role in the circulation, and laid the foundation of our knowledge of the venous system.
- *Tomasso Rima.* In the late 1700s, this Swiss surgeon recognized the crucial role of venous reflux at the level of the saphenofemoral junction in the pathogenesis of truncal varicosities, deducing that the logical treatment of this disorder should be high ligation of the saphenous vein.
- *Charles Gabriel Pravoz.* This French surgeon attempted to thrombose arterial aneurysms in 1851, using an injection syringe and the first sterile needles.

- ▶ *Delore.* In 1896, Delore postulated that, for lasting effects, a sclerosant must lead not only to thrombus formation but also to the production of venous endothelial damage.
- ▶ *Fredrich Trendelenburg.* Trendelenburg described the diagnostic test that bears his name and also helped to popularize the practice of high ligation of the greater saphenous vein.
- ▶ *Paul Linser.* During World War I, Linser popularized the injection of lower extremity varicosities. At first he injected sublimate and later hypertonic saline. He is known as a co-father of sclerotherapy.
- ▶ *Jean Sicard.* This French phlebologist began injecting at the same time hypertonic sodium salicylate solution for treatment of lower extremity varicose veins. He is known, along with Linser, as a co-father of sclerotherapy.
- ▶ *Raymond Tournay.* Having refined the technique of and indications for sclerotherapy, he was the first to employ puncture incisions for the treatment of intravascular clots. Tournay developed a school of sclerotherapy and wrote the treatise *La sclerose des varices.*
- ▶ *Karl Sigg.* This German sclerotherapist advocated widespread treatment of large varicose veins by means of sclerotherapy. His major treatise is entitled *Varicose Veins, Lower Extremity Ulcers and Thrombosis.*
- ▶ *William Foley.* In the 1950s, Foley popularized the technique of sclerotherapy in the United States. He employed "Heparasol," a heparin–hypertonic saline compound.
- ▶ *Robert Muller.* This Swiss dermatologist, in the 1950s, described a technique for varicose vein avulsion through multiple stab incisions. He called it *la phlebectomie ambulatoire.*
- ▶ *Mitchell Goldman.* An American phlebologist who helped to make sclerotherapy a science in the United States. Goldman wrote a text entitled *Sclerotherapy Treatment of Varicose and Telangiectatic Leg Veins.* This became the standard text used by those who were learning the technique in this country. In 1994, he described the utilization of a noncoherent light source or "Photoderm" for the treatment of small-diameter veins.

The treatment of cosmetic and symptomatic varicose vein disease has evolved into an field of specialization unto itself. In order to understand the various techniques employed in the treatment of venous disease, we must have an understanding of the anatomy and pathophysiology of the superficial and deep venous systems.

The present text provides the clinical phlebologist with such a background. It includes a detailed discussion of practical phlebology, beginning with patient evaluation, indications for vascular testing, and clinical approaches to the treatment of veins of varying size.

A complete review of sclerosing agents, technique modifications, and therapeutic approaches equips the reader with the tools to treat all types of venous problems, from cosmetic telangiectasis and reticular veins to truncal varicosities, perforating veins, and axial venous incompetence.

The manual continues with a thorough discussion of complications encountered in sclerotherapy practice to aid in understanding, minimizing, and managing them appropriately.

The final chapter is devoted to new technologies for treating venous problems, including laser and flash-lamp technology, ambulatory phlebectomy, echosclerotherapy, and endovascular vein obliteration.

It is hoped that this book will take the reader to a higher level of sophistication in managing his or her patients with venous pathology. It presents a simple, clinically oriented, practical approach that will enable phlebologists to incorporate the information it offers into their daily practice.

As we approach the millennium, the information provided in this text will bridge the gap between traditional sclerotherapy and the phlebology of the future.

Neil S. Sadick, M.D.

ACKNOWLEDGMENTS

I would like to acknowledge the late William Foley, M.D., my first teacher, who evoked my interest in the field of phlebology; as well as my wife, Amy, and my daughter, Sydney, whose inspiration enabled this text to come to fruition.

CHAPTER 1

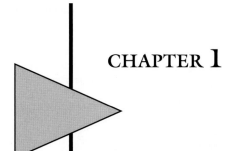

INTRODUCTION TO THE VENOUS SYSTEM

Varicose veins and the small-vessel proliferative ectasias known as *telangiectasias* (commonly referred to as "spider veins") are common problems that not only affect one's appearance but may also affect quality of life and, in their most extreme presentations, lead to disabling sequelae such as thrombophlebitis, ulceration, stasis dermatitis, hyperpigmentation, refractory edema, and lipodermatosclerosis. In many patients, these symptoms may be severe enough to curtail or limit work or leisure activities. However, as we approach the twenty-first century, there are multiple sclerotherapeutic, surgical, laser, and broad flash-lamp light sources that are helpful in treating venous disease and are the focus of this practical guide. In order to institute these therapeutic options, one must have a thorough understanding of the anatomy and pathophysiology of the venous system, which is the subject of the present chapter.

Anatomic Considerations

The venous system of the legs is divided into two channels. The first is the deep venous system, consisting of the veins that lie within the muscular system. The second consists of superficial veins distributed outside of the muscular compartment. These two channels run parallel with the long axis of the lower extremities and are connected or have interfascial connections through a number of perforating veins (Fig. 1-1).

Approximately 90% of venous blood leaves the legs by the deep veins through the action of muscular compression. This system of retrograde blood flow is termed the *calf-muscle pump,* or *peripheral heart.* Thus there exists an orderly drainage pathway of the venous system where superficial cutaneous veins drain into superficial large veins, which are external to the muscular fascia. Subsequently

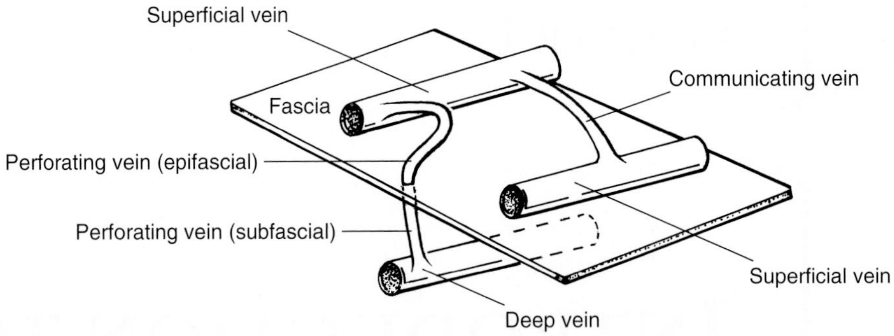

Figure 1-1

Diagram of the venous system. The superficial venous system is connected to the deep venous system (subfascial) by a number of connecting (epifascial) conduits called *perforating veins.*

the deeper veins drain the superficial venous system via the fascial perforating veins or via the major communicating veins of the superficial venous system, the greater or lesser saphenous veins (Fig. 1-2). The alternative pathways of venous outflow are summarized as follows:

1. Subcutaneous veins → long/short saphenous vein → saphenofemoral/popliteal junction → deep venous system
2. Subcutaneous veins → long/short saphenous veins → perforators → deep venous system
3. Subcutaneous veins → perforators → deep venous system
4. Subcutaneous veins → "alternative pathways"—i.e., sciatic drainage (posterior thigh), lateral subdermal drainage (lateral thigh) → pelvic veins.

Deep Venous System

The deep venous system (Fig. 1-3) begins with three paired veins, the anterior and posterior tibial and the peroneal veins at the level of the lower leg, which join to form the popliteal vein, usually at the level of the knee joint. As one moves toward the thigh, the popliteal vein courses proximally into the superficial femoral vein. After it is joined by the deep femoral vein, it becomes the common femoral vein (CFV). Subsequently, as the CFV passes beneath the inguinal ligament, it becomes the external iliac vein, which is joined by the internal iliac vein to become the common iliac vein. This then empties into the inferior vena cava (IVC).

Superficial Venous System

The major conduits of the superficial venous system (Fig. 1.4a and 1.4b) are the long saphenous vein (LSV) and the short saphenous vein (SSV). These are the major pathways connecting the superficial and deep venous systems. The long LSV begins in the foot with the medial dorsal arch veins and runs superiorly, in front

Figure 1-2

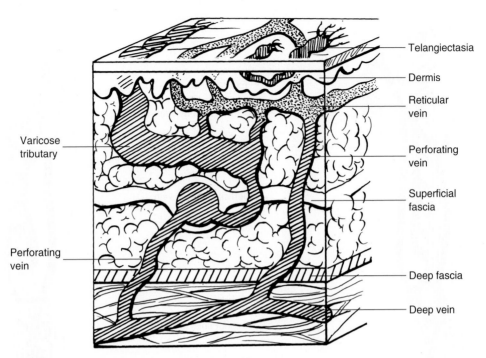

Anatomic representation of the venous system. The deep venous system drains the superficial venous system, which, in turn, is fed from the skin surface by telangiectasias in the dermis, which drain via reticular veins into the larger venous channels located in the reticular dermis and subcutaneous compartments.

of the medial malleolus and behind the femoral condyle, to empty into the femoral vein at the saphenofemoral junction (SFJ), which is normally located two finger-breadths below the anterior superior iliac spine at the fossa ovalis. Up to 25% of individuals may have variations of this anatomic location or may have accessory saphenous veins, which may lead to variance in this important anatomic anastomotic landmark. At the SFJ, the LSV is joined by the superficial circumflex iliac, superficial inferior epigastric, and superficial external pudendal veins as well as other unnamed veins before entering the fossa ovalis. The LSV receives several important tributaries as it ascends the leg, including the anterior superficial tibial and posterior arch veins in the calf and the anterolateral and posteromedial superficial veins in the thigh.

The other major drainage conduit of the superficial venous system is the SSV. It begins in the foot along the lateral malleolus with the dorsal venous arch vein and then traverses superficially along the contour of the calf upward and medially. In approximately 60% of patients, it joins the popliteal vein within 8 cm of the knee joint. Other sites of termination vary and include an anastomosis more than 8 cm above the knee as well as drainage into the LSV via the oblique arch vein (the Giacomini vein) in the superficial thigh, into the superficial or deep femoral veins, or into tributaries of the internal iliac veins.

Other important superficial veins serve as anatomic landmarks in evaluating the patient with venous disease (Table 1-1). These include:

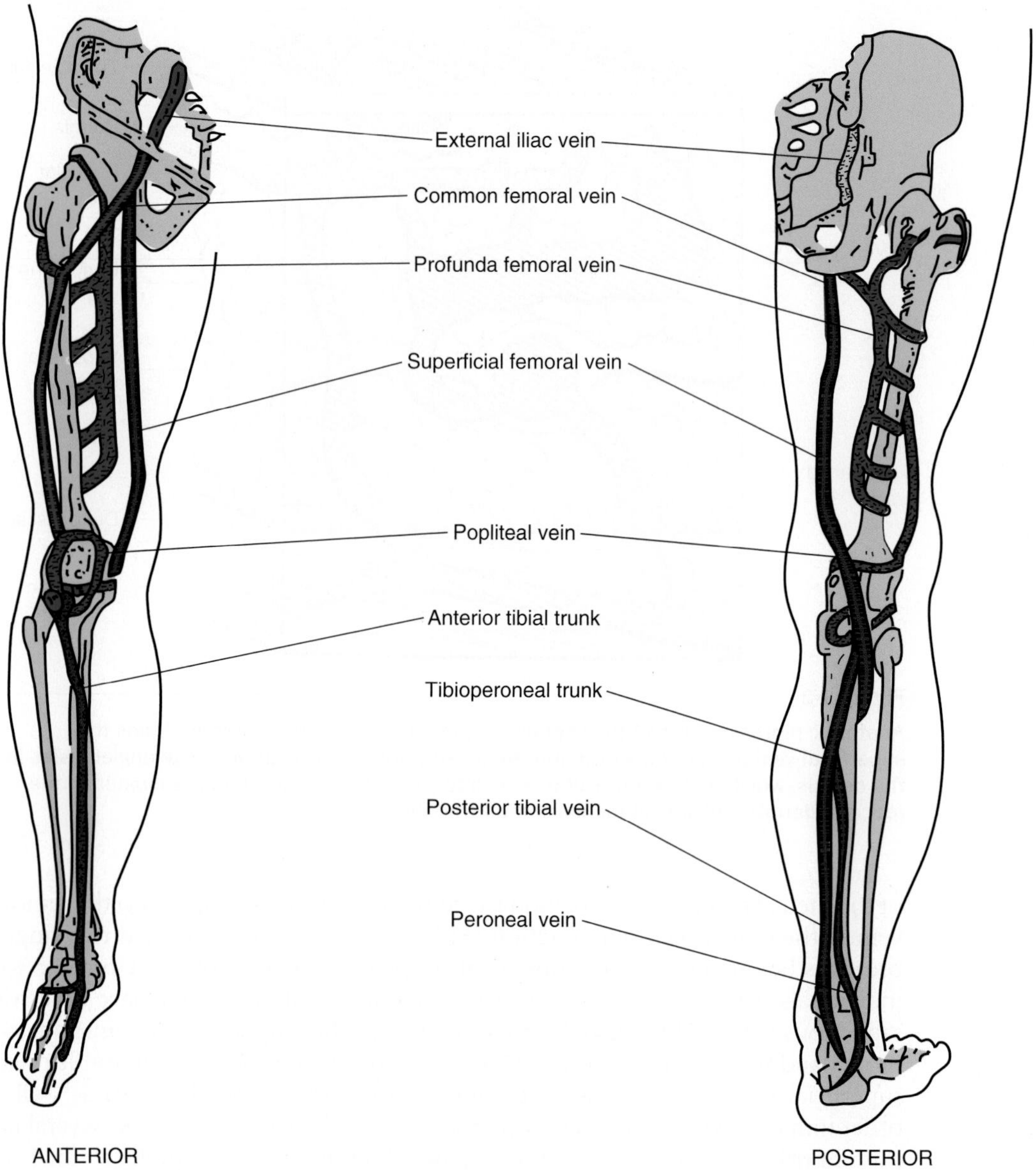

Figure 1-3

Deep venous system. The major drainage vessels below the knee is the popliteal vein, while the femoral vein is the major portal of drainage in the inguinal area of the groin (long saphenous distribution).

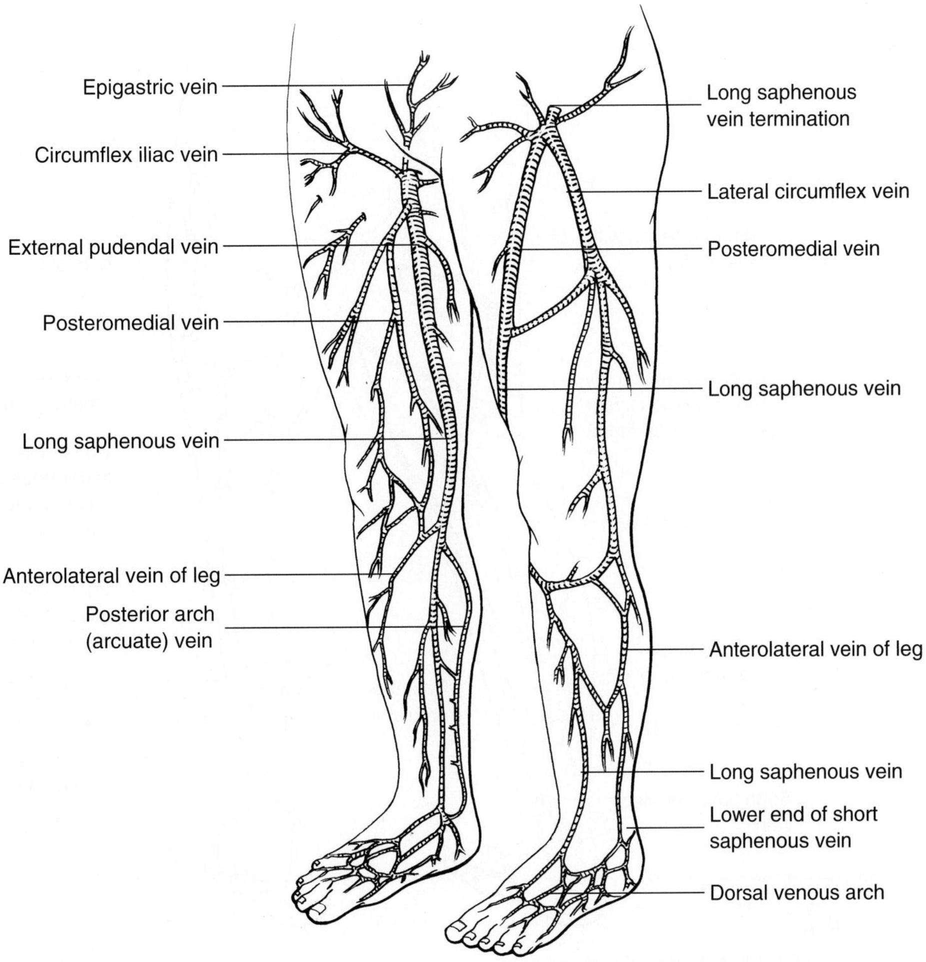

Figure 1-4

Superficial venous system: (A) anterior and (B) posterior distribution of the major axial trunks of the superficial venous system, the greater and lesser saphenous veins, and associated tributaries. ***(continued)***

1. The accessory saphenous vein, which, when present, runs from the lateral knee to the saphenofemoral junction.
2. The anterior crural veins, which traverse the lower calf to the medial knee.
3. The infragenicular veins, which provide drainage around the knee.
4. The lateral subdermal system (Albanese veins). These fetal remnants are commonly located on the lateral thigh and lateral calf. They are often noted in association with eruptive telangiectasis in these areas and serve as the "high pressure" feeding vessels to the smaller telangiectatic vessels.

In addition to the aforementioned veins, the superficial vasculature is composed of multiple connecting reticular veins that bridge surface reticular telangiectasia with underlying larger superficial vessels. In the setting of high-pressure deep venous reflux, these veins may appear varicose in nature.

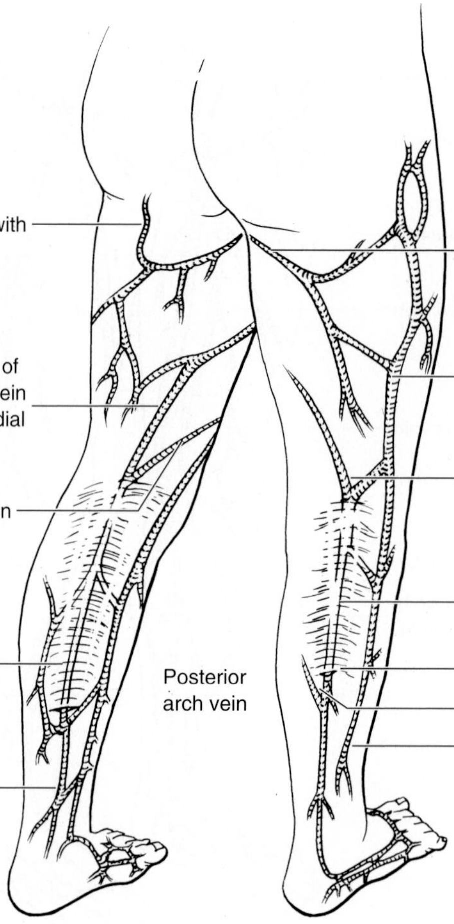

Figure 1-4 (Continued)

Communicating (Perforating) Venous System

Perforating communicating veins (Fig. 1-5) are the "connectors" between the superficial and deep venous systems. Perforating veins may be "direct," in which case the communication is from the LSV or SSV or a tributary to the deep vein, or "indirect," in which case the communication is through one of the muscular sinusoidal channels. The direct perforating veins are thought to be more constant in position and hemodynamically more important than indirect veins. There are more than 100 perforating veins in each leg, the majority of which are located below the knee. Valvular orientation directs the blood from superficial to deep through these veins except in the foot, where the perforating veins have no valves. Although most veins are unnamed, there are several perforating veins that take on anatomic importance in approaching the patient for possible sclerotherapy and/or surgical treatment.

1. *Thigh perforators.* Hunterian perforators, located in the midthigh. These are common causes of medial thigh varicose veins in patients with a competent SFJ. In addition, these perforators may be unaffected by vein

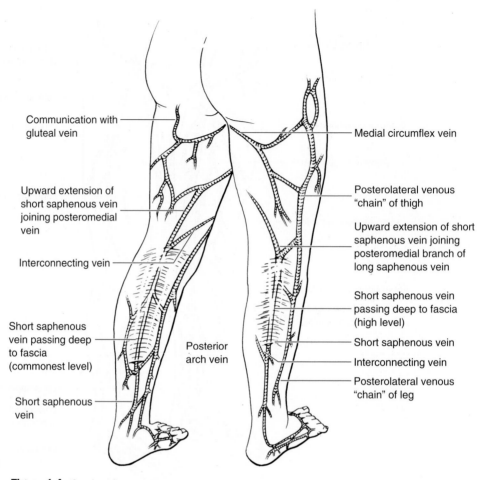

TABLE 1-1. ANATOMIC CLASSIFICATION OF VENOUS STRUCTURES

Superficial veins
Telangiectases/reticular veins
Greater (long) saphenous (GSV)
above knee
below knee
Lesser (short) saphenous (LSV)
Nonsaphenous
Deep veins
Inferior vena cava
Iliac
common
internal
external
Pelvic—gonadal, broad-ligament, other
Femoral
common
deep
superficial
Popliteal
Crural—Anterior tibial, posterior tibial, peroneal (all paired)
Muscular—gastrocnemial, soleal, other
Perforating veins
Thigh
Calf

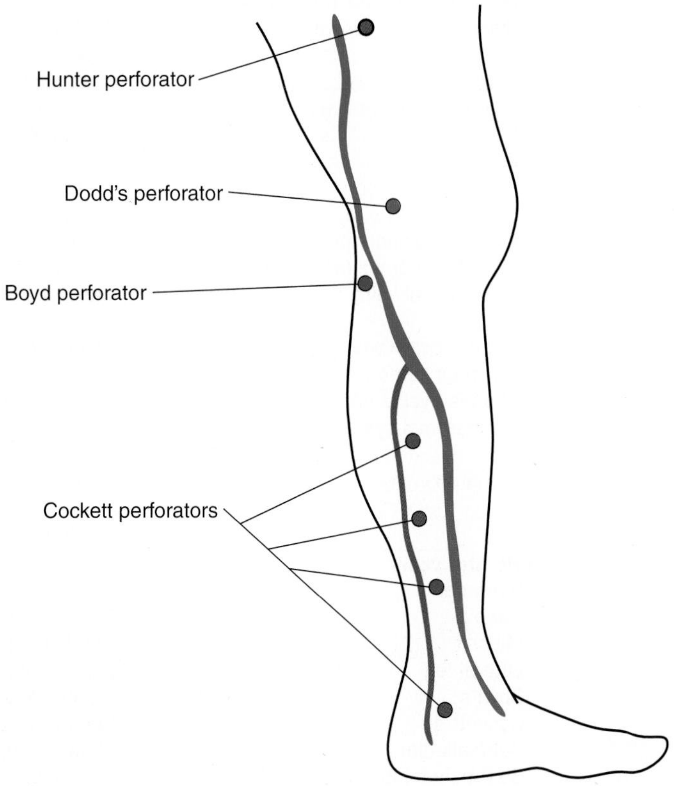

Figure 1-5

Perforating (communicating) veins of major importance commonly associated with truncal varicosities of the lower extremity.

stripping and are thus a common source of postoperative recurrence. There are also Dodd's perforators, located in the distal thigh.

2. *Knee perforators.* Boyd's perforators, located along the medial knee and anteromedial calf. These vessels connect the LSV to the crural veins. They are the most common site for the development of primary varicose veins.
3. *Leg/ankle perforators.* Cockett's perforators, located along the medial aspect of the calf, and the submalleolar vein, on the medial aspect of the ankle. These perforators are important in the pathophysiology of venous ulcers in this anatomic region. An anatomic classification of superficial and deep veins is presented in Table 1-1.

Anatomic Warning Zones

At all locations, veins lie in proximal association with the arteries and nerves. During sclerotherapy and surgical procedures such as ligation/stripping, endoscopic fulguration/resection, or ambulatory phlebectomy, these anatomic considerations must be kept in mind. A summary of important axial and communicating (perforating) venous landmarks is presented in Table 1-2.

TABLE 1-2. ANATOMIC VENOUS LANDMARKS OF IMPORTANCE

Name	Location
Axial veins and their tributaries	
Greater saphenous vein	Dorsum of the foot → medial malleolus → medial calf → popliteal space → medial thigh → groin → terminates in the femoral veins
Lesser saphenous vein	Lateral aspect of the foot → dorsal venous arch → lateral malleolus → midline of calf → popliteal fossae → popliteal vein (may penetrate the deep fascia) at any point from the middle third of the calf upward
Accessory saphenous vein	Lateral knee → saphenofemoral junction
Vein of Giacomini (ascending superficial vein)	Popliteal fossa—connects the lesser saphenous vein to the greater saphenous vein on the upper thigh
Anterior crural veins	Low lateral calf → medial knee
Genicular vein	Drains the skin around the knee
Albanese veins (lateral subdermal system)	Arise from the infragenicular and paraperoneal veins. (produce telangiectatic flares in the lateral thigh and calf)
Leonardo vein	Medial leg lies posterior and parallel to the lesser saphenous vein, connects to the posterior tibial vein via Cockett's perforators
Perforator veins	
Hunterian	Proximal to medial midthigh
Dodd's	Medial distal thigh, 2–6 cm above knee joint
Midcalf	Soles and gastrocnemius zones
Lateral leg	Lateral leg, 4 cm above to 6 cm below knee joint
Boyd's	Medial, 4–10 cm below knee
Cockett's	Medial, 7, 12, and 18 cm above medial malleolus
Submalleolar	Medial, retromalleolar
Gastrocnemius	Posterior, 5 and 12 cm above os calcis

In performing these procedures, caution zones involving the *nerves* include the following:

1. The saphenous nerve, which courses along with the LSV. Vulnerable areas of injury include (a) the knee where it emerges from the substorial canal and (b) the medial dorsal aspect of the foot where it lies alongside or adherent to the saphenous vein.
2. The sural nerve, which may be damaged when sclerosant is injected into the dorsal foot.

Caution zones involving the *arteries:*

1. The superficial external pudendal artery, which lies in close proximity to the LSV and the SFJ and may be inadvertently cannulated with injections at this site or injured with surgical ligation of the LSV at this junctional landmark.
2. The gastrocnemius artery, which may be injured with sclerotherapy of the LSV or SSV within the calf.
3. The lesser saphenous artery, which may be injured by sclerotherapy in the calf of the associated SSV.
4. The perforating arteries/nerves, which lie in close proximity to the perforating veins and may be injured when associated veins are injected by sclerotherapy techniques.

Structural Components of the Venous System

Vein Wall Components

Veins are made up of three basic components (Figure 1-6):

1. Adventitia—composed of smooth muscle fibers and collagen. Nutrition to veins is provided by the vasa vasorum, which are arteriovenous connections located in the blood vessel wall.
2. Media—composed primarily of myocytes aggregated into three muscular layers. At this level as well, one may notice bundles of organized collagen fibers as well as aggregates of elastic fibers.
3. Intima—composed of intricately organized elastic fibers and a layer of endothelial cells.

The venule is the first part of the venous system serving as a conduit for capillaries, the major linkage between the arterial and venous circulation. Capillaries average from 20 to 40 μm in the upper dermis to 200 to 400 μm in the deeper dermis and subcutaneous tissue. Above this size they become more clearly defined as class I or II venulectasia, with corresponding enlargement of the media and adventitial collagenomuscular layers.

The smaller postcapillary venules then drain into collecting veins in the deeper dermis. These veins evolve a more continuous muscular coating.

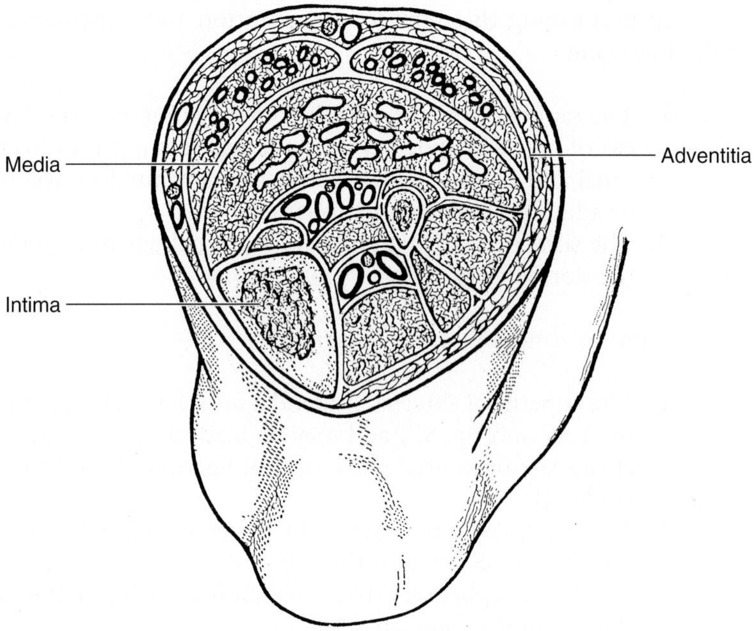

Figure 1-6

Veins are made up of three major components: adventitia, composed of smooth muscle and collagen; media, composed of myocytes; and intima, composed of elastic fibers and endothelial cells.

Clinically apparent telangiectasias are dilated vessels in the superficial dermis usually lined by a single endothelial cell layer and thin muscular and adventitial components. These bluish to red telangiectasias are most likely dilated venules that serve as connecting tributaries to larger veins of the lower extremities.

Valves

One-way valves are located in the deep venous system, the saphenous vein system (superficial venous system), and the communicating perforator veins. Valves assure that venous blood flows from the superficial venous system into the deep venous system (via the calf muscle pump) and then proximally toward the heart (Fig. 1-7). Venous valves are composed of a thin layer of collagen and variable amounts of smooth muscle covered on both surfaces by endothelium. These relatively avascular structures contain free-moving cusps that assist in preventing bidirectional flow.

Valves in the proximal LSV and SSV prevent reflux from the deep to the superficial veins. As previously stated, venous blood may also travel from the superficial to deep veins via communicating perforating veins. These veins also have valves that prevent reflux from the deep to the superficial system except in the foot, where blood may flow in either direction. The valves of these perforators are located subfascially.

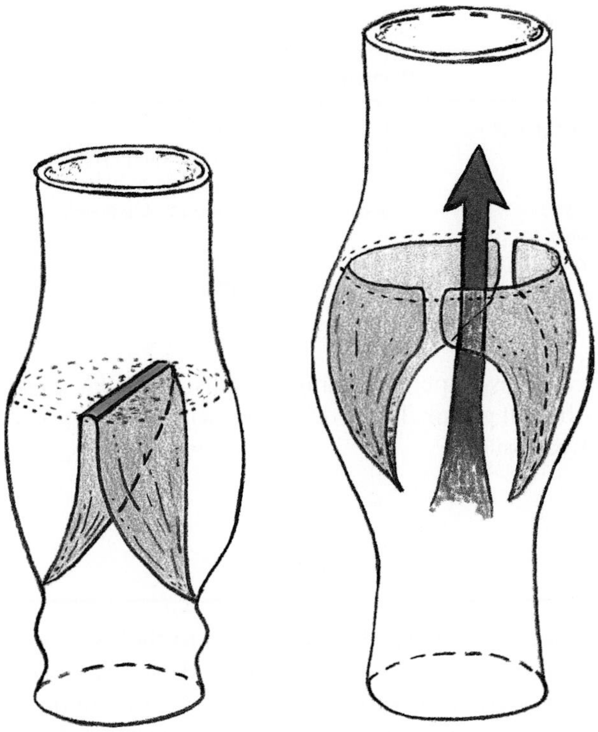

A, B

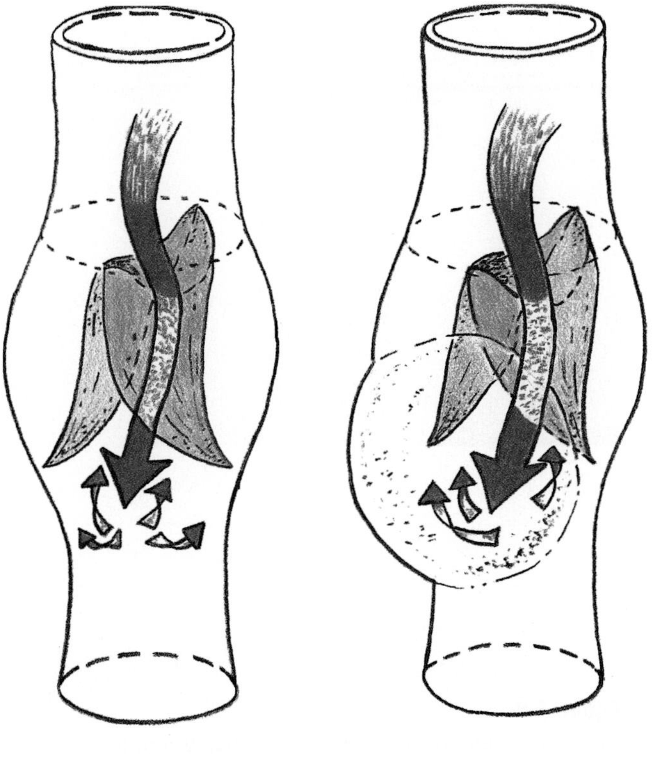

C, D

Figure 1-7

Normal valve function produces leaflet closure during inspiration and (**A**) antegrade flow during expiration (**B**). Retrograde flow (**C**) may occur during all phases of the respiratory cycle when diseased valves are present.

TABLE 1-3. VESSEL CLASSIFICATION

Type	Vessel Class	Diameter	Color
I	Telangiectasis "spider veins"	0.1–1 mm	Red
II	Venulectasia	1–2 mm	Violaceous, cyanotic
III	Reticular veins	2–4 mm	Cyanotic to blue
IV	Nonsaphenous varicose veins (usually related to incompetent perforators)	3–8 mm	Blue to blue-green
V	Saphenous varicose veins	7–8 mm	Blue to blue-green

The deep veins (popliteal veins, superficial femoral veins, and CFVs) constitute the outflow tract from the calf pump. These deeper vessels lie unsupported in the loose subfascial connective tissue.

Vessel Classification

Varicose veins and telangiectasia may be classified according to their size and appearance (Table 1-3). Type I red telangiectasia (Fig. 1-8) and type II violaceous venulectasia (Fig. 1-9) are the vessels most commonly seen for treatment on a cosmetic basis. Telangiectasia of the legs may occur in several patterns: (a) linear or

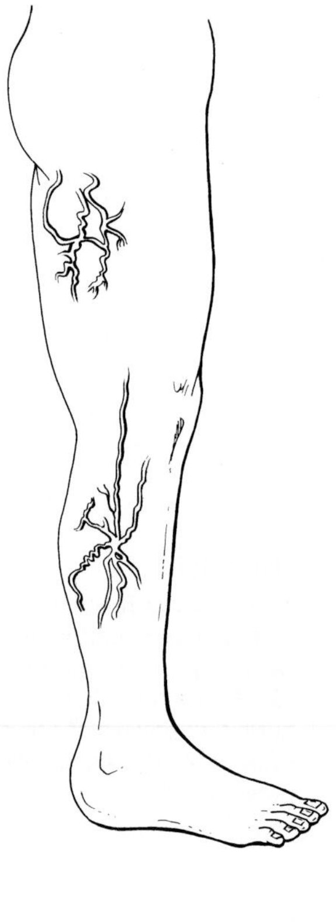

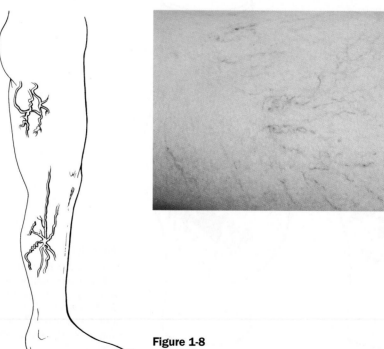

Figure 1-8
Type I red spider telangiectasia (less than 2 mm in diameter).

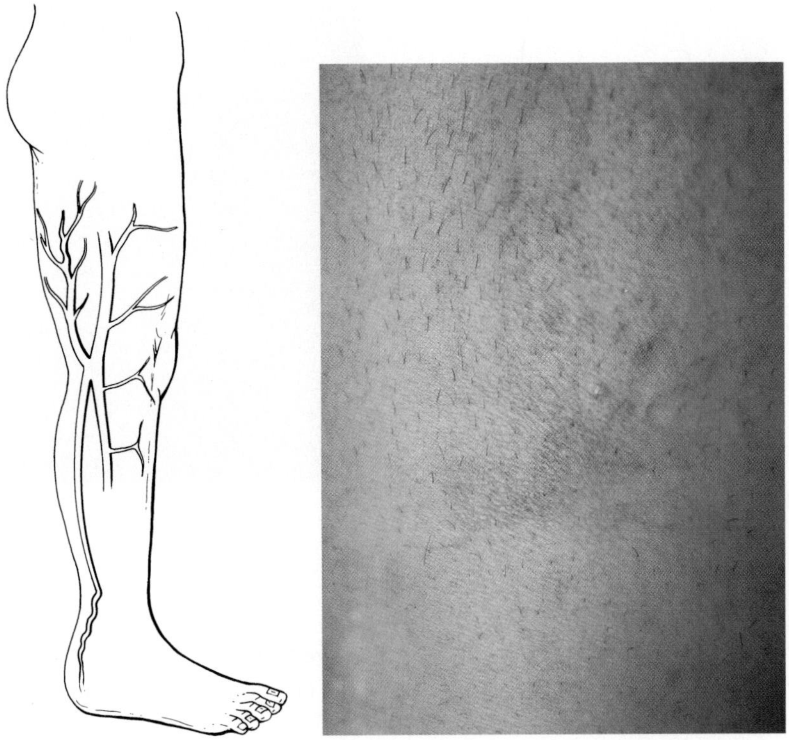

Figure 1-9

Type II blue venulectasia (less than 2 mm in diameter) containing an increased amount of deoxyhemoglobin.

simple, (b) arborizing, (c) papular, or (d) starburst ("spider veins"). The papular pattern is commonly associated with genetic conditions or collagen vascular diseases. The other three patterns are those for which patients most commonly seek sclerotherapy.

Type III vessels (Fig. 1-10) are reticular veins, which are 2 to 4 mm in diameter, cyanotic to blue in color, and usually feed arborizing foci of telangiectasia and venulectasia. Class IV veins are nonsaphenous truncal varicosities (Fig. 1-11). They are usually 3 to 8 mm in diameter, blue to blue-green, and are the majority of clinically evident varicose veins noted on physical examination of the lower extremities. In addition, they are usually related to incompetent perforators.

Finally, type V varicose veins are those of the greater and lesser saphenous systems (Fig. 1-12). They are 7 to 8 mm in diameter and of blue to blue-green hue. These veins, as described previously, are the major communicating conduits of the superficial and deep venous systems.

It is important for physicians performing sclerotherapy to understand the classification scheme outlined above so that they may communicate on physical examination results and treatment approaches in a uniform and consistent fashion.

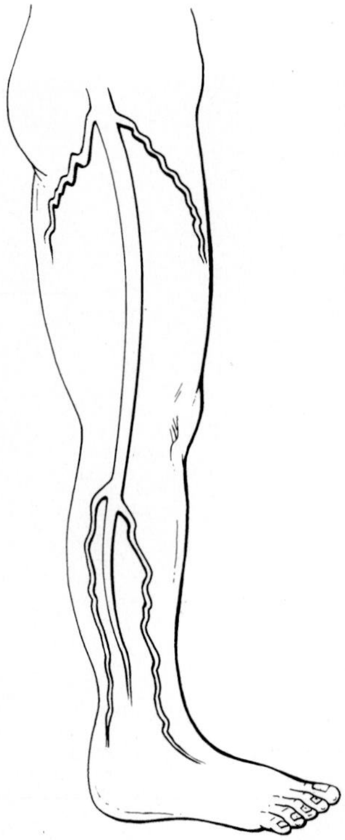

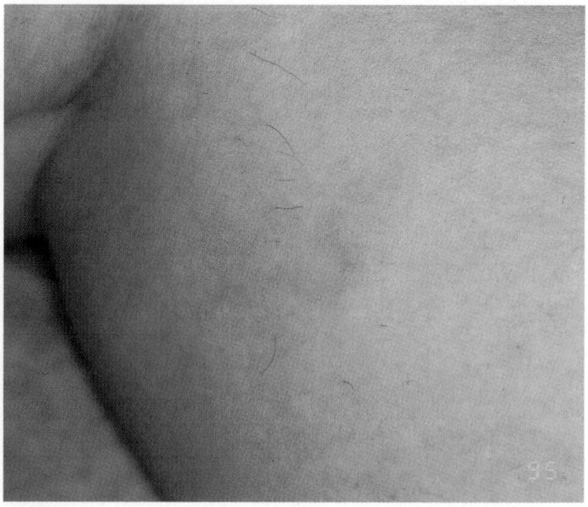

Figure 1-10

Type III reticular veins 2–4 mm in diameter with cyanotic hue.

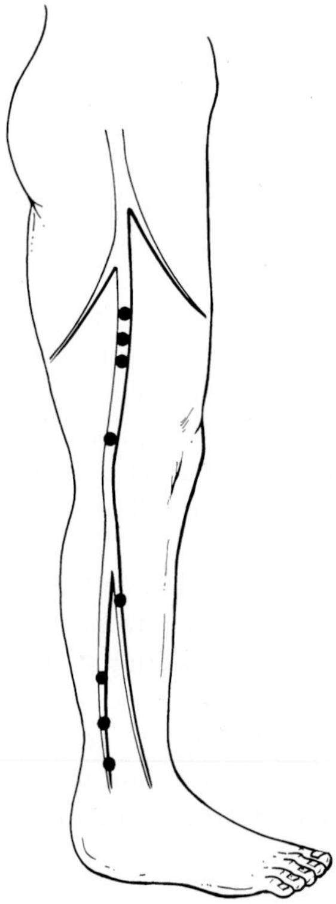

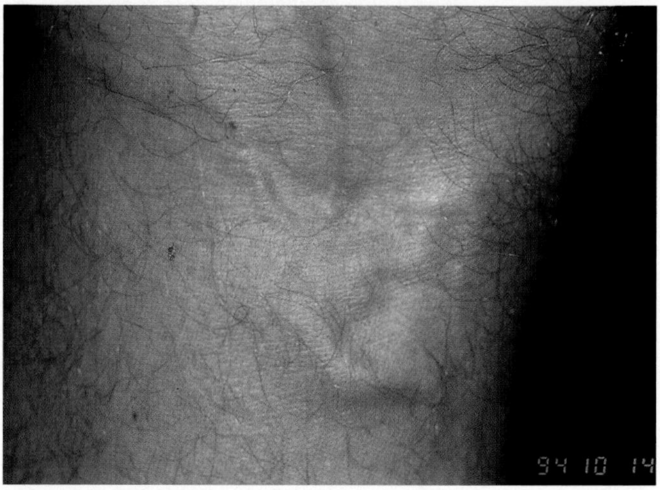

Figure 1-11

Type IV nontruncal saphenous varicosities and perforating veins usually 3–8 mm in diameter.

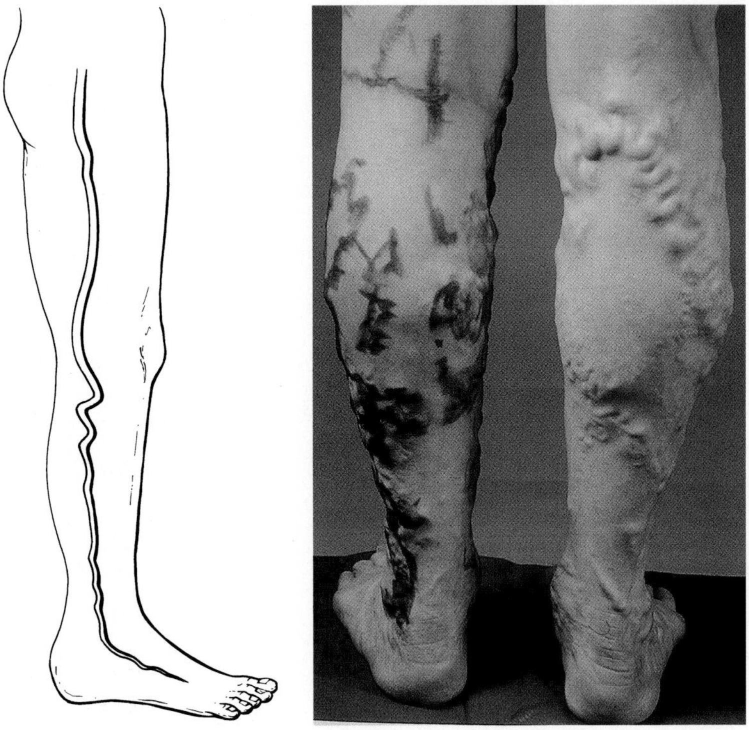

Figure 1-12
Axial varicose veins of the greater or lesser saphenous systems, usually 7–8 mm in diameter.

Conclusion

Presented in this chapter is an overview of the anatomy and structural considerations of the venous system, which is essential to an understanding of the logical diagnostic and treatment approaches to venous problems presented in the remainder of this text. In addition, descriptive criteria regarding vessels and uniform classification will help the sclerotherapist to communicate in a uniform and standardized fashion.

BIBLIOGRAPHY

Ad Hoc Committee at the American Venous Forum 6th Annual Meeting 22–25 February 1994, Maui, Hawaii. Classification and grading of chronic venous disease in the lower limbs: a consensus statement. *Phlebology* 1995; 10:42–45.

Goldman MP, Bennett RG. Treatment of telangiectasia: a review. *J Am Acad Dermatol* 1987; 17:167–182.

Goldman MP, Weiss RA, Bergan JJ. Diagnosis and treatment of varicose veins: a review. *J Am Acad Dermatol* 1994; 31:393–413.

Somjen GM. Anatomy of the superficial venous system. *Dermatol Surg* 1996; 21:35–45.

Weiss RA, Goldman MP. Advances in sclerotherapy. *Cos Derm* 1995; 13:431–445.

CHAPTER 2

Epidemiology and Pathophysiology of Varicose and Telangiectatic Leg Veins

Incidence of Telangiectasia/Varicose Veins

An estimated 30% to 60% of adults have varicose veins, and the incidence increases with age. Varicose veins may occur with exponentially increased frequency over an individual's lifetime. Previous studies estimate the following prevalence:

	Ages	Prevalence
Women	20–29	8%
	50–59	41%
	70–79	72%
Men	20–29	1%
	50–59	24%
	70–79	43%

The lower incidence in men may reflect underreporting, as males may not be as concerned with the physical appearance of their lower extremities. In addition, the incidence of telangiectasias (type I) and venulectasias (type II)—which are more commonly asymptomatic—is far greater than indicated by the data presented here, which represent true varicose vein disease. It is likely that vascular abnormalities in some form affect almost all individuals at some point in their lives; however, it is only those patients with either symptomatic disease, those with sequelae of venous insufficiency (i.e., stasis dermatitis, ulcers, lipodermatosclerosis, etc.), or patients who seek medial help for cosmetic concerns who actually come to the attention of the practicing phlebologist.

It is of interest that, in selected cases, varicose veins may occur in childhood. This occurrence presents most commonly in three settings: (a) where there is a strong family history of varicose vein disease, (b) in the setting of underlying vascular malformations such as Klippel–Trenaunay or Sturge–Weber syndrome, and (c) in the setting of childhood collagen vascular diseases—i.e., dermatomyositis.

In summary, the more we are aware, through careful physical examination, of our patients' venous abnormalities, the more exactly the incidence of varicose and telangiectatic leg veins will be defined in the future.

Predisposing Factors

The etiology of varicose and telangiectatic veins (Table 2-1) remains an enigma. Genetic factors have been felt to play a major role. In previous studies published by the author, approximately 80% of patients with telangiectasia or varicose veins had at least one family member with telangiectasia or varicose veins. In this group of patients, 80% noted the familial occurrence on the maternal side, suggesting a possible sex-linked, autosomal dominant inheritance pattern. In vivo studies by the author are presently in progress, with direct in-office examination of family pedigrees in the hope of providing more accurate clinical data in the future.

Other possible etiologic factors that have been shown to be associated with venous abnormalities include anoxia, infection, physical factors [i.e., sunlight (ultraviolet irradiation)], chemicals, hormonal influences (pregnancy, oral contraceptive therapy), constipation, and "collagen dysplasia" manifest by fibrillar irregularities and altered proteoglycan function mediated through lysosomal enzyme function. Angioproliferative factors are also felt to be possibly involved in the pathophysiology of venous ectasias. Studies presently in progress in the author's

TABLE 2-1. PREDISPOSING FACTORS FOR TELANGIECTATIC/VARICOSE VEINS

Positive family history
Pregnancy onset
  Onset in first trimester
  Onset in second to third trimester
  Onset following pregnancy
Oral contraceptive usage (estrogen and/or progesterone)
Standing vocation (>6 h/day)
Obesity (>20% over ideal weight)
X-ray/ultraviolet exposure
History of thrombophlebitis
Infection/anoxia of the lower extremity
Chronic increased intraabdominal pressure (chronic constipation, straining on defecation or urination)
Wearing tight clothing (corsets, girdles)
Prolonged sitting in chairs (compression of veins)
Sitting with one leg crossed over the other (habitual)

laboratory are intended to define the possible role of endothelial and fibroblastic growth factors in the development of varicose and telangiectatic vein dysfunction.

Pregnancy is felt to be the second most common predisposing factor in the development of venous disease. It is noteworthy that varicose and telangiectatic veins may occur early in first trimester of pregnancy, before significant uterine enlargement occurs, suggesting that increased hydrostatic pressure is not the sole mechanism underlying development of telangiectasia and varicose veins in this setting. Other factors—i.e., hormonally mediated angioproliferative factors—may also play a role in the setting. Previous studies by the author have failed to isolate estrogen or progesterone receptors in either pregnant or non-pregnant patients with telangiectases.

Finally, past studies have implicated additional factors such as standing vocations (greater than 6 hours per day), obesity (greater than 20% over ideal weight), x-ray/ultraviolet exposure, history of thrombophlebitis, and infection/anoxia of the lower extremity as contributing factors in the development of varicose/telangiectatic veins. Predisposing factors of varicose/telangiectatic veins are summarized in Table 2-1.

In conclusion, the etiology of telangiectatic and varicose veins is probably multifactorial. Genetic predisposition is probably the most important single factor. An understanding of the predisposing factors for development of telangiectatic and varicose veins may help to prevent their future progression after sclerotherapy, laser/flash-lamp surgery, or other surgical intervention is performed. By educating patients, we may help to slow the progression of vascular proliferative disease in genetically susceptible individuals.

Complications of Venous Disease

The complications of venous disease include the following:

- Pigmentation
- Stasis dermatitis
- Cellulitis
- Lipodermatosclerosis
- Ulceration
- Bleeding
- Thrombophlebitis

Pigmentation

Pigmentation (Fig. 2-1) is caused by persistent venous hypertension with subsequent capillary hyperpermeability, permitting proteinaceous fluid and red blood cells to escape into the subcutaneous tissue. Pigmentation from hemosiderin deposition ensues secondary to pressure-force vector-related extravasation of erythrocytes. The most common predisposed area is the distal third of the leg extending onto the ankle. Treatment of varicosities may allow this pigmentation to slowly resolve.

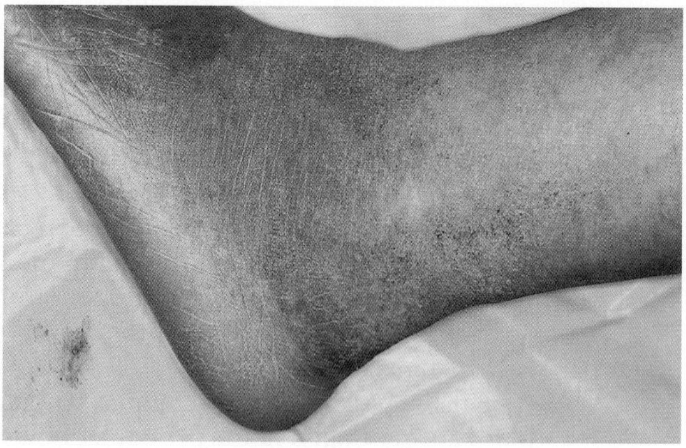

Figure 2-1
Pigmentation related to chronic venous insufficiency is secondary to backflow pressure–related extravasation of erythrocytes, leading to hemosiderin deposition.

Stasis dermatitis

Chronic venous hypertension may lead to release of inflammatory mediators such as cytokines, which produce a dermatitis manifesting as dry, scaly patches or plaques (Fig. 2-2).

Cellulitis

Pruritus may lead to excoriation with subsequent skin breakdown, which may eventuate in subacute or acute cellulitis (Fig. 2-3). Redness, tenderness, and induration may envelope the lower one-half to one-third of the leg, requiring leg elevation, external compression, moist dressings of aluminum acetate solution 1%–5% (Domeboro Solution) (Bayer Corporation, West Haven, CT, U.S.A.) and systemic antibiotics.

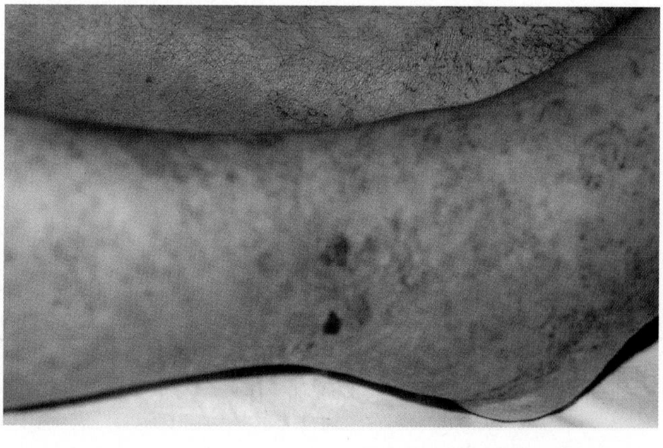

Figure 2-2
Stasis dermatitis manifests as dry, scaling plaques, often pruritic on the distal legs, often associated with chronic deep venous insufficiency.

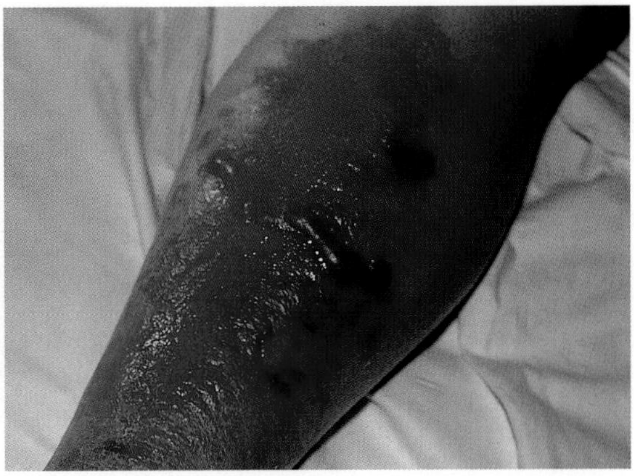

Figure 2-3

Cellulitis manifests as tenderness, redness, and induration most often involving the distal limb; it is most commonly related to microfissuring due to secondary dermatophytosis, chronic deep venous insufficiency, or pruritus-related secondary necrotic excoriation.

Lipodermatosclerosis

As extravasated proteins and red blood cells organize, the subcutaneous tissue begins to undergo fibrosis, leading to lipodermatosclerosis (Fig. 2-4), a condition characterized by fibrotic hyperpigmented plaques at the ankle.

Ulceration

Ulcers (Fig. 2-5) may occur either spontaneously or owing to superficial abrasion or minor trauma. The present theory of venous ulceration is that capillary occlusion by polymorphonuclear leukocytes occurs, with release of proteolytic enzymes causing tissue destruction.

Bleeding

This rare but serious complication occurs from an erosion through a varicosity's wall. Spontaneous hemorrhage can be a medical emergency, but blood loss is not usually severe. After the acute bleeding is stopped by pressure and elevation, the

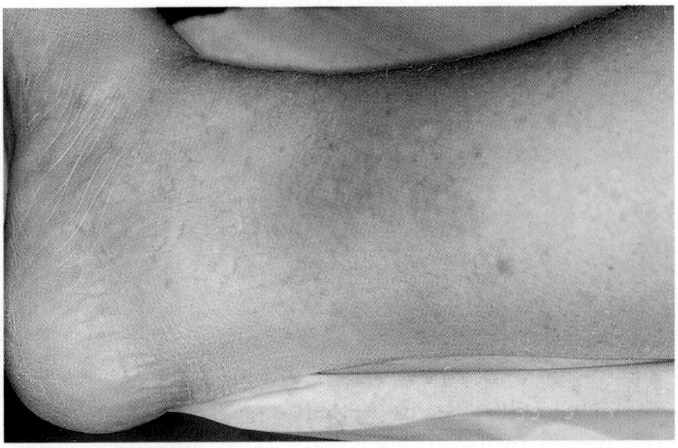

Figure 2-4

Lipodermatosclerosis. Chronic inflammation may lead to the development of fibrotic, hyperpigmented plaques, most commonly noted at the ankle.

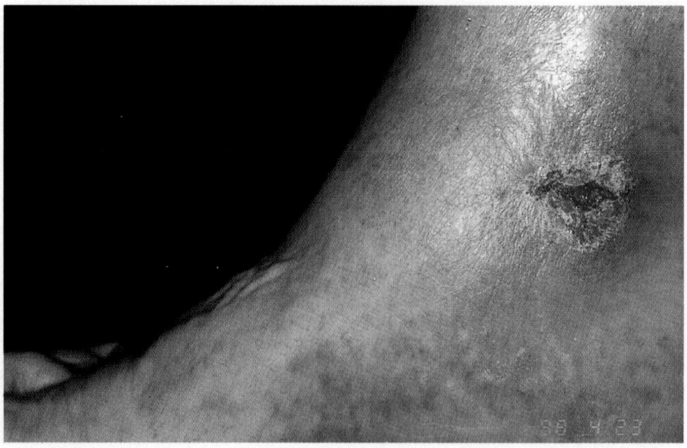

Figure 2-5
Ulceration. Cytokine- and protease-mediated factors in the setting of an altered microcirculation may lead to the development of well-demarcated ulcerations, most commonly noted at the medial malleolus.

offending vein should be treated preferably by injection/compression sclerotherapy.

Thrombophlebitis

Usually presenting as redness, tenderness, and induration that may occur after a trivial injury to a prominent varicose vein, superficial thrombophlebitis (Fig. 2-6) may be treated conservatively with compression and nonsteroidal antiinflammatory drugs or through early surgical avulsion of the thrombosed varicosity. Rarely, extension upward into the saphenous vein or deep venous system may occur, which may require more aggressive anticoagulant therapy.

Nonsurgical Approaches Helpful in Slowing the Progression of Venous Disease

Damage caused to the venous wall by insufficiency of the venous valves and subsequent increase in volume is irreversible. Prophylactic measures merely prevent progression of the existing disease.

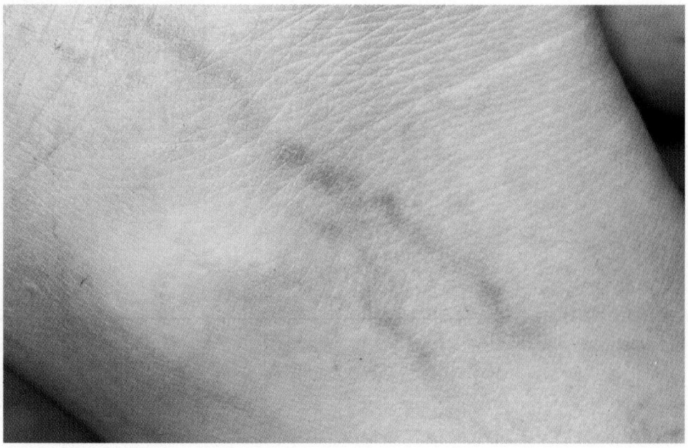

Figure 2-6
Thrombophlebitis usually presents as a red, tender, indurated cord along a given vein segment.

Pathophysiologic factors such as reduced rate of flow and increase in blood volume can be positively influenced by the following measures:

Compression hosiery

Exercise—specific exercises to activate the pump in the calf veins and ankle
- Sports
  - Hill walking
  - Dancing
  - Cross-country skiing
  - Golf
  - Swimming
  - Cycling
- Weight reduction
- Elevation of the legs several times daily for 5 to 10 minutes
- Orthopedic inserts for flat/splay feet
- Cold shower of the feet several times daily for 3 to 5 minutes
- Drug therapy
  - Medications that increase venous tone
- Compression therapy

The fundamental effect of compression therapy is to improve venous flow. This is accomplished by four basic mechanisms:

1. Reduction in pathologic distention of veins
2. Approximation of insufficient venous valves, thus restoring their functional effectiveness
3. Reduction of the volume in the veins, thus increasing the rate of blood flow in them
4. Increasing fibrinolytic activity of the venous wall, thus reducing the risk of thrombosis

Compression Bandaging

Compression bandaging is used to counteract complications induced by edema or venous hypertension. Compression bandaging produces short-term measured compression of both the superficial and deep venous systems. Congestion is reduced by high working pressures and movement. For compression bandaging to be effective, it is essential that the correct technique be used when applying firm, limited-stretch bandages to produce graduated pressure that reduces in a distal-to-proximal direction. Either crepe or tape bandages may be chosen.

Examples of tape bandages are as follows:

1. 3M Microfoam Surgical Tape
   3M Medical Surgical Division
   St. Paul, MN, U.S.A.

2. Tubigrip Tubular Support Bandage
   Seaton Products Inc.
   Montgomeryville, PA, U.S.A.
3. Coban Tape
   3M Medical Surgical Division
   St. Paul, MN, U.S.A.

An example of a crepe bandage is

Medi-Rip Bandage
Conco Medical Company
Bridgeport, CT, U.S.A.

The following general rules of bandaging need to be followed for clinical efficacy:

1. Every bandage should be applied with the foot dorsally flexed to avoid folds in the ankle region.
2. The compression bandage must reach the toe joints and include the heel.
3. The pressure of the bandage must be highest in the ankle region and decrease continuously proximally.
4. During bandaging, the bandage roll should be fed along the surface of the limb.
5. Plane regions should be upholstered.
6. The compression bandage must follow the outline of the leg.
7. Only bandages with low elasticity should be used.

Compression stockings are less effective than compression bandages in the treatment of venous ulcers because of their lower ambulatory pressure.

Compression Hosiery

Unlike compression bandaging, with its high working pressure, compression hosiery exerts a resting pressure that varies depending on the garment's class of compression. Pressure is controlled by the limited ability of the hosiery to stretch, thereby approximating incompetent venous valves, accelerating venous return, increasing fibrinolytic activity of the venous wall, and thus reducing the risk of thrombosis.

In general, compression hosiery is better tolerated and easier to put on than compression bandages, thus increasing patient compliance. Compression hosiery is made of a two-way-stretch fabric; that is, the stocking is elastic both lengthwise and widthwise. The stockings have graduated pressure, decreasing from the ankle upward.

Compression Issues

1. Are there any contraindications?
   a) Arterial occlusive disease
   b) Peripheral Doppler pressure below 70 mmHg

2. When should compression hosiery be prescribed?
   a) After edema is minimized
   b) After treatment of cutaneous abnormalities
3. Which compression class is most appropriate? (Table 2-2)
   Class I (20 to 30 mmHg)
   - Telangiectasia
   - Clinical heaviness or tiredness
   - Pregnancy prophylaxis

   Class II (30 to 40 mmHg)
   - Varicose veins
   - Moderate edema
   - After minor ulcers have healed
   - After sclerotherapy and varicose vein operations

   Class III (40 to 50 mmHg)
   - Chronic (postthrombotic) venous insufficiency
   - Severe edema
   - Atrophie blanche
   - Dermatosclerosis
   - Reversible lymphedema

   Class IV (50 to 60 mmHg)
   - Chronic severe venous insufficiency
   - Severe ulceration

TABLE 2-2. GUIDELINES FOR DETERMINATION OF COMPRESSION THERAPY

Compression Class	Vessel Type	Associated Symptoms/Conditions
Class 1: 20–30 mmHg	Telangiectasia	Heaviness, tiredness in the legs
Class 2: 30–40 mmHg	Varicose veins	Moderate edema Pregnancy varicosities After healing of minor ulcers After sclerotherapy After ambulatory phlebectomy
Class 3: 40–50 mmHg	Varicose veins	Chronic (postthrombotic) venous insufficiency Severe edema Atrophie blanche Dermatosclerosis
Class 4: 50–60 mmHg	Varicose veins	Severe venous insufficiency Lymphedema

Determination of compression class based on venous filling time of PPG (LRR)
20–25 sec: class 1
20–20 sec: class 2
<20 sec: class 3–4

PPG, photoplethysmography.
LLR, light reflection rheography.

TABLE 2-3. HOSIERY LENGTHS

Length	Type
Below knee (calf)	A–D
Above knee (midthigh)	A–F
Thigh length	A–G
Pantyhose	A–M
Maternity tights	A–MU

- ▶ Severe dermatosclerosis
- ▶ Severe lymphedema

4. What length should the stockings be? (Table 2-3) Thigh-level stockings are indicated if the thighs are also affected by varicosities or if thrombophlebitis develops at that level. Medical compression pantyhose should be prescribed for venous insufficiency that extends up into the groin.
5. What are aids in keeping stockings up?
   - ▶ Roll-on adhesive for half-thigh or thigh-length stockings
   - ▶ Half-thigh or thigh length stockings with grip-top pantyhose
   - ▶ Thigh-length stockings (left or right) with waist attachment
6. What information should a prescription for compression hose contain?
   a) Model number and brand
   b) Compression class
   c) Diagnosis

SAMPLE PRESCRIPTION FOR MEDICAL COMPRESSION STOCKINGS

Please supply ____________ pair/s (BRAND) graduated compression stockings.

Style	Compression in mmHg 20–30	30–40	40–50	50–60
□ Calf	□	□	□	□
□ Half thigh	□	□	□	□
□ Thigh		□	□	□
□ Thigh with waist attachment		□	□	
□ Panty	□	□		
□ Panty, maternity	□	□		
□ Male tights		□		

Diagnosis: ________________________________

Drug therapy of Venous Insufficiency/Ulceration

1. Fibrinolytic therapy

   Based on the rationale that venous insufficiency and ulceration lead to skin hypoxia secondary to an oxygen diffusion block caused by pericapillary fibrin

- ► Stanazol (anabolic steroid) (Winstrol, Sanofi Pharmaceuticals, New York, NY, U.S.A.)

  Side effects—masculinization, menstrual irregularity, weight gain, headache
- ► Defibrotide

2. Hydroxyrutisides

   Restore the barrier properties of the fiber matrix between capillary endothelial cells
   - ► O-(B-hydroxyethyl)-rutoside (HR)
3. Prostaglandins

   Properties making these agents effective in the treatment of peripheral vascular disease include vasodilation, inhibition of platelet aggregation, and inhibition of neutrophil activation
   - ► Prostaglandin (PGE_1)
4. Methylxanthines

   Their role in venous insufficiency is based on a reduction of white cell aggregation activation and mild fibrinolytic activity
   - ► Pentoxifylline (400 mg tid) (Trental, Hoechst-Roussel Pharmaceuticals, Kansas City, MO, U.S.A.)
5. Others
   - ► Gingko biloba (Pharmanex Inc., Simi Valley, CA, U.S.A.)

     A flavonoid that decreases free-radical formation from activated leukocytes and protects fibrous components of the veins against proteolytic degradation
   - ► Daflon

     A semisynthetic flavonoid that prevents inflammation by interfering with the generation of prostaglandins and the production of H_2O_2 and thromboxane A_2 as well as decreasing the release of histamine from mast cells. It is also a free-radical scavenger.
   - ► Low-dose urokinase (Abbokinase, Abbott Laboratories, North Chicago, IL, U.S.A.)

     Reduces pericapillary fibrin cuff.

All of the agents require further research to establish their role in the management of patients with venous insufficiency.

Pathophysiology

Varicose Veins

There are three major components to the venous system, which cycle through a triphasic sequence of rest → contraction → relaxation (Fig. 2-7):

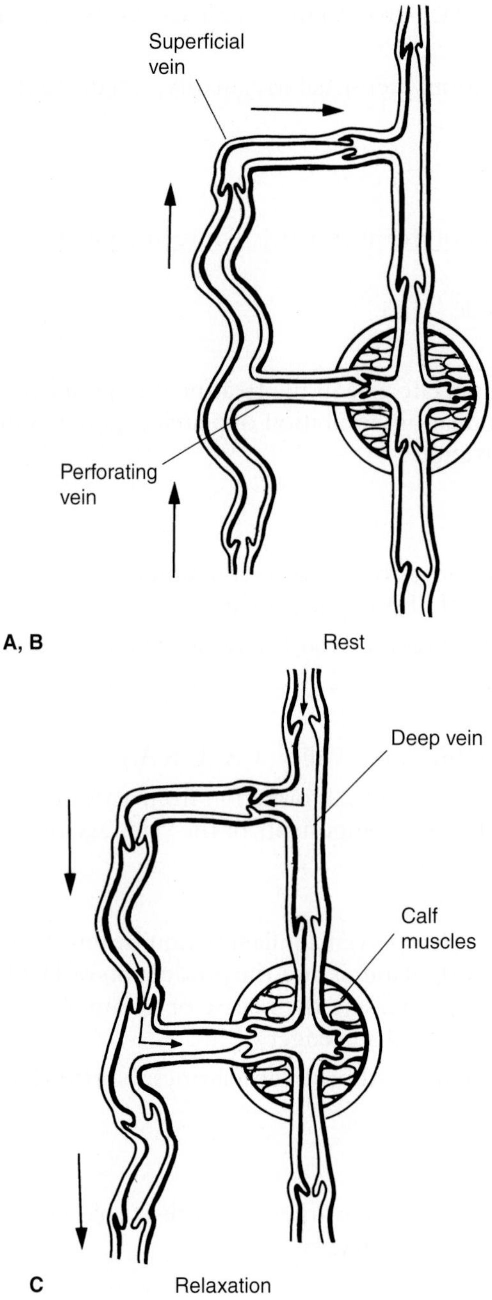

Figure 2-7

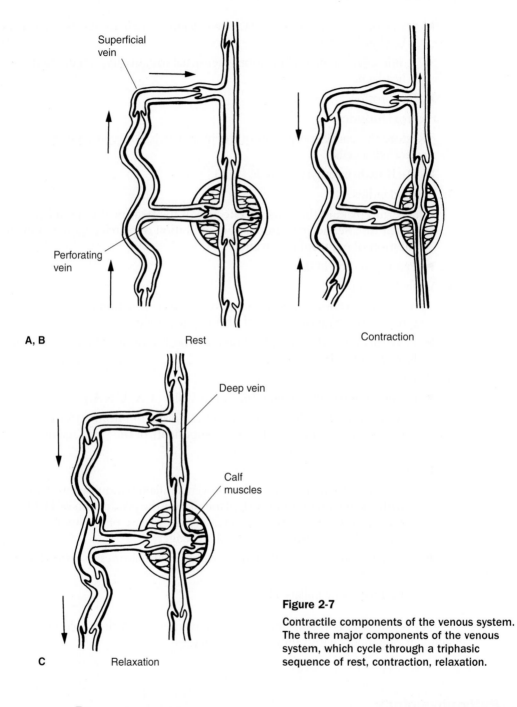

Contractile components of the venous system. The three major components of the venous system, which cycle through a triphasic sequence of rest, contraction, relaxation.

Deep venous system
Superficial venous system
Perforating system—connects the superficial and deep venous systems

The deep venous system lies subfascially in the deep muscular layer. The majority of deoxygenated blood that is returned from the legs is transported to the

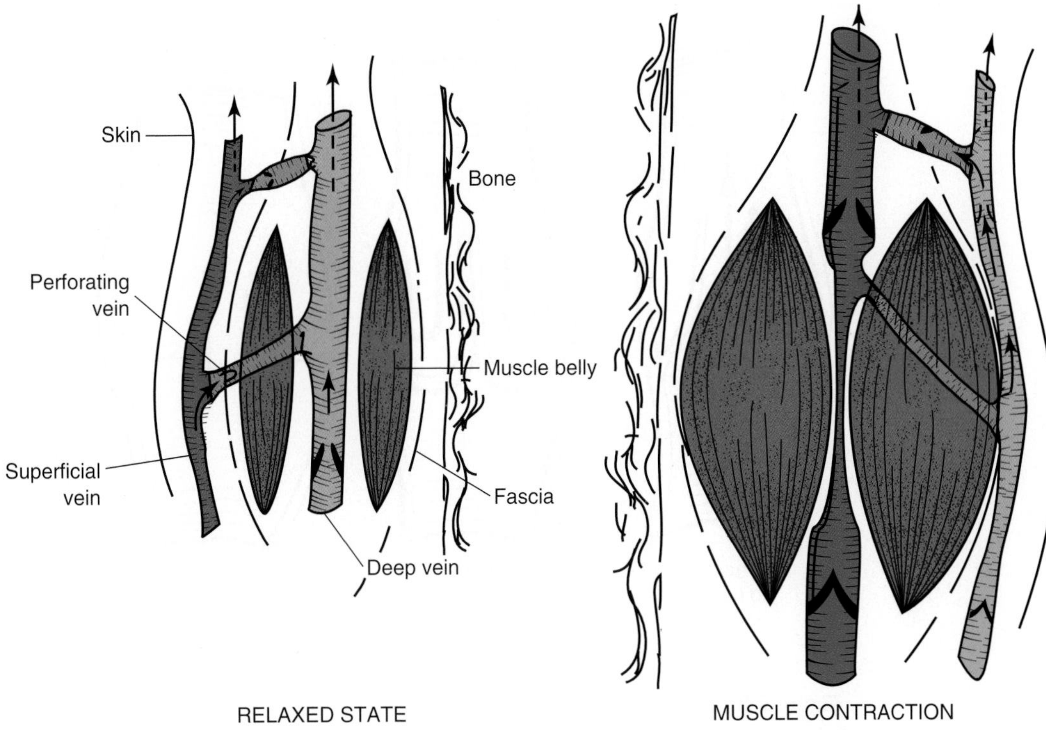

Figure 2-8

The calf-muscle pump, or "peripheral heart," is located primarily in the calves. During inspiratory muscle contraction, compression of veins transports blood to the heart by means of the deep venous system.

heart by the deep venous system. The mechanism by which this movement occurs is mediated through muscular compression of veins and is thus called the *muscular pump system* or *peripheral heart,* which is located primarily in the calves. (Fig. 2-8).

The superficial venous system is located outside the muscles. Only about 10% of the blood is transported by the superficial veins. The main function of superficial vessels is drainage of venulectasis and telangiectasis of the skin.

The third interconnecting channel is the perforating venous system; it connects interfascially the superficial and deep venous systems, which run parallel with the long axis of the lower extremities.

During leg muscle relaxation, backflow of blood (reflux) is prevented by means of passive one-way venous valves (Fig. 2-9). For example, the superficial saphenous veins have from 6 to 10 valves spaced approximately 8 to 10 cm apart. Transport of blood from the superficial to the deep veins occurs via the perforating veins during muscle relaxation, when the pressure in the deep veins falls below the pressure in the superficial veins. On average, the hydrostatic pressure in the lower legs is approximately 100 mmHg or more at rest (compared with 35 mmHg in the distal arm). However, when the calf muscle contracts during walking or exercise, the pressure generated can reach 200 to 300 mmHg. In the set-

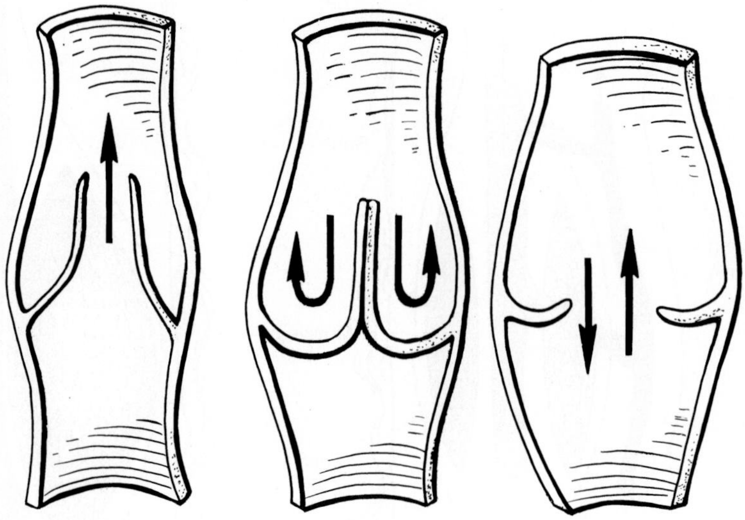

Figure 2-9

Venous valve function. With normal venous valve function (A), there is normal blood flow to the heart. Normal valve apposition (B) prevents distal retrograde flow. Abnormal valve function (C) may lead to backward flow of blood, over time leading to the development of dilated or "varicose" veins.

ting of valvular incompetence, chronic backflow-induced elevated venous pressure leads to venous distention (varicose sacculation) "blowout phenomena" (Fig. 2-10).

Three major factors are felt to be responsible for the development of varicose veins from a pathophysiologic perspective:

- Increased venous pressure
- Valve problems
- Hereditary venous dysplasia

Major causes of these contributing factors are listed in Table 2-4.

The major unanswered question is whether distention of the vein wall precedes the development of varicose veins or occurs as a consequence of long-standing valvular incompetence. It is felt that failure of the vein wall is due to an intrinsic defect of connective tissue regulation. It has been shown that there are reduced amounts of collagen and elastin in varicose veins as compared with controls. It has also been shown that venous valve failure begins with depression of the valve at the vein wall's connecting point or commissure; this leads to expansion of the valve cusps and subsequent impaired apposition, leading to "valvular incompetence."

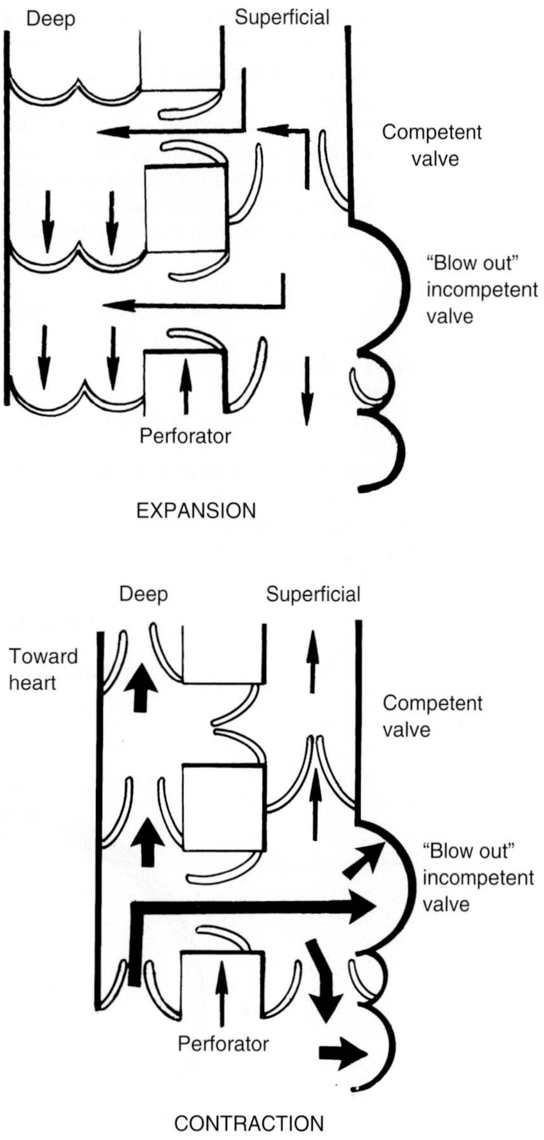

Figure 2-10

Valve blowout phenomena. In the setting of valvular incompetence, chronic backflow-induced elevated venous pressure leads to venous distention, or "blowout phenomena."

Telangiectasis/Venulectasia

Telangiectasias are made up of the smallest vessels treated by sclerotherapists (0.1 to 1 mm). They represent distended arterioles or capillaries, tend to have a reddish hue, and are generally blush with the skin surface. Venulectasias are small vessels arising from the venous side of capillary loops; they tend to be slightly elevated from the skin surface and have a bluish hue (Fig. 2-11). The major theoretical issue in terms of these small vessels is whether they arise as a result of increased venous pressure in larger vessels or whether various angiogenic factors play a role in

TABLE 2-4. PATHOPHYSIOLOGIC FACTORS IN THE DEVELOPMENT OF VARICOSE VEINS

Increased venous pressure
- Proximal
  - Pelvic obstruction (tumors, pregnancy)
  - Increased intraabdominal pressure (i.e., obesity, constrictive clothing, high-impact exercise, Valsalva maneuvers)
  - Saphenofemoral incompetence
  - Venous obstruction (tumors, thrombotic disease states)
- Distal
  - Perforator abnormalities
  - Venous obstruction (thromboembolic disease states)
  - Arteriovenous anastomoses

Valve problems
- Acquired
  - Secondary to chronic thromboembolic disease (deep venous thrombophlebitis)
- Congenital
  - Congenital absence of venous valves
  - Decreased number of venous valves

Hereditary venous dysplasia
- Impaired regulation of venous connective tissue metabolism (collagen, elastin)

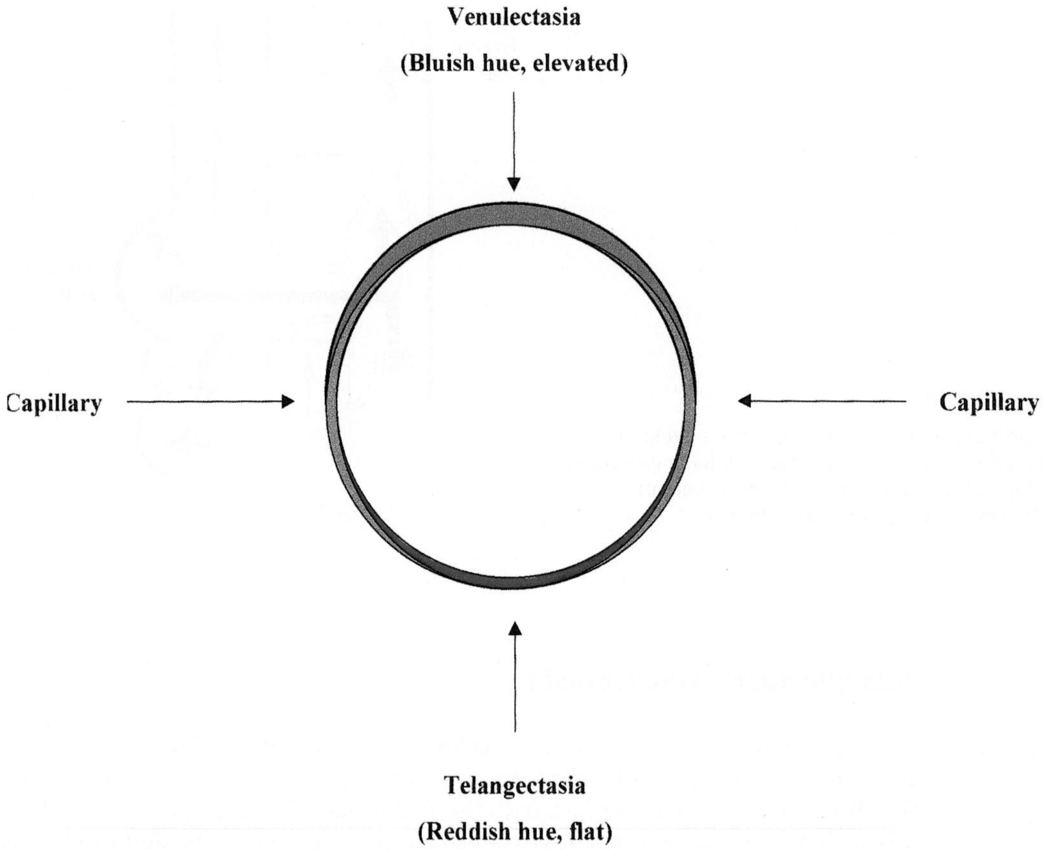

Figure 2-11

Schemata—Capillary loop with evolution of elevated venulectasia (bluish in hue) and flat telangiectasia. (reddish in hue)

TABLE 2-5. PATHOPHYSIOLOGIC FACTORS IN THE DEVELOPMENT OF TELANGIECTASIS

Genetic diseases/proliferations
Nevus flammeus and associated genetic disease states
Klippel–Trenaunay syndrome
Congenital poikilodermas
Rothmund–Thomson syndrome
Bloom's syndrome
Hemangiomas and associated disease states
Maffuci's syndrome
Hereditary states
Essential progressive telangiectasia
Cutis marmorata telangiectasia congenita
Acquired diseases
Collagen vascular diseases
Mastocytosis
Human immunodeficiency virus (HTLV III)
Pigmentary purpuric dermatoses
Malignant atrophic papulosis (Degos' disease)
Necrobiosis lipoidica diabeticorum
Hyperthyroidism
Keratosis lichenoides chronica
Atrophoderma
Physical/hormonal factors
Pregnancy/hormonal therapy
Steroid atrophy
Chronic UVB exposure (poikiloderma of Civatte)
Traumatic scarring
Infection/hypoxic states
Radiodermatitis
Heat/infrared exposure (erythema ab igne)

HTLV, human T-cell leukemia/lymphoma virus; UBV, ultraviolet B.

their development. Regardless of etiology, these small-diameter vessels occur as a manifestation of three major etiological states:

1. Genetic diseases/proliferations
2. Acquired diseases
3. Physical/hormonal factors

A summary of these factors is listed in Table 2-5.

Conclusion

Having a basic understanding of the epidemiology and pathophysiology of telangiectasis and varicose veins, the sclerotherapist may approach the patient with venous disease in terms of history taking and physical examination in an erudite manner.

BIBLIOGRAPHY

Abu-Own, Scurr JH, Coleridge-Smith PD. Effect of compression stockings on the skin microcirculation in chronic venous insufficiency. *Phlebology* 1995;10:5–11.

Christopoulos D, Nicolaides AN, Belcaro G. The long term effect of elastic compression on the venous hemodynamics of the leg. *Phlebology* 1991;6:85–93.

Cornu-Thenard A, Boivin P, Baud JM, DeVincenzi I, Carpenter PH. Importance of the familial factors in varicose disease. *J Dermatol Surg Oncol* 1995;20:318–326.

Pardes JB, Nemeth AJ. Adverse sequelae of venous hypertension. *Semin Dermatol* 1993;12:66–71.

Sadick NS. Predisposing factors of varicose and telangiectatic leg veins. *J Dermatol Surg Oncol* 1992;18:883–886.

CHAPTER 3

IN-OFFICE EVALUATION OF TELANGIECTATIC AND VARICOSE VEINS

Focused History Taking

The physician who aspires to achieve expertise in performing sclerotherapy of varicose and telangiectatic leg veins must understand that a detailed history and careful physical examination are necessary before treatment can proceed. It is an established fact that the severity of signs and systems often does not correlate with the severity of underlying venous disease. Therefore, it is prudent to assume that "there is more than meets the eye" when one is evaluating patients with varicose veins and telangiectasias. And although the extent of underlying disease may prove to be relatively minor, the potential consequences of inappropriate evaluation and treatment warrant a cautious and complete systematic approach. A complete historical documentation of the patient with lower extremity venous complaints should include the following phlebology history:

1. Vascular history
   a. Varicose vein problems
   b. Phlebitis
   c. Blood clots
   d. Pulmonary embolism
   e. Leg ulcer
   f. Leg fractures

   g. Cellulitis
   h. Leg swelling
2. Spectrum of leg pain
   a. Resting pain
   b. Resting cramps
   c. Night cramps
   d. Tiredness
   e. Heaviness in the legs
   f. Numbness
   g. Burning sensation
3. Previous vein treatments
   a. Sclerotherapy
   b. Laser therapy/Flash lamp
   c. Electrocauterization
   d. Surgery (vein stripping, ligation)
   e. Ambulatory phlebectomy
4. Medications
   a. Aspirin
   b. Blood thinners (anticoagulants)
   c. Pain killers
   d. Arthritis medications such as nonsteroidal antiinflammatory drugs (NSAIDs)
   e. Insulin
   f. Corticosteroids
   g. Oral contraceptives (birth-control pills)
   h. Hormone replacement (estrogen, progesterone)

History taking should be geared to elicit factors predisposing patients to varicose vein disease, as discussed in Chapter 2. Of greatest importance, patients should be questioned about a family history of varicose veins and telangiectasia and any related venous disease states. A positive family history of varicose vein disease makes truncal or axial vein disease more likely in the patient questioned, which would subsequently lead to a more comprehensive approach on physical examination and decision making concerning further laboratory testing. This information should also document the age of onset of any such condition. A history of deep venous thrombosis (DVT), arterial occlusive disease, or diabetes mellitus is also of importance. The phlebologist should also determine the circumstances surrounding any exacerbation of signs or symptoms. For example, an increase in the size or number of varicose veins or in associated symptoms may be the result of previously undiagnosed DVT—the likelihood of which would increase if these exacerbations occurred following events such as surgery, periods of immobilization, or traumatic injuries such as fractures.

The history should also include questions about underlying excerbating conditions, which may reveal the source of venous dilation. These factors include pregnancy, changes in bowel habits (i.e., chronic constipation), habitual high-impact exercise, occupations requiring prolonged standing or sitting, current or past obesity, or usage of constrictive tight clothing, all of which result in chronic increased intraabdominal pressure. Habitual leg crossing may also be a source of increased venous pressure in the legs.

A detailed history of any previous laboratory/imaging examinations and previous treatment for venous conditions is also of relevance. This should include sclerotherapy, surgical intervention (ligation, stripping, ambulatory phlebectomy, radiofrequency obliteration) or laser and noncoherent light-source modalities. Patients in whom varicosities have recurred during treatment may have had incomplete treatment or may have underlying sources of reflux that may have not been adequately addressed.

Signs and symptoms should be thoroughly discussed and documented. Careful questioning may be necessary to pinpoint the onset of signs and symptoms as well as activities or circumstances leading to their exacerbation or alleviation. Of importance, the use of support hose should be elicited. Many patients may self-prescribe support hose prior to presenting to the physician. Improvement of symptoms with the use of support hose points to venous problems as the source of lower extremity discomfort.

Documentation of a patient's medication history is also of significance. Major classes of drugs that may affect the outcome of sclerotherapy—in terms of bruising or lack of results—include:

- Aspirin
- Anticoagulants
- Persantine
- NSAIDs
- Corticosteroids
- Hormones—estrogen, progesterone

A complete review of systems should also include information concerning easy bruisability or collagen vascular disease related symptomatology (i.e., Raynaud's phenomenon), which may elicit an underlying state of hypercoagulability or vascular fragility such as the following:

- Antiphospholipid antibody (anticardiolipin antibody) syndrome
- Protein C deficiency
- Protein S deficiency
- Coagulation factor deficiency
- Platelet defects

The taking of a complete phlebology history may also be facilitated by questionnaires, which will help the patient to concentrate on these issues prior to the interview with the physician. A sample form is presented in Fig. 3-1.

PHLEBOLOGY PATIENT QUESTIONNAIRE

I. ARE YOU SEEKING TREATMENT FOR:
A. Cosmetic reasons (solely for improvement of appearance) ______
B. Medical reasons (relief of pain, swelling, aching, or cramps
C. Both ______

II. VASCULAR HISTORY - General
Do you have a history of:
Varicose vein problems ______
Phlebitis ______
Blood clots ______
Pulmonary embolism ______
Leg ulcer ______
Leg fractures ______
Cellulitis ______

III. VASCULAR HISTORY - specific
Indicate which of these problems you have had:

	Right leg	Left leg	How many years
a) Pain in your:			
Lower limbs	___	___	___
Thigh	___	___	___
Calf		___	___
Leg	___	___	___
b) Swelling of the legs	___	___	___
c) Skin or ulcer problems	___	___	___
d) Others			

Specify: ______

If you experience pain in your lower limbs:

	No	Yes
a) Is the pain exacerbated by:		
Extended periods in position	___	___
Heat	___	___
Menstrual periods	___	___
Exercising and/or walking	___	___
Medication	___	___
Others		
Specify: ______		
b) Is the pain alleviated by:		
Elevation of the limbs	___	___
Elastic stockings	___	___
Walking and/or exercising	___	___
c) Indicate the type of pain:		
Resting pain	___	___
Resting cramps	___	___
Night cramps	___	___
Tiredness	___	___
Heaviness in the legs	___	___
Pain in specific areas	___	___
Numbness	___	___
Burning sensation	___	___

Additional comments:
______

Have you ever been treated for one of the following:
a) Phlebitis (inflammation of a vein) ______ ______
Right leg ___ Left leg ___
Hospitalization ______
b) Leg ulcer ______ ______
Right leg ___ Left leg ___
Hospitalization ______
c) Pulmonary embolism (blood clots in legs) ______ ______
Hospitalization ______
d) Deep vein thrombosis (blood clots in legs) ______ ______
Hospitalization ______

Have you ever been treated for varicose veins with:
a) Sclerotherapy ______ ______
b) Laser therapy ______ ______
c) Photoderm ______ ______
d) Electro-cauterization ______ ______
e) Surgery (vein stripping) (ligation) ______ ______
f) Ambulatory phlebectomy ______ ______

IV. PAST MEDICAL HISTORY
Have you had any of the following: Check if yes
Heart murmurs ______
Heart trouble (chest pain, palpitations, congestive heart failure) ______
High blood pressure ______
Pregnancy (indicate number) ______
Diabetes ______
Seizures or convulsions ______
Fainting or dizzy spells ______
Stroke ______
Nervous breakdown ______
Psychological illness (e.g. depression) ______
Frequent infection of boils ______
Hepatitis ______
Abnormal or prolonged bleeding ______
Easy bruising ______
Difficult skin healing or abnormal scarring ______
Blood disease (e.g. leukemia) ______
Blood transfusions ______
HIV infection or AIDS ______
Exposure to HIV or AIDS ______
Colitis or other bowel disease ______
Breathing problems (any) ______
Asthma ______
Hives ______
Kidney disease ______
Autoimmune disease (e.g. lupus) ______
Severe arthritis ______
Weight gain ______
Anything else you have suffered from that is not listed above - please specify: ______

V. SURGICAL HISTORY:
List any operations you have had and their approximate dates. Please mention any complications you experienced.

Surgery	Year	Complications

Figure 3-1

Sclerotherapy questionnaire. A complete phlebology questionnaire to be filled out by the patient may be helpful in the collection of historical and symptomatic data when patients present for evaluation of venous problems. It may also serve as a time-saving mechanism. *(continues)*

PHLEBOLOGY PATIENT QUESTIONNAIRE (CONTINUED)

VI. MEDICATIONS:

Do you take any of the following: Check if yes

	Check if yes
Aspirin	______
Blood thinner (anticoagulants)	______
Pain killers (e.g. Ibuprofen)	______
Arthritis medications	______
Insulin	______
Cortisone (steroids)	______
Oral contraceptives (birth control pill)	______
Estrogen, Progesterone, or other hormones	______

List all medications that you take regularly or occasionally.

VII. ALLERGIES: ____________________

VIII. PERSONAL ACTIVITIES LIST:

Does your work requires a:	No	Yes
a) Prolonged standing position	___	___
b) Prolonged sitting position	___	___

In the course of a normal day, how much time is spent in standing position:

a) 10% of the day ______
b) 20% of the day ______
c) 30-50% of the day ______
d) More than 50% ______

	No	Yes
Do you wear elastic support stockings	___	___
Do you exercise regularly (high impact)	___	___
Do you smoke:	___	___
If yes, how many per day ___		
Do you drink:	___	___
If yes, how many drinks per day ___		
Ultraviolet exposure	___	___

IX. PREVIOUS LABORATORY EVALUATIONS
(Please include years)

Have you ever had your veins examined by:

a) Doppler ultrasound examination ___ ___
b) Light Rheography (L.R.R.) ___ ___
c) Photoplethysmography (P.P.G.) ___ ___
d) Pneumoplethysmography ___ ___
e) Venography ___ ___
f) Duplex ultrasound ___ ___

Figure 3-1 *(Continued)*

Signs and Symptoms of Varicose Veins and Telangiectasias

The majority of patients presenting to the phlebologist do so for esthetic reasons. However, there is often a combination of reproducible symptoms and signs that may be associated with venous incompetence. Symptoms may include pain, cramping, fatigue, dull aching, restlessness of the legs, stinging, burning, and a sensation of heaviness in the legs (Table 3-1). If pain is the major symptom, there may be a concomitant problem such as musculoskeletal pain, radicular neuropathy, or mixed arterial insufficiency. Distinguishing symptoms of arterial versus venous disease of the lower extremities are outlined in Table 3-2. Pain and other symptoms are frequently relieved with walking or wearing graduated class II 30- to 40-mm Hg support hose and worsen with prolonged standing, sitting, or inactivity. Nighttime exacerbations may be related to impaired venous outflow dur-

TABLE 3-1. SIGNS AND SYMPTOMS OF VARICOSE VEINS

Burning
Cramping
Dermatitis
Edema
Heaviness
Hemorrhage
Hyperpigmentation
Leg fatigue
Pain/throbbing
Pruritus
Restless leg
Stinging
Skin induration
Thrombophlebitis of superficial vessels
Ulceration

ing the day, leading to an accumulation of acidosis-inducing metabolites. Symptoms may be exacerbated during pregnancy, menstruation, or sexual intercourse.

It has been shown in several studies that symptoms are not directly related to either the number or diameter of varicose veins. Weiss and Weiss reported that 53% of patients in their 215-patient series who sought sclerotherapy for varicose veins complained of symptoms in the areas of the visibly involved vessels. Of this symptomatic subset, 60% sought treatment for varicosities less than 1 mm in di-

TABLE 3-2. DISTINGUISHING FACTORS OF ARTERIAL VERSUS VENOUS DISEASE OF THE LOWER EXTREMITIES

Signs and Symptoms	Arterial Disease	Venous Disease
Pain		
Ambulation	Worsens	Improves
Limb dependency	Improves	Worsens
Limb elevation	Worsens	Improves
Location	Calf or foot	Aching, burning
		Cramping or pruritus at site of varicosity
Compression hose	Worsens	Improves
Limb temperature	Cool	Warm
Ulceration sites	Lateral malleolus	Medial malleolus
	Distal toes	Lower calf
	Dorsal foot	Lower ankle
Ulceration characteristics	Ulceration necrosis	Erythematous
	Dry eschar	Moist
		Granulation tissue
		Often present
Cutaneous findings	Shiny atrophic skin	Eczematoid dermatitis
	Xerosis	Hyperpigmentation
	Diminished hair	Lipodermatosclerosis
	Growth	
	Nail dystrophy	
	Atrophie blanche	

I. Define sources of reflux, proximal to distal
    A. Determine patterns of origin of telangiectasis and clusters of varicosities.
II. Classify the type of varicosities present in a given patient. These can be subdivided clinically into two groups:
    A. Large varicose veins
        1. Axial varicosities
            a. Greater saphenous vein
            b. Lesser saphenous vein
        2. Truncal varicosities
        3. Branch varicosities
        4. Incompetent perforators
    B. Small varicose veins
        1. Reticular varicosities
        2. Venulectasias
        3. Telangiectasias
III. Look for signs of venous insufficiency.
    A. Regions of pigmentation
    B. Corona phlebectasia
    C. Scars from healed ulcerations or past surgical procedures
    D. Induration
    E. Local warmth
    F. Stasis dermatitis
    G. Ulcerations
    H. Atrophie blanche

A flowchart may be employed to summarize findings of the physical examination (Fig. 3-4).

Specific points in physical examination are as follows:

1. Palpation of arterial pulses. If arterial pulses are absent, an ankle–brachial index must be calculated. This is performed by obtaining a systolic blood pressure while the patient is in the supine position, with the cuff about the ankle. The systolic blood pressure obtained is then compared with the brachial systolic pressure. The normal ankle brachial index is greater than 1. If the index obtained is lower or the systolic blood pressure at the ankle is below 100 mm Hg, arterial disease is likely present. Therefore compression stockings may be contraindicated and sclerotherapy treatment should proceed with extra caution.
2. Palpation of veins. This gives a rough estimate of the pressure within veins, which may influence choice of sclerosant. Both the long (Fig. 3-5) and short (Fig. 3-6) saphenous veins may be palpated and may reveal evidence of palpable thrills with distal compression if incompetent.

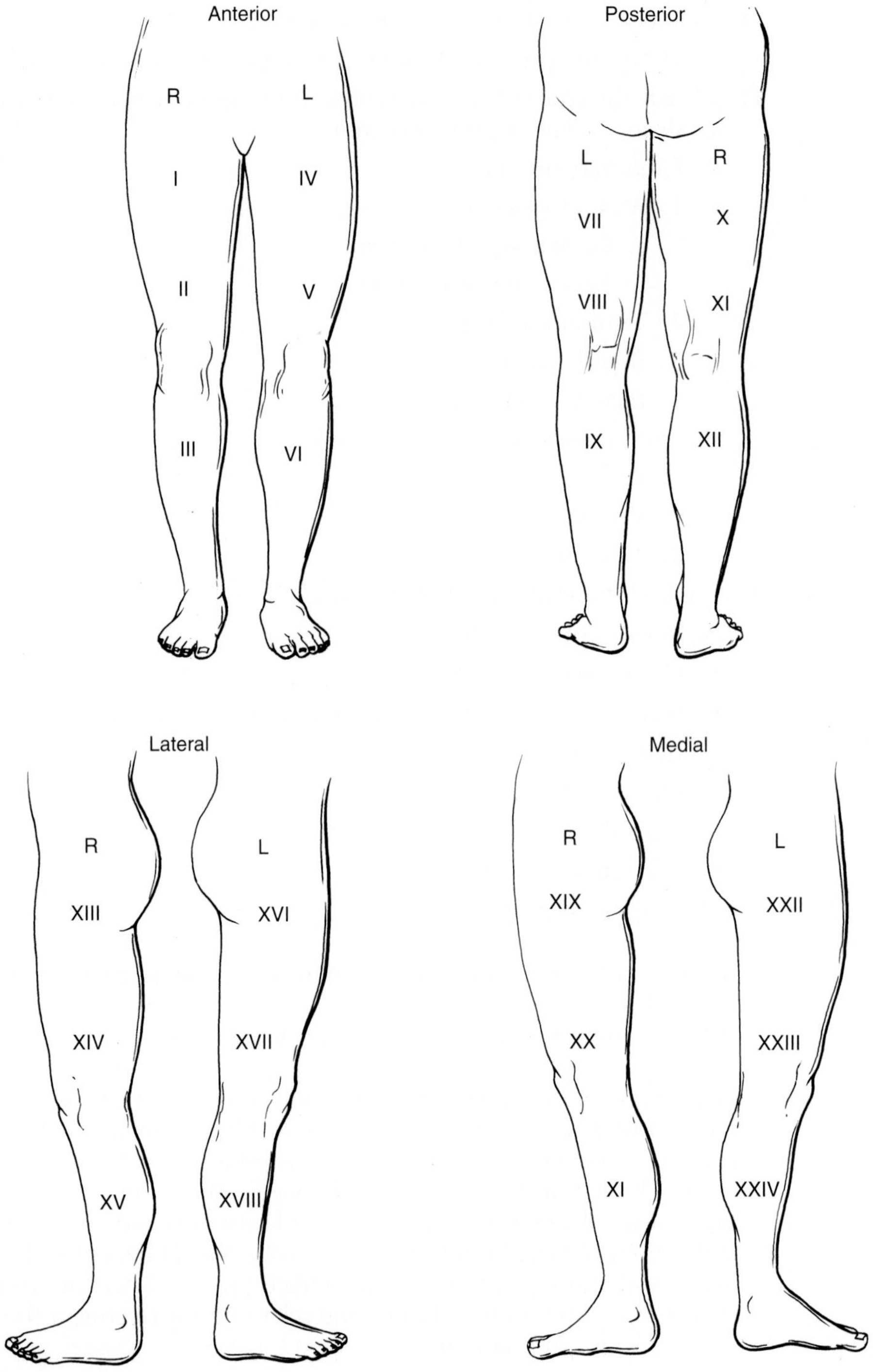

Figure 3-4

Phlebology physical examination flowchart. This may help the phlebologist to record physical examination data concerning the size and location of varicose veins and associated signs of venous insufficiency.

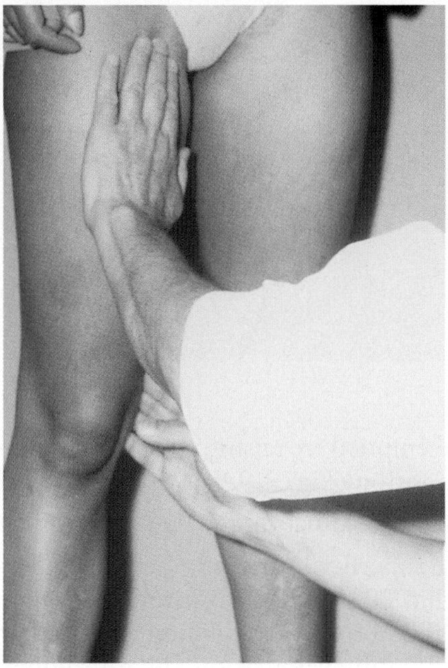

Figure 3-5

Palpation of greater saphenous vein. A palpable thrill may indicate incompetence at the saphenofemoral junction in the groin.

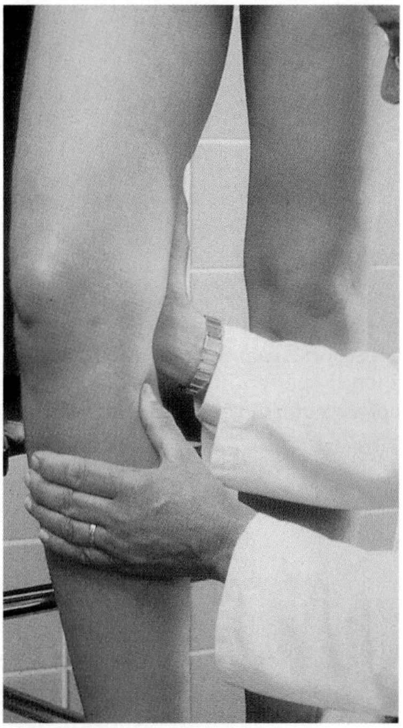

Figure 3-6

Palpation of lesser saphenous vein. A palpable thrill may indicate insufficiency of the lesser saphenous system (saphenopopliteal junction) at the level of the popliteal fossa.

Facial gaps (areas of easy compressibility) may be felt and are often associated (50% to 70% of the time) with perforator veins. Examination is performed with a soft-gloved finger running along the course of the varicose vein (Fig. 3-7) and *areas of dysfunction may be appropriately marked.* This diagnostic maneuver is performed with the patient in the supine position. If, when the patient subsequently stands, a perforator is present, the vein will refill only upon release of pressure. This technique will help identify the source of proximal perforator incompetence.

3. Ancillary diagnostic tests include the Schwartz test (cough test) (Fig. 3-8), which is used to diagnose vein incompetence (most commonly of the greater saphenous vein at the saphenofemoral junction, or SFJ).
    a. The examiner places a hand over the proximal portion of the long saphenous vein (LSV).
    b. The patient is then asked to cough or perform a Valsalva maneuver.
    c. The occurrence of a palpable impulse indicates the presence of valvular insufficiency at the SFJ and at any valve between that point and the site of palpation.
4. The Trendelenburg test (Fig. 3-9) may be used to diagnose incompetence of the SFJ.

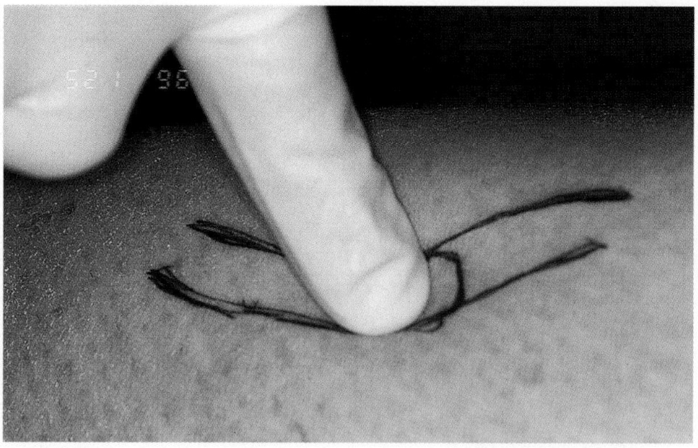

Figure 3-7

A soft-gloved finger marks fascial gaps in perforating veins. Identification of fascial gaps (areas of easy compressibility) may help to identify perforating veins as sources of superficial venous reflux.

a. The superficial veins of the leg are emptied by raising the leg 60 degrees above the horizontal in a supine position (Fig. 3-9A).
b. A hand or tourniquet is placed at the proximal thigh (Fig. 3-9B).
c. The patient then stands, and if the superficial varicosity below the hand or the tourniquet fails to refill within 20 seconds (positive test result), the reflux likely comes from the SFJ (Fig. 3-9C). Rapid filling (in less than 20 seconds) denotes incompetent perforating veins below the tourniquet.

5. The Perthes test (Fig. 3-10) detects degree of valvular insufficiency, obstruction to the deep venous system, or perforator vein incompetence.
   a. While the patient is standing, a tourniquet is applied to the upper portion of the thigh.
   b. The patient is then instructed to walk.

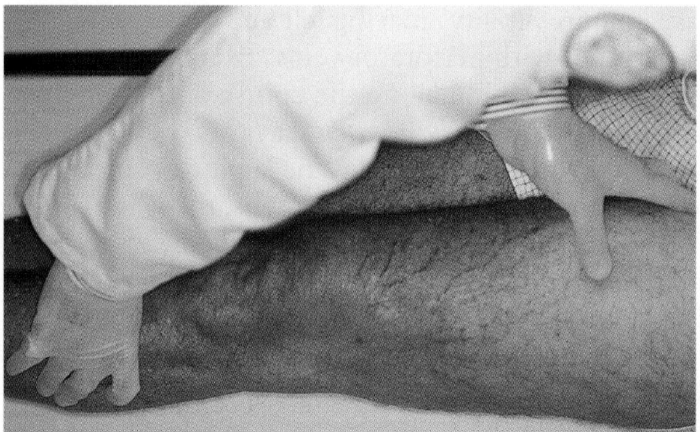

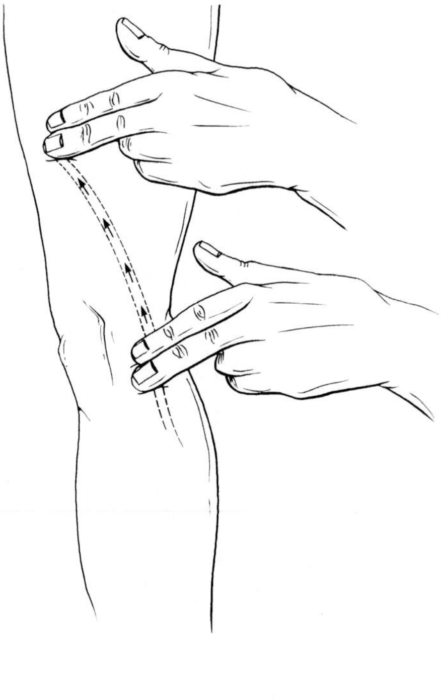

Figure 3-8

Schwartz test. A palpable thrill produced by tapping over the surface of the vein indicates an abnormally large volume of blood being displaced by the tap, suggesting significant reflux. This can be useful for mapping the course of the reflux to the highest point.

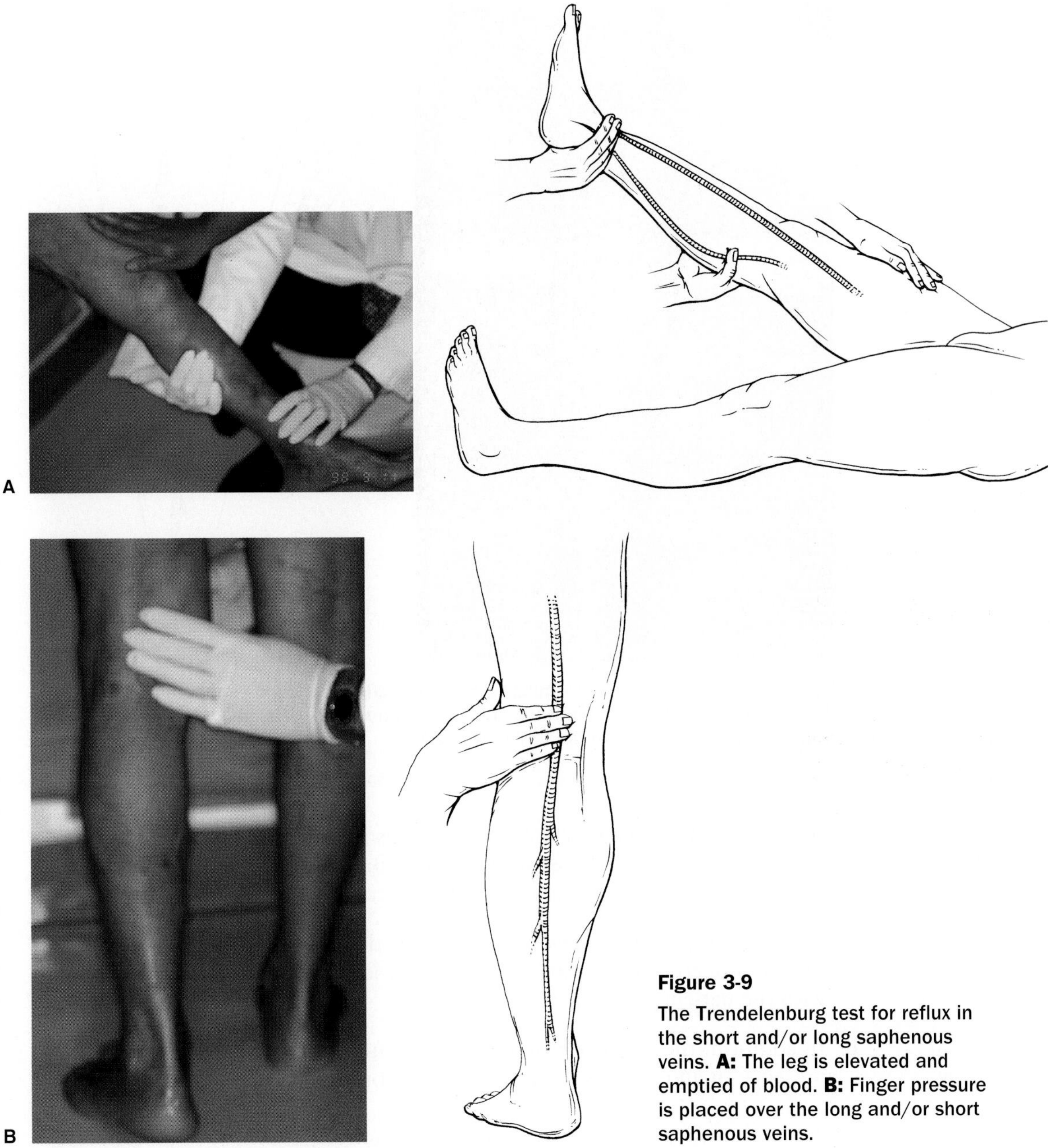

Figure 3-9

The Trendelenburg test for reflux in the short and/or long saphenous veins. **A:** The leg is elevated and emptied of blood. **B:** Finger pressure is placed over the long and/or short saphenous veins.

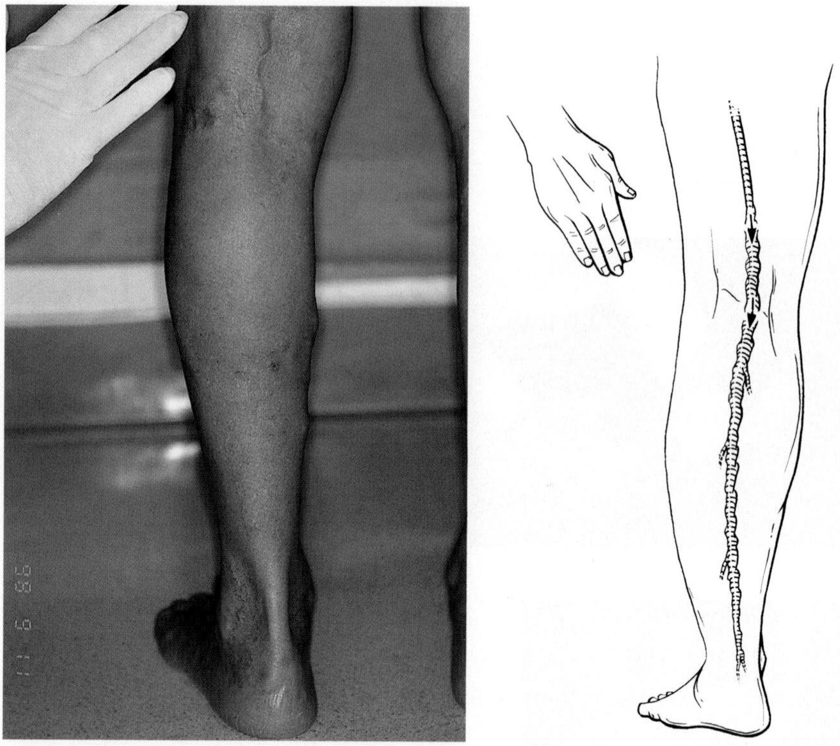

C

Figure 3-9 C: Finger release—bulging indicates reflux in the long saphenous vein (LSV). Concomitant dilatation of the short saphenous vein (SSV) indicates transmission of reflux from the LSV to the SSV.

c. A decrease in the diameter of varicose veins indicates that these veins are emptying efficiently by means of the calf muscle pump and that the deep venous system is not the source of the varicosities.

d. In a patient with incompetent perforators, deep vein thrombus, or other causes of deep venous insufficiency, the varicose veins will increase in size with the patient walking.

e. In addition, the onset of pain or venous claudication indicates the presence of an obstruction in the deep venous system.

Other techniques employing manual obstruction, tourniquet placement, palpation, and patient positioning have been used in the past; however, the above clinical tests are less employed with the advent of noninvasive vascular testing. However, inspection and palpation remain important parts of the approach the phlebologist must take in initially encountering a patient with varicose veins and these techniques will guide his or her approach to further vascular testing. Although a significant number of false-positive and false-negative results are elicited, expertise in physical examination will enable the practicing phlebologist to direct the therapeutic plan appropriately.

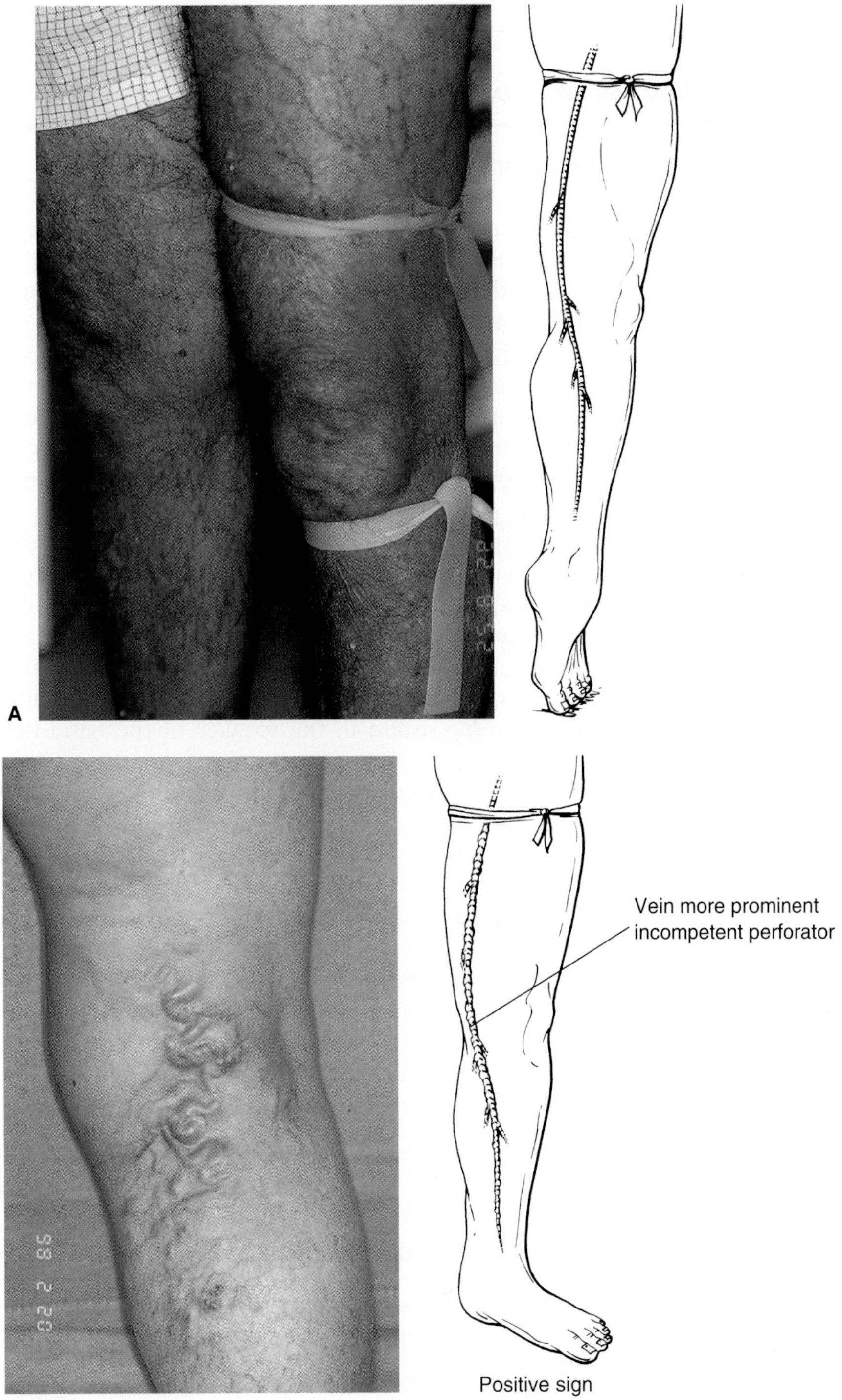

Figure 3-10

Perthes test. Detection of incompetence of a perforating vein. **A:** The patient rises up on his or her toes to exercise the calf muscles. A tourniquet is placed to block the superficial venous system and the patient exercises again. A negative test is manifest by decreased vein distention, indicating competent valves and perforator competence. **B:** Positive test: the superficial veins become more distended if the perforator is incompetent, indicating reflux from the deep to the superficial system through the incompetent valves of the perforating vein.

Vascular Laboratory Testing Options

Doppler Evaluation

Once the physical examination has been completed, a decision must to be made concerning the need for further vascular testing. General guidelines that may help to determine the need for vascular testing prior to the institution of sclerotherapy are listed in Table 3-4.

Once a decision has been made that vascular testing is indicated, the next decision concerns the order in which to proceed. With the understanding that the goal of treatment of a varicose vein of any size is to stop the leak or reflux at its origin, the simplest, most convenient, and most reliable way to detect the leak or reflux is by using Doppler ultrasound. This will help the clinician to determine the appropriate injection sites for a rational sclerotherapy sequence.

The Doppler instrument is the "stethoscope" of the phlebologist and should be present at every venous examination. The Doppler handpiece contains a probe with two mechanisms: a sensing crystal and a transmitting crystal (Fig. 3-11). The transmitting crystal sends sound waves that are reflected off red blood cells moving through the examined blood vessel. The moving erythrocytes cause a frequency shift, which is detected by the receiving crystal. This shift is subsequently translated into an audible sound in the speaker of the hand-held Doppler unit (Fig. 3-12).

There are two basic types of Doppler units:

1. Unidirectional. This is the standard Doppler, which detects blood flow in either direction across the sensing probe. No readout is available. This type of Doppler is used in presclerotherapy evaluation or to assess the results of treatment. It is considered part of the routine evaluation and is not insurance-reimbursable.
2. Bidirectional. This type of Doppler also detects blood-flow shifts in either direction across the sensing probe. In addition, it can give a graphic readout that traces blood flow either toward or away from the sensing probe. This type of Doppler can also produce waveform analysis of arterial signals.

TABLE 3-4. INDICATIONS FOR VASCULAR TESTING

1. Asymptomatic telangiectasia greater than 4 mm in diameter
2. Any varicosity greater than 2 mm in diameter extending throughout the calf or thigh
3. "Starburst" cluster of telangiectasia when present over points of perforating veins (mid–posterior calf, medial knee, medial midthigh, medial distal calf)
4. Reticular varicosities
5. Perforating veins
6. Varicose veins, truncal or saphenous origin
7. Clinical signs of venous insufficiency
8. Symptomatic veins of any diameter
9. History of deep venous thrombosis and/or thrombophlebitis
10. History of previous venous surgery or sclerotherapy with poor results or recurrence of varicosities

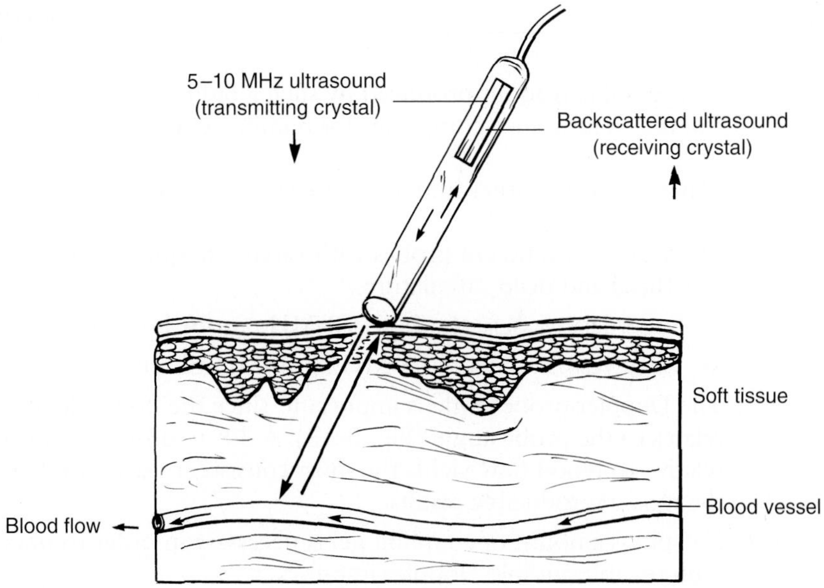

Figure 3-11

Doppler principles. The Doppler handpiece contains a probe with two mechanisms: a sensing and a transmittal crystal. The transmitting crystal sends out acoustic waves which are reflected from moving erythrocytes. Moving erythrocytes cause a frequency shift that is detected by the receiving crystal and translated into an audible sound by a hand-held speaker.

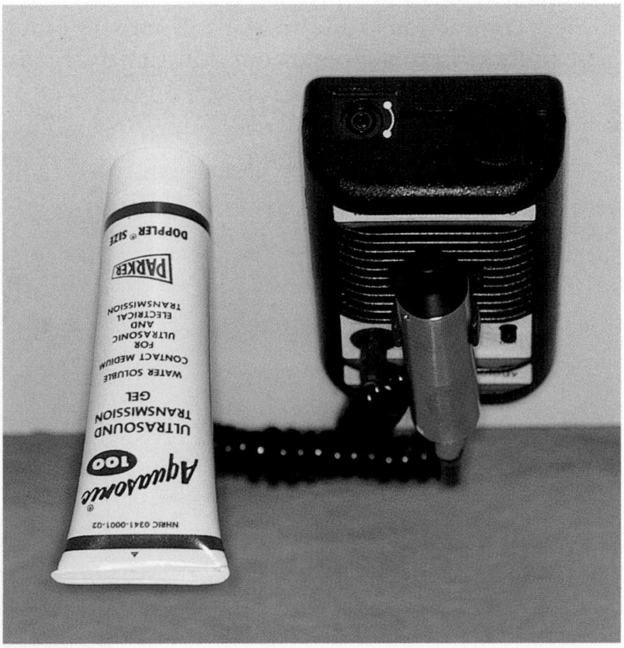

Figure 3-12

Doppler/clinical examination of superficial vessels is carried out with an 8- to 10-MHz probe. Deep vessels are examined with a 4- to 5-MHz probe.

The graphic readout produced by such a bidirectional device may be submitted to insurance companies for reimbursement consideration.

There are three other important considerations in Doppler examination:

1. There are two different probes with varying frequency for examining the superficial and deep vasculature.
   a. Superficial vessels: the 8- to 10-MHz probe is utilized.
   b. Deep vessels: the 4- to 5-MHz probe is utilized.
2. The Doppler probe angle is important, since the flow-velocity waveform relates to the probe angle (Fig. 3-13). A 30- to 45-degree probe angle relative to blood flow yields the most consistent waveform height and thus the most reproducible results.
3. A copious amount of coupling gel is necessary in order to obtain clear, reproducible audible Doppler impulses.

In utilizing the Doppler, two basic sounds are recognizable, spontaneous sounds and augmented sounds.

Spontaneous sounds are unidirectional signals whose intensity increases when the patient exhales and decreases on inhalation (i.e., the signals synchronize with the changes in intraabdominal pressure, which occur when the diaphragm rises or falls).

In contrast to the arterial system, which is a constant high-pressure conduit, the venous system is a low-pressure pathway with forward momentum generated by muscle contractions (due to the calf muscle pump) at irregular intervals. Because of these factors spontaneous flow signals are inaudible by Doppler ultra-

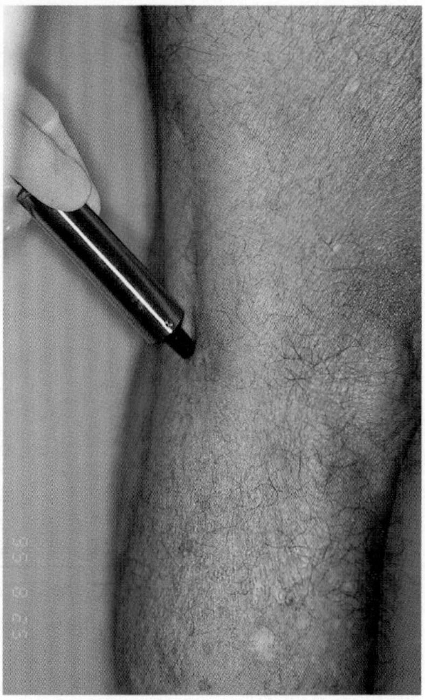

Figure 3-13

Doppler probe angle. A 30–45 degree probe angle relative to blood flow yields the most consistent waveform height and the most reproducible results.

TABLE 3-5. VENOUS DOPPLER CHARACTERISTICS

*S*pontaneous
*U*nidirectional
*P*hasic with respiratory cycle
*N*onpulsatile
*A*ugmented

sound with the patient at rest. Exceptions are large veins in the groin (femoral vein) communicating with abdominal veins, which are influenced by excursions of the diaphragm, and cases of right-sided heart pressure elevation.

Augmented sounds are audible signals produced by maneuvers that augment venous blood flow (i.e., manual compression of the calf muscle pump). These sounds, particularly those in the superficial system at the groin, may be augmented by Valsalva maneuvers. The venous Doppler characteristics are summarized in Table 3-5.

Two basic maneuvers are performed in Doppler testing—proximal and distal compression (Fig. 3-14).

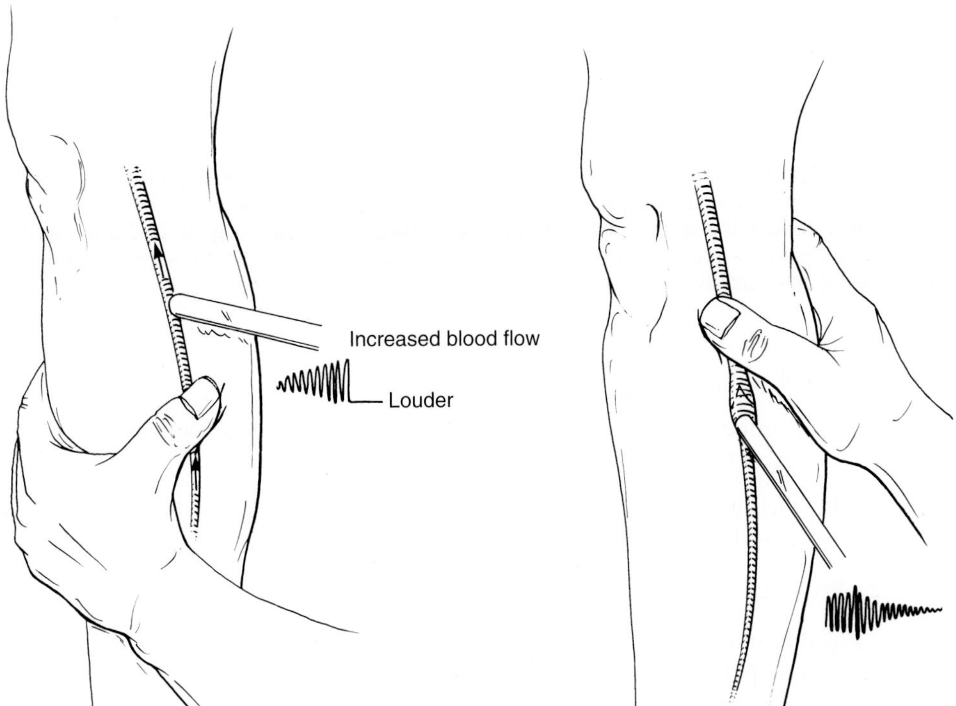

A, B

Figure 3-14

Schematic Doppler principles—normal responses to ultrasound maneuvers: A: Compression distal to the probe forces blood proximally, augmenting the Doppler signal. B: Compression proximal to the probe obliterates the venous flow and the Doppler signal as competent valves snap shut.

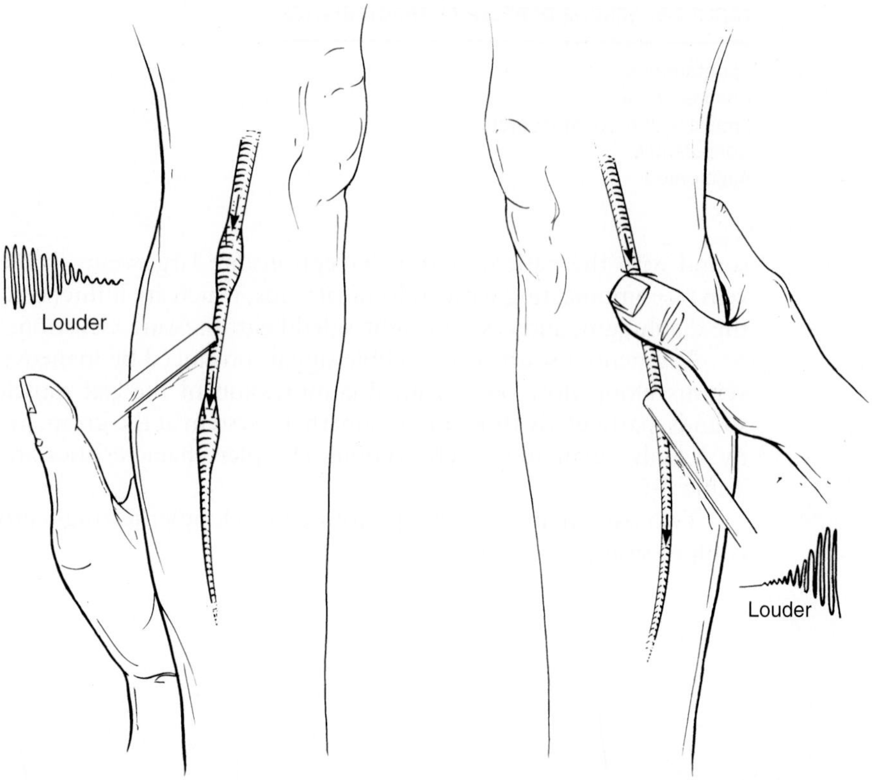

C, D

Figure 3-14 (*continued*) **C:** Schematic Doppler principles—reflux responses to ultrasound maneuvers: On release of elastic compression, the enlarged volume of blood refluxes back down through the incompetent valves, augmenting the Doppler signal. **D:** Compression proximal to the probe increases reflux down through the incompetent valves, augmenting the Doppler signal.

1. Distal compression
   a. Competent vein produces a short sound with cessation within 5 to 10 seconds as valves shut.
   b. Incompetent vein (reflux). Continuous flow manifest by a "whooshing" sound is elicited.
2. Proximal compression
   a. Competent vein. Brief sound that stops within 2 to 5 seconds as competent valves snap shut is provided.
   b. Incompetent vein. Prolonged whooshing sound as blood flows through incompetent valves is elicited.

Like other clinical evaluations, Doppler examination should proceed on an orderly, systematic fashion (Table 3-6) (Fig. 3-15). A suggested examination sequence is as follows:

TABLE 3-6. DOPPLER LOCATIONS TO BE EXAMINED

I.	Deep veins (4- to 5-MHz probe)
	Posterior tibial vein: posterior to medial malleolus
	Popliteal vein: popliteal fossae
	Superficial femoral vein: midthigh
	Common femoral vein: below inguinal ligament
II.	Superficial veins (8- to 10-MHz probe)
	Greater saphenous vein: below inguinal ligament
	Lesser saphenous vein: lower posterior thigh to the popliteal fossa
	Perforators: isolated as compressible fascial defects
	Reticular veins: look for associated areas of telangiectatic flares

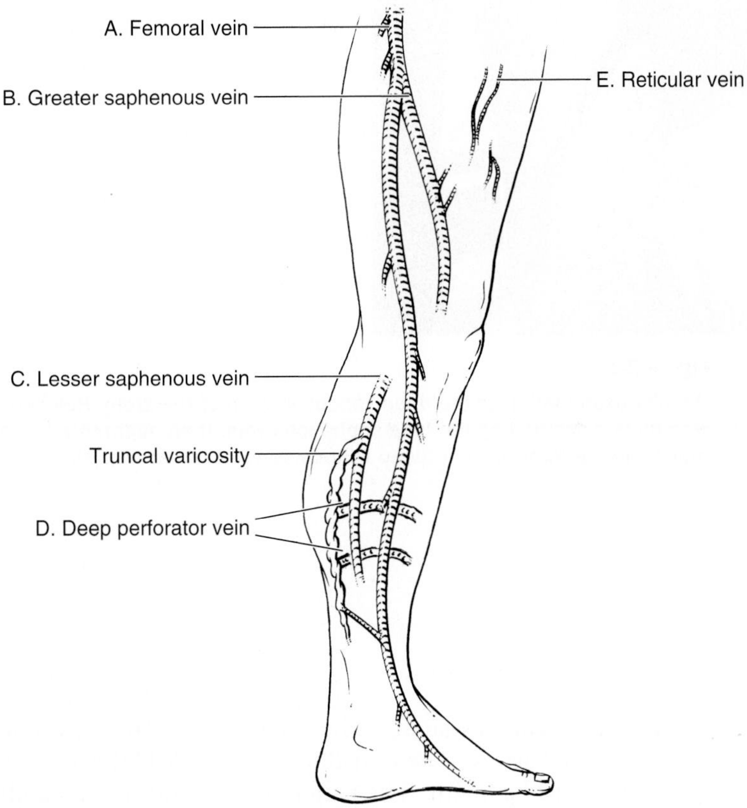

Figure 3-15

Sequence of Doppler evaluation (schematic) **A:** Deep venous system at the groin. **B:** Superficial venous system at the groin. **C:** Popliteal fossa. **D:** Perforators/truncal varicosities. **E:** Reticular veins.

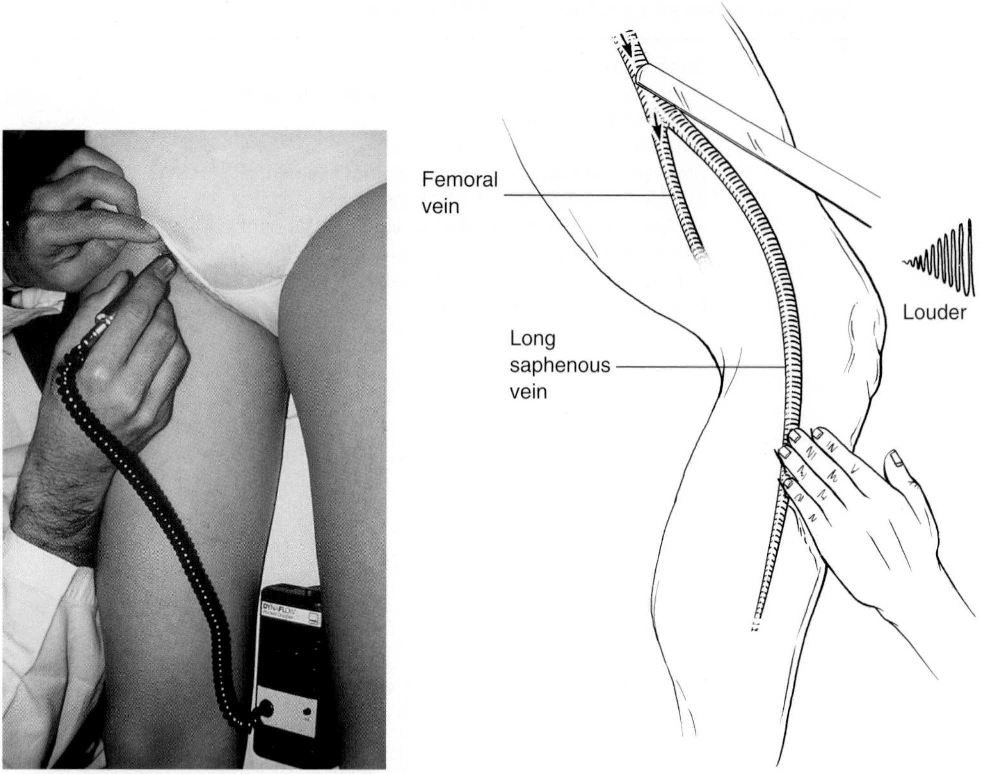

Figure 3-16

Doppler examination of the deep venous system of the groin. Release of distal compression with fingers obstructing the long saphenous vein. If an augmented signal is heard, the reflux may be in the femoral vein (deep venous system) rather than the saphenofemoral junction.

1. Deep venous system at the groin (Fig. 3-16). Femoral vein medial to the femoral artery. The transducer (4 to 5 MHz) is placed below or at the inguinal ligament. The patient may be sitting or standing.
2. Superficial venous system at the groin (Fig. 3-17). Greater saphenous vein, femoral vein junction. An 8- to 10-MHz transducer is used, as the SFJ is located 1 to 4 cm below the inguinal ligament. The patient may be sitting or standing. If incompetence is heard, the release of the distal compression maneuver is repeated with fingers obstructing the LSV. If an augmented signal is still heard, the reflux may be in the femoral vein rather than the SFJ.
3. Popliteal fossa/knee (Fig. 3-18). The lesser saphenopopliteal junction (SPJ). The site of the SPJ, sought with an 8- to 10-MHz probe is vari-

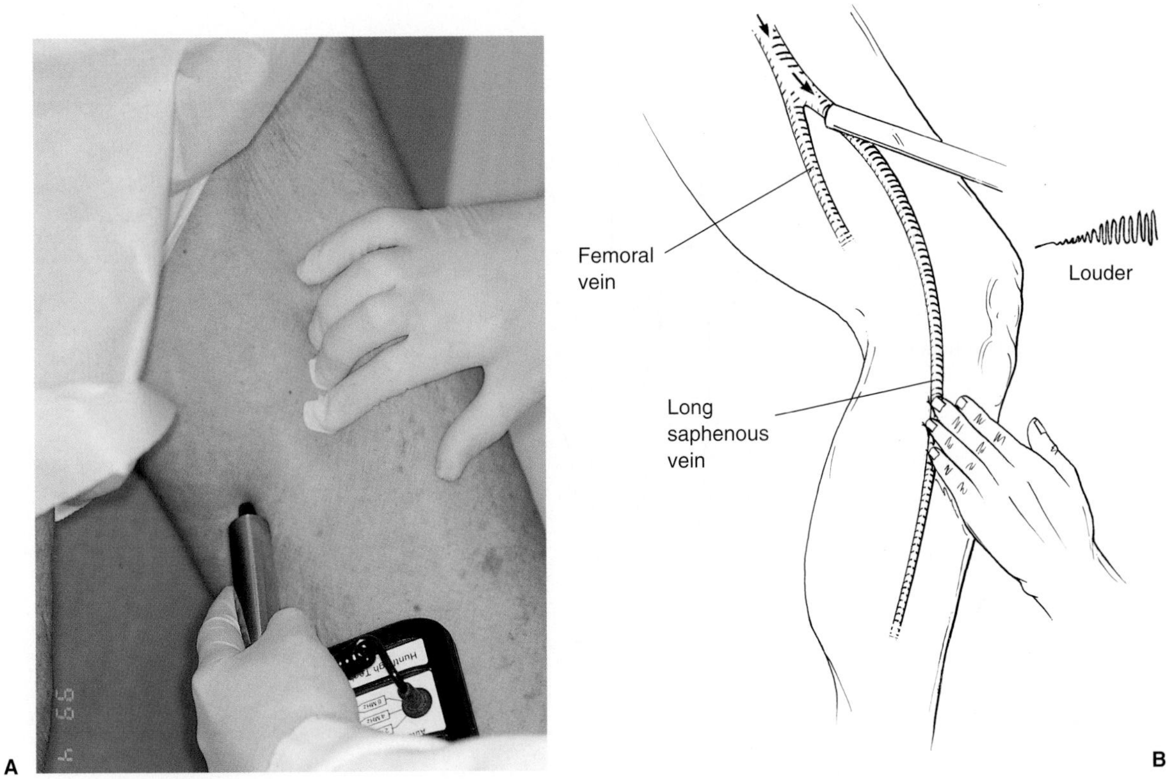

Figure 3-17

Doppler evaluation of the superficial system at the groin. **A:** Reflux at the saphenofemoral junction (SFJ) with the probe placed just below the SFJ. **B:** A loud, prolonged signal with release of distal compression is suggestive to reflux.

able and may appear anywhere from the lower posterior thigh to the popliteal fossa. The SPJ lies adjacent to the popliteal artery and is found just lateral to the arterial signal. By switching to a 4- to 5-MHz probe, one may identify deep reflux in the popliteal or gastrocnemius veins. If a loud signal indicative of reflux is heard in this anatomic zone, the physician should repeat the maneuver, releasing the distal compression while his or her fingers obstruct the SSV. If an augmented signal is still heard, the reflux may be in the popliteal vein itself rather than the SPJ. In examining this area two points of importance should be considered: (a) spontaneous sounds may be heard, as in the femoral vein, and (b) this part of the examination is usually performed in the standing dorsiflexed position.

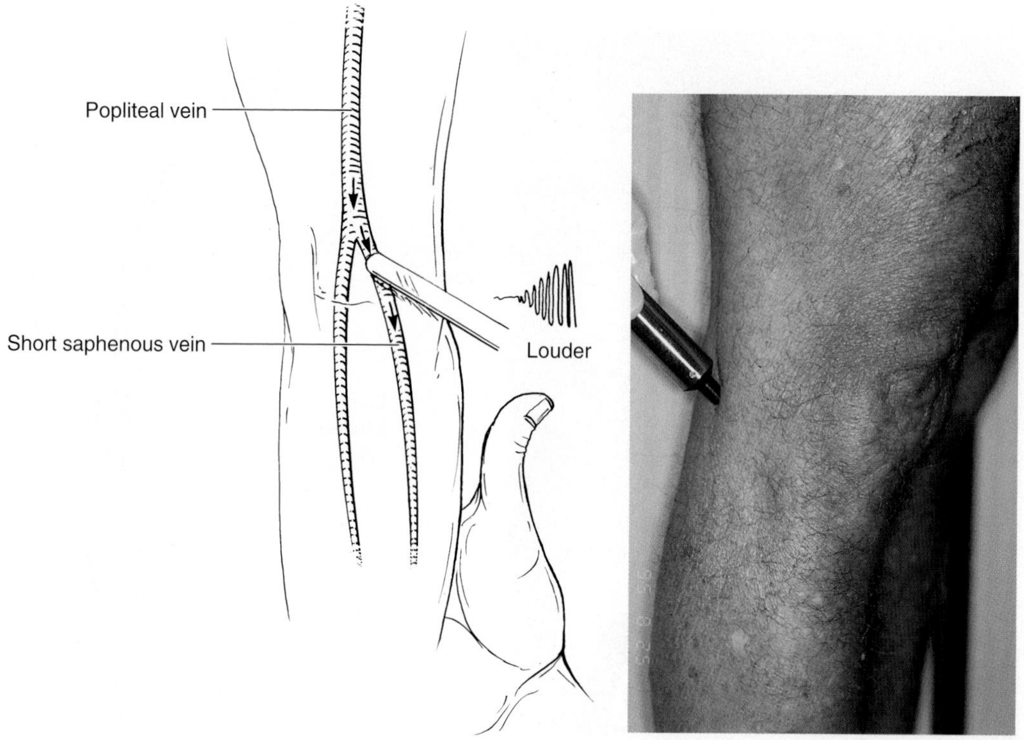

A

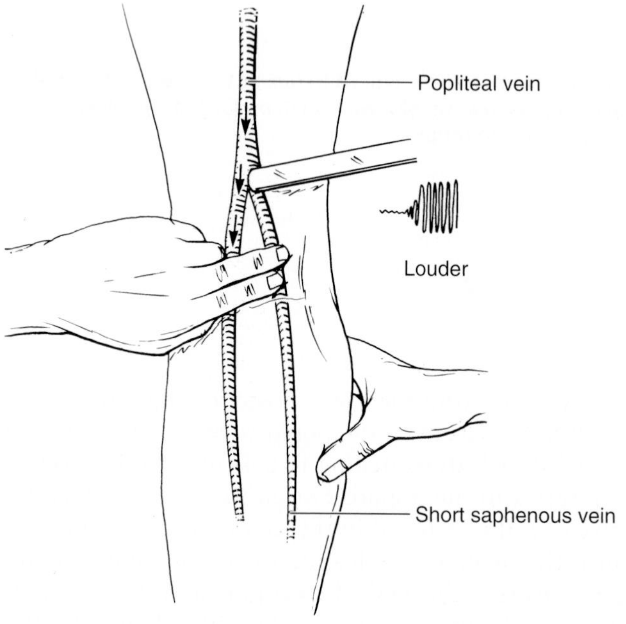

B

Figure 3-18

Doppler examination of the popliteal fossa. **A:** With the probe placed just below the saphenopopliteal junction, a loud signal heard at the release of distal compression is indicative of reflux. **B:** The release of distal compression is repeated with a finger obstructing the short saphenous vein. If an augmented signal is persistent, reflux may be in the popliteal vein (deep venous system) rather than the saphenopopliteal junction.

4. Perforators (Fig. 3-19). Perforators are located by palpation as fascial gaps, manifesting as areas of easy compressibility, as previously described. An 8- to 10-MHz probe placed over these bulging points with the patient in a standing position will produce audible sounds with augmented maneuvers. Alternately, with tourniquets blocking the superficial system, proximal compression results in an augmented signal only if there is reflux from the deep system through an incompetent perforator.
5. Reticular veins. The Doppler is used particularly to isolate reticular veins, which are a source of reflux and associated with flares of telangiectasia on the thigh (lateral subdermal complex of Albanese) or calf. These venous reflux points are more difficult to appreciate. They are isolated utilizing an 8- to 10-MHz probe with extremely light pressure, using the method of distal compression release. The patient may be sitting or standing.

Information obtained on Doppler ultrasound examination may be summarized in a flowchart, as in Fig. 3-20.

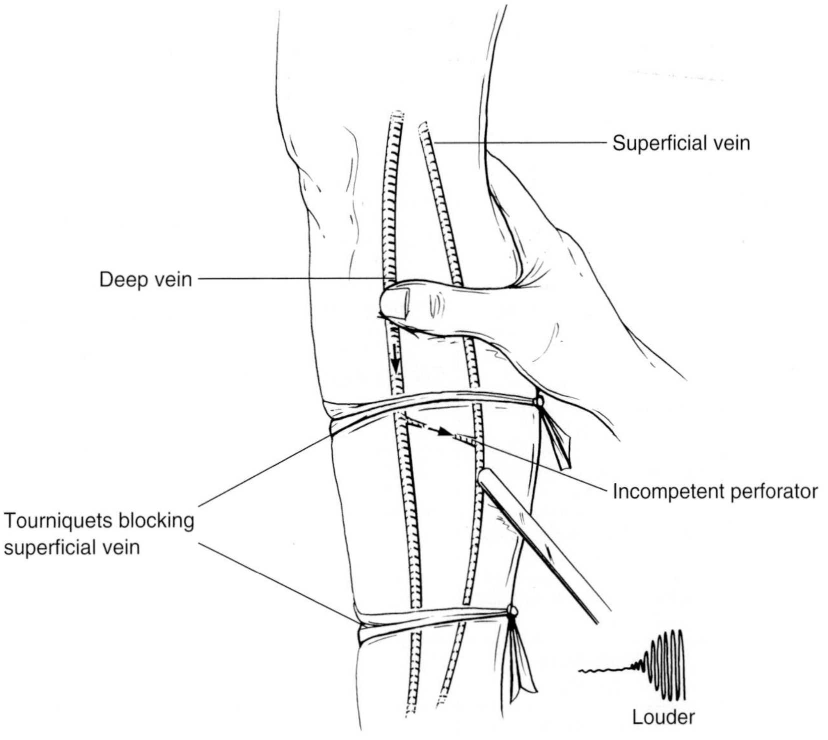

Figure 3-19

Doppler examination of perforators. With tourniquets blocking the superficial system, proximal compression results in an augmented signal if there is reflux from the deep venous system through an incompetent perforator.

DOPPLER EXAMINATION

Patient Name (Last, First, Middle Initial)

Date

Right Leg

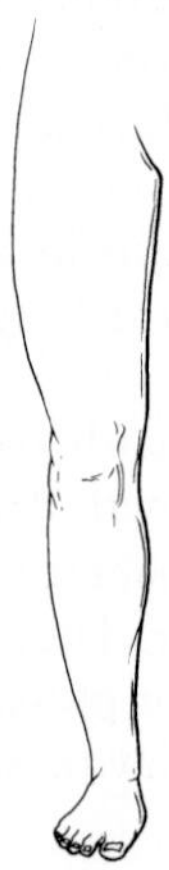

ANTERIOR

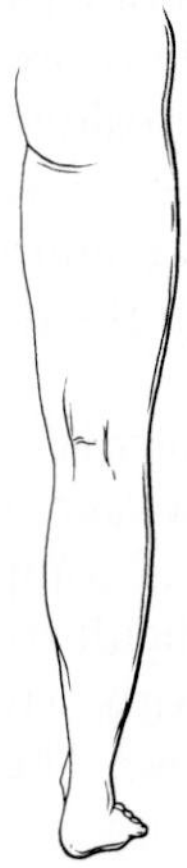

POSTERIOR

Left Leg

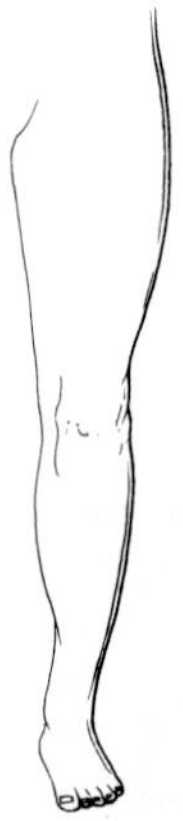

ANTERIOR

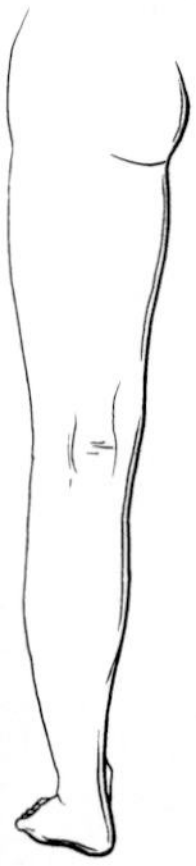

POSTERIOR

Support hose

Predisposing factors

Symptoms

Other Vascular Tests

L.R.R./P.P.G.

Duplex ultrasound

Air plethysmography

Perforator Locations Noted on Leg Diagram

	Distal Compression Release	Proximal Compression Phase	Valsalva Maneuver
Saphenofemoral Junction RIGHT			
Saphenofemoral Junction LEFT			
Saphenopopliteal junction RIGHT			
Saphenopopliteal Junction LEFT			
Perforators RIGHT			
Perforators Left			
Reticular veins Right			
Reticular veins Left			

The accuracy of Doppler evaluation relies on the experience of the user. Previous studies state a 49% to 96% accuracy as compared with more sophisticated imaging methods, such as duplex ultrasound evaluation.

In summary, the Doppler evaluation is an integral part of the sclerotherapy evaluation. It is used to identify sources of reflux that are to be treated first in the sequence of treatment design. It may also demonstrate physiologic sites of increased venous pressure subsequent to reflux in small-caliber vessels, such as telangiectasia (associated with underlying perforators or reticular veins), which might not otherwise be evident. In addition, it may also be used to enhance sclerotherapy treatment by locating minor perforators, which may be the best source of injection sites. It may also be utilized to treat veins not obvious on the surface of the skin with the patient in a standing or supine position (echosclerotherapy; see Chapter 14). Finally, it may be used to assess the results of sclerotherapy treatment by substantiating points of obliteration of venous reflux.

Photoplethysmography/Light-Reflective Rheography

Although Doppler ultrasound detects sites of valvular incompetence, photoplethysmography (PPG) and light-reflective rheography (LRR) allow quantification of the function of the leg muscle pump by means of simple examination. They both augment the physiologic significance of Doppler findings and, by a series of tourniquet applications, can distinguish between superficial and deep venous insufficiency.

Also of importance is the fact that these tests are not highly dependent on clinician skills. Thus, although false-positive and false-negative results range from 1% to 3%, there is less user variability than with Doppler ultrasound evaluation.

Indications for PPG and LRR evaluation are as follows:

1. Distinguishing superficial from deep venous insufficiency
2. Quantification of the degree of venous insufficiency
3. Observing the pumping ability of the deep venous system
4. Evaluating the results of sclerotherapy treatment

With the PPG, a single photoelectric light source illuminates a small area of skin while an adjacent photoelectric sensor measures the reflectance of light. The light source emits near infrared light (940 nm), which measures blood in the intradermal venous plexus approximately 2 mm deep and is minimally absorbed by the epidermis (15%). The measuring probe is attached to the medial aspect of the lower leg. During movement, venous pressure falls and accordingly the venous plexus become more translucent. The resulting light reflection is measured by photoelectric cells and recorded (Fig. 3-21). Recently a digital PPG (D-PPG, ELCAT, Wolfratshause, Germany) has been devised that is portable and has a

Figure 3-20

Doppler flowchart. Used to document the result of Doppler ultrasound evaluation and to enable the sclerotherapist to identify points of reflux that will serve as initial points of therapeutic intervention.

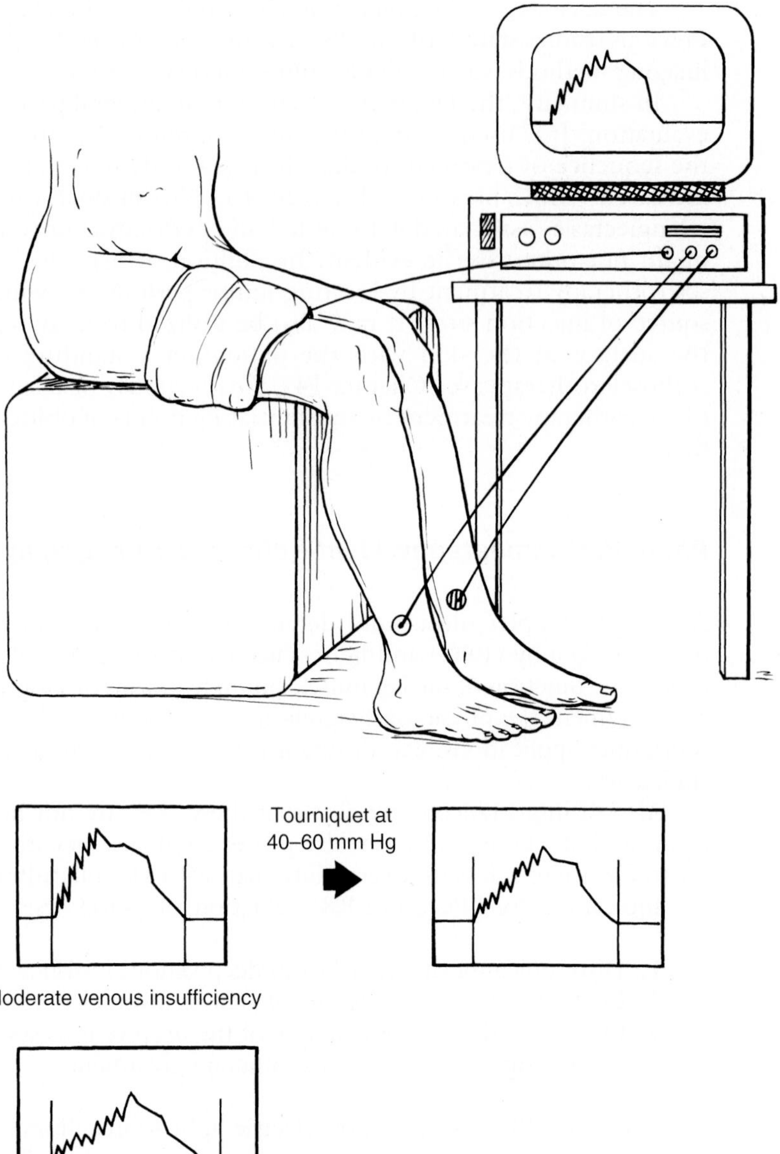

Figure 3-21

Photophethysmography (PPG). This venous measuring device emits near infrared light (940 nm) by means of a photoelectric sensing electrode that, by means of light reflection, measures venous pressures, calibrated as venous refill times. As shown, the measuring probe is attached to the medial aspect of the lower leg.

dedicated microprocessor which standardizes the signal received by the photoelectric sensor, leading to reproducible baselines independent of skin thickness or pigmentation. This makes it possible to obtain quantitative venous pump measurements (Fig. 3-22).

LRR includes three light diodes, rather than one, to illuminate the whole venous plexus of a small area of skin, with a single sensor measuring light reflectance and an additional sensor measuring skin temperature. The amount of reflectance is then related to the blood volume in the area of the probe (Fig. 3-23).

PPG and LRR results are relatively equal and both are approved by the U.S. Food and Drug Administration (FDA) for the testing of venous insufficiency. The LRR and PPG (noninvasive) curves are the two-dimensional mirror images of the venous pressure (invasive) curve (Fig. 3-24).

The testing protocol for the D-PPG and LRR is as follows:

1. The patient sits relaxed with knees bent 110 to 120 degrees.
2. The probe containing light-emitting and sensory diodes is taped to the medial aspect of the lower leg 8 to 10 cm (4 inches) above the medial malleolus (Fig. 3-25).
3. After a resting period of 3 to 5 minutes to establish a resting venous baseline, the patient dorsiflexes the foot 10 times (eight times for D-PPG). This activates the calf muscle pump and empties the calf's deep venous system with decreasing venous pressure. The venous plexus of the skin empties, yielding an increased reflectance of light. This is

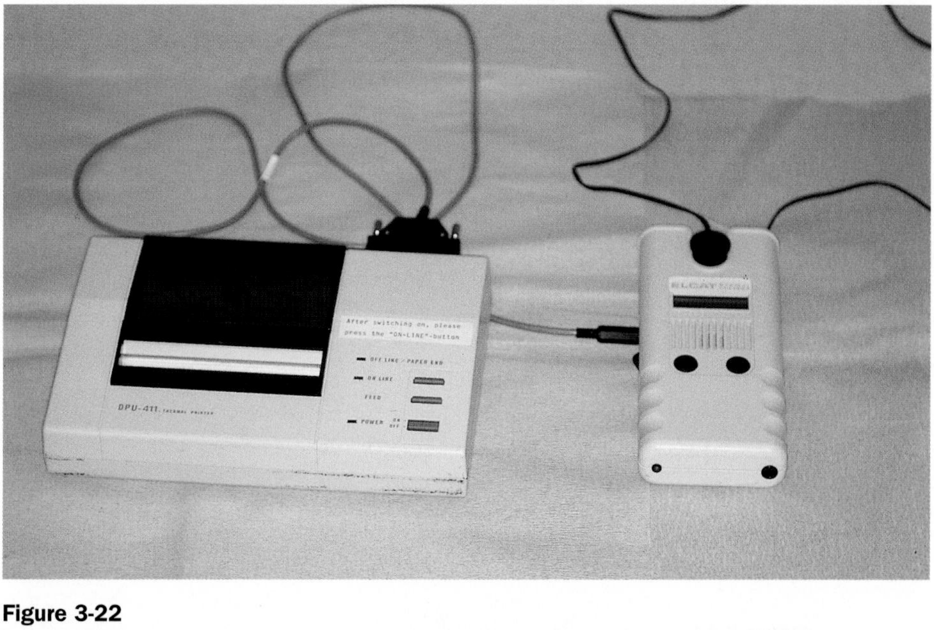

Figure 3-22

Digital PPG-ELCAT. The newly introduced digital PPG (D-PPG ELCAT, Wolfrathause, Germany) is equipped with a dedicated microprocessor that standardizes the photoelectric sensor signal, leading to standardized results independent of skin thickness or pigmentation. Quantitative venous pump measurements are thus readily obtainable.

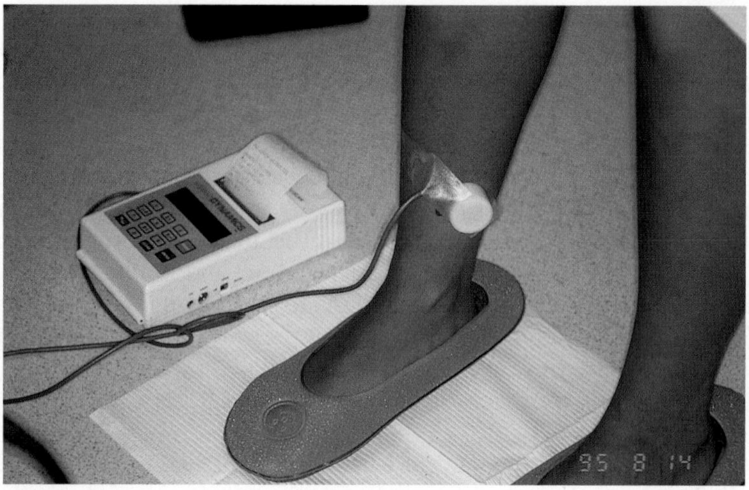

Figure 3-23

Light-reflective rheography (LRR) testing includes three light diodes that measure both light reflectance and skin temperature. Reflectance is related to blood volume and is presented as a readout on a monitor apparatus.

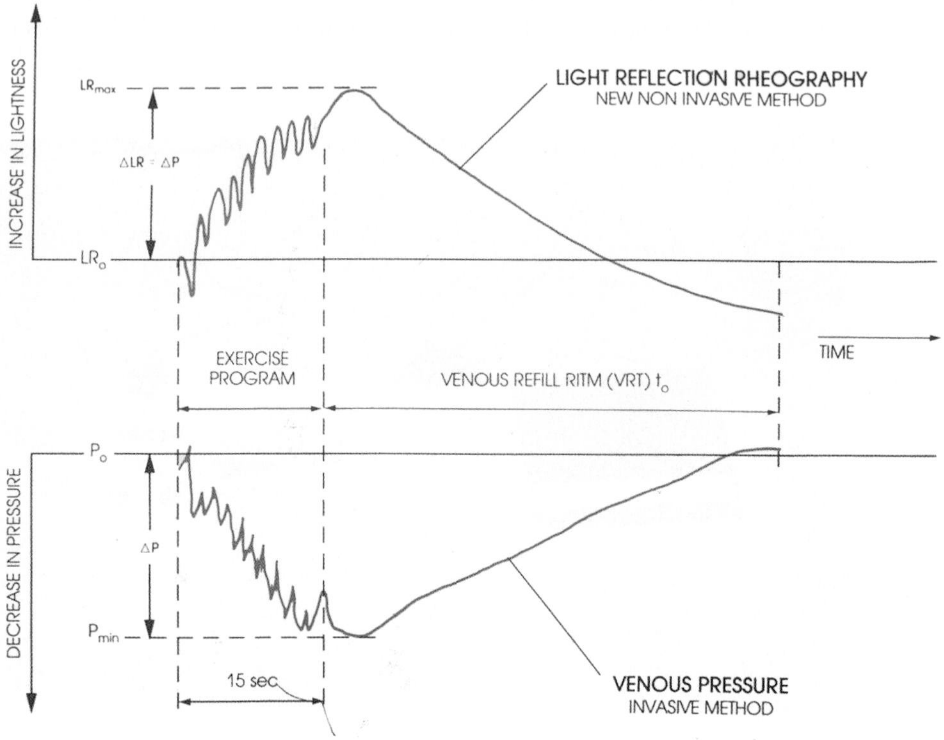

Figure 3-24

Light-reflective rheography (LRR) refilling curve the LRR and photoplesythmography (noninvasive) curves are the two-dimensional mirror images of the in vivo venous pressure (invasive) refilling curves.

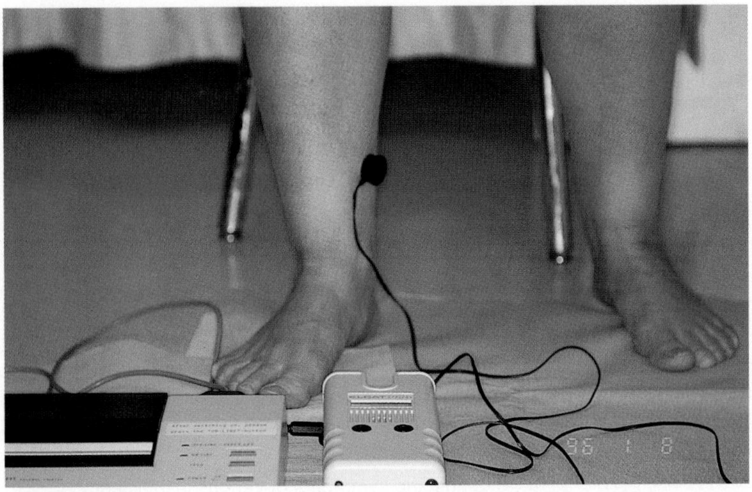

Figure 3-25

Testing protocol for photoplesythmography (PPG). Light-emitting and sensory diode containing probe is taped to the medial aspect of the lower leg 8 to 10 cm above the medial malleolus. After a resting period of 3 to 5 minutes to establish a resting venous baseline, dorsiflexion of the foot 10 times (8 times for the digital PPG) is carried out, which activates the calf muscle pump and empties the calf deep venous plexus, yielding an increased reflectance of light. This is shown on a tracing supplied by an attached printout device.

shown on a tracing as the change in reflected light from the skin under the probe.

4. After the calf muscle pump stops, blood refills the skin plexus, which absorbs increasing amounts of light as venules fill.
5. A direct relationship is postulated between the filling of deep leg veins and filling of measured veins in the skin.
6. The PPG (LRR) tracing slowly returns to its initial baseline as the calf veins fill.

It is generally understood that a refilling time of less than 25 seconds indicates venous valvular insufficiency, while refilling times longer than 25 seconds indicate normal venous valve function. This test can also quantitate the degree of venous insufficiency as follows: class I (mild), 19 to 24 seconds refill time, up to class III, less than 10 seconds refill time (severe insufficiency) (Table 3-7).

TABLE 3-7. QUANTITATIVE REFILL TIMES OF PHOTOPLETHYSMOGRAPHY/LIGHT-REFLECTIVE RHEOGRAPHY

Class	Refill Time	Degree of Venous Insufficiency
0	>25 sec	Normal
I	19–24 sec	Mild insufficiency
II	10–18 sec	Moderate insufficiency
III	<10 sec	Severe insufficiency

If the initial test shows a refill time of less than 25 seconds, the following maneuvers can be performed to localize the source of vascular incompetence (Fig. 3-26).

1. Apply above-the-knee tourniquet (Fig. 3-27).
   a. This occludes the superficial system.
   b. If refill time is normalized to greater than 25 seconds, the source of reflux is at the SFJ or midthigh perforators.
   c. One may now proceed with sclerotherapy or surgical treatment.
   d. If the refill time is still less than 25 seconds, one proceeds to step 2.

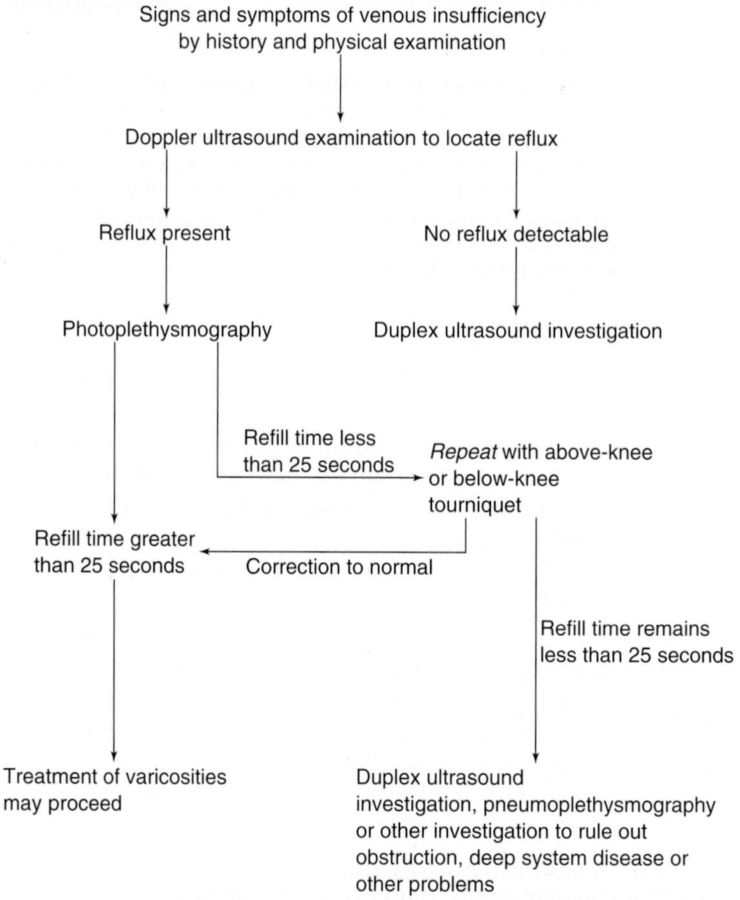

Figure 3-26

Protocol flowchart for digital photoplesythmography. Sequence of maneuvers including tourniquet placement that can be performed in order to localize the source of vascular incompetence.

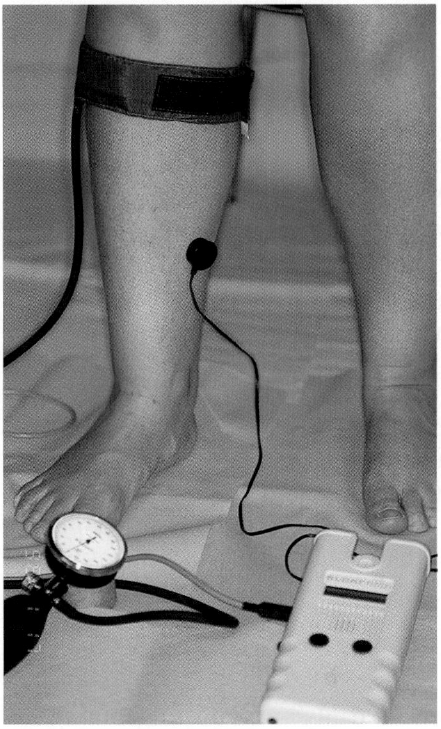

A

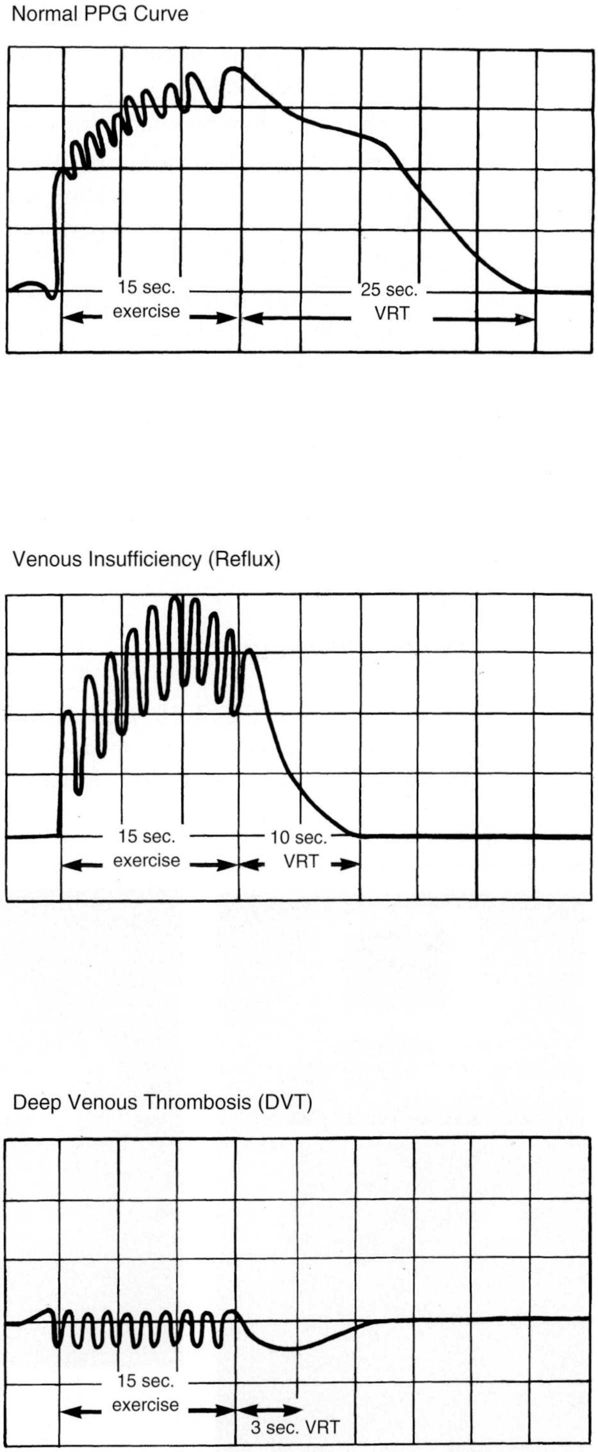

B

Figure 3-27

Tourniquet maneuvers with digital photoplesythmography (D-PPG). **A:** Application of an above-the-knee tourniquet utilizing the D-PPG or light-reflective rheography will occlude the superficial venous system. If reflux time normalizes to greater than 25 seconds, the source of reflux is at the saphenofemoral junction or midthigh perforators. If the reflux time remains less than 25 seconds, a below-the-knee tourniquet may be applied. Correction may indicate calf perforators. Lack of correction with both above- as well as below-knee perforators indicates deep venous insufficiency. **B:** Refill curves showing the normal condition, venous insufficiency (reflux), and deep venous thrombosis.

2. The tourniquet is applied below the knee.
   a. If the refill time normalizes, reflux is in the superficial system, usually in the calf perforators.
   b. One may then proceed with sclerotherapy.
3. If the refill time does not normalize with the above- or below-the-knee tourniquet, one is usually dealing with deep venous insufficiency and sclerotherapy should not be performed without further evaluation, such as duplex ultrasound.
   a. False results may be obtained in patients with impaired ankle joint mobility or arterial occlusive disease that prevents normal cutaneous blood flow.

In summary, PPG/LRR can localize primary sources of reflux. They can also measure treatment success as well as predict the outcome of the elimination of varicosities requiring external compression to correct them before treatment.

More sophisticated quantitative testing, such as pneumoplethysmography, is available in vascular laboratories but beyond the scope of this text.

Duplex Ultrasound

Duplex scanning (Fig. 3-28) is a relatively new modality in the investigation of venous diseases. By combining accurate assessment of anatomic structure and functional evaluation of blood flow, it has become the standard by which other inves-

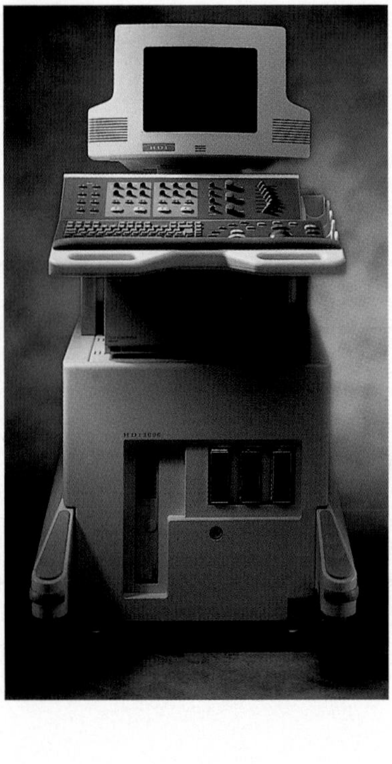

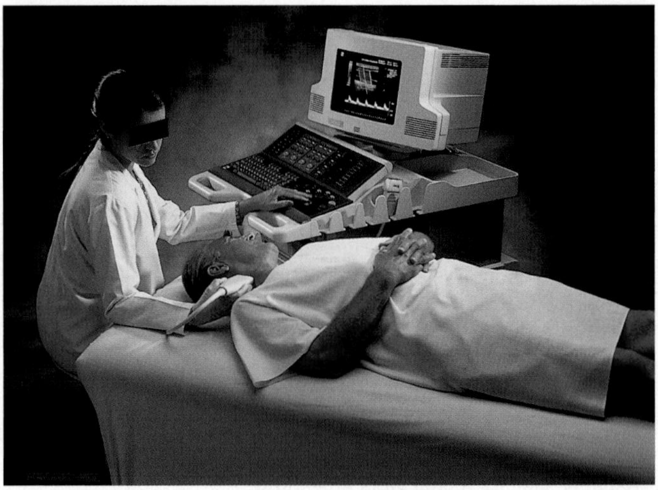

Figure 3-28

Duplex ultrasound combines B-mode imaging of the deep and major superficial veins with directional pulsed Doppler to assess blood flow.

tigations are judged. It is expensive technology and should be utilized in appropriate situations where clinical information cannot be obtained by less expensive modalities. In addition, it requires extensive training in order to gain significant proficiency. A comparison of Doppler and duplex ultrasonography is presented in Table 3-8.

Indications for the use of duplex ultrasound are as follows:

1. Evaluation of the deep venous system for evidence of thrombosis
2. Evaluation of the superficial venous system for
   a. Quantification of junctional reflux
   b. Localization of perforating veins
3. To aid the sclerotherapist in placing sclerosing solutions accurately during treatment
   a. Treatment of SFJ incompetence
   b. Treatment of SPJ incompetence
   c. Treatment of incompetent veins audible by Doppler evaluation but not visible with the patient in a supine or standing position

   In these settings, duplex-guided sclerotherapy may reduce the incidence of intraarterial injection.
4. Augmentation maneuvers to determine if effective sclerosis occurs with injection
5. Postsclerotherapy evaluation of the degree of endofibrosis and recanalization in sclerosed veins

There are three basic physical principles of duplex venous ultrasound.

TABLE 3-8. A COMPARISON OF DOPPLER ULTRASOUND AND DUPLEX SCANNING IN THE PRESCLEROTHERAPY EVALUATION

	Doppler	**Duplex**
Portability	Portable	Not easily portable; "luggable" units available
Ease of use	Requires a short period of training and experience	Requires a longer period of training
Cost (approximate)	Unidirectional: $300 Bidirectional: $2,500	Gray scale: $40,000 and up Color: $150,000 and up
Information obtained	1. Patency, competence of venous valves 2. Deep venous thrombosis in thigh (? calf)	1. Patency, competence of venous valves 2. Deep venous thrombosis with greater accuracy 3. Velocity of reflux 4. Anatomy and anomalies of venous system 5. Termination of short saphenous vein 6. Thrombosis versus sclerosis
Reliability	Less reliable because of blind, nonpulsed sound beam	More reliable because of actual visualization of vein being examined

1. B-mode imaging of the deep and major superficial veins. Ultrasound imaging frequencies are similar to those of the conventional Doppler.
   a. A 7.5- to 10-MHz probe is used to visualize superficial and perforating veins.
   b. A 5.0- to 7.5-MHz probe is utilized for imaging deep veins.
2. Directional pulsed Doppler assessment of blood flow.
3. Color duplex imaging superimposes blood flow information onto the B-mode ultrasound image, permitting the visual assessment of blood flow (Fig. 3-29).

A summary of duplex findings is shown in Table 3-9.

Although this modality is not part of most practitioners' armentarium at this time, the phlebologist performing sclerotherapy should be familiar with their indications so that appropriate referrals can be instituted. If one is going to inject axial junctions (the SFJ or SPJ) or include ambulatory phlebectomy as a part of one's therapeutic armentarium, duplex ultrasound should be an integral part of the practice setting in such cases.

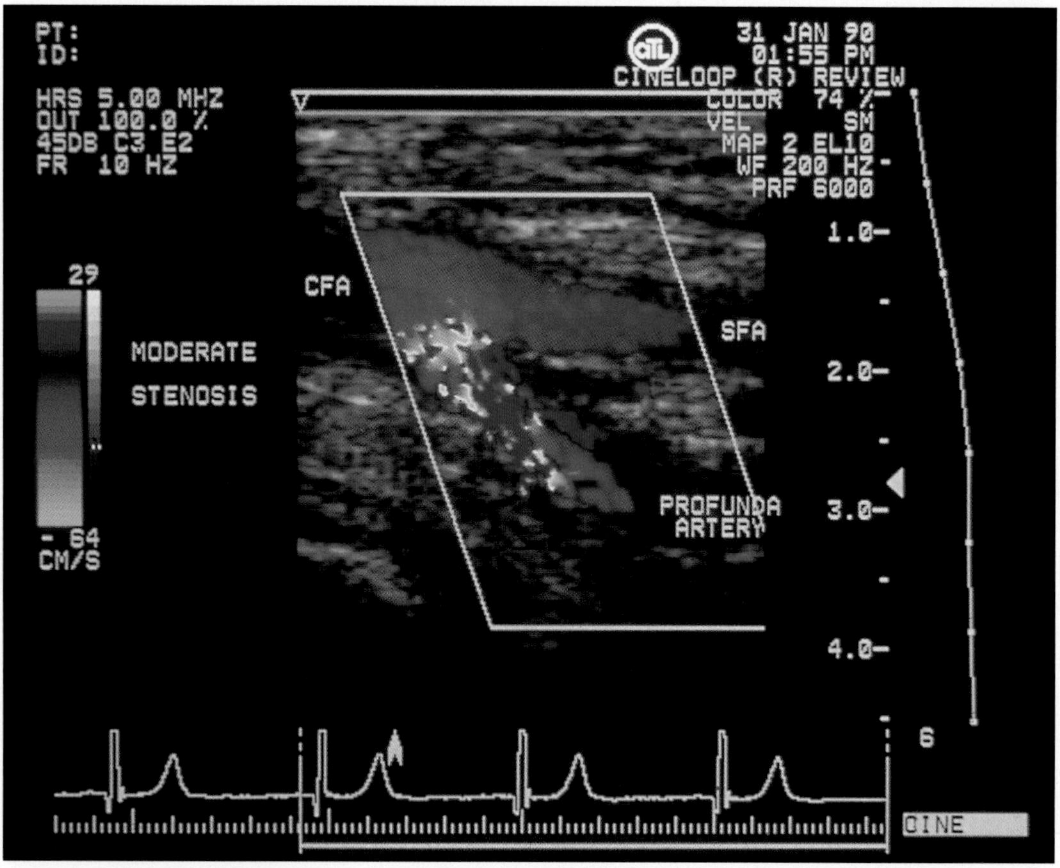

Figure 3-29

Color duplex ultrasound. Color duplex imaging superimposes blood flow information onto the B-mode ultrasound image, permitting the visual assessment of blood flow.

TABLE 3-9. DUPLEX FINDINGS IN NORMAL AND VARICOSE VEINS

Normal Veins	Varicose Veins
Usually echo-free (high-resolution gray scale instruments may show smooth blood flow on the B-mode image)	Turbulent flow Moderate to marked echogenicity Reflux flow Collateral flow
Thin-walled veins	Irregular vein wall
Visualization of venous valves	Venous distention
Valve cusps move freely and symmetrically	Valve abnormalities
Easily compressible by a small amount of pressure with the ultrasound probe	Incompressible

Conclusion

As can be seen from the preceding pages, appropriate history taking, physical examination, and laboratory testing are essential in defining an individual's specific venous problem (i.e., cause and location of reflux pathology). Only by defining the specific local or venous aberrations can one go on to institute the appropriate sclerotherapeutic and/or surgical intervention and thus administer the most optimal care to the patient. As in all fields of medicine, diagnosis remains the cornerstone of appropriate, effective therapy.

Venous evaluation identifies sources of increased pressure transmitted by incompetent valves to surface veins, causing varicosities and telangiectasias. Doppler ultrasound permits sites of reflux (incompetent valves) to be localized, whereas plethysmography (PPG) and light-reflective rheography (LRR) enable physiologic measurements and sources of incompetent valves to be analyzed. With tourniquet placement, accurate localization of superficial versus deep venous disease may be elucidated. When the answer is still not apparent with these modalities, anatomic and functional precision can be achieved with duplex ultrasound testing.

BIBLIOGRAPHY

Butie A. Clinical examination of varicose veins. *Dermatol Surg* 1995;21:52–56.

Fronek A. Photoplethysmography in the diagnosis of venous disease. *Dermatol Surg* 1995;21:64–66.

Isaacs MN. Symptomatology of vein disease. *Dermatol Surg* 1995;22:321–323.

Neumann NAM, Boersma I. Light reflection rheography: A non-invasive diagnostic tool for screening venous disease. *J Dermatol Surg Oncol* 1992;18:425–430.

Somjen GM, Ziegenbein, DMU, Johnston, AN, Royle JP. Anatomical examination of leg telangiectasias with Duplex scanning. *J Dermatol Surg Oncol* 1993;19:940–945.

Thibault PK. Duplex examination *Dermatol Surg* 1995;21:77–82.

Weiss RA. Evaluation of the venous system by Doppler ultrasound and photoplethysmography or light reflection rheography. *Semin Dermatol* 1993;12:78–87.

Weiss RA. Vascular studies of the legs for venous or arterial disease. *Dermatol Clin* 1994;12:175–189.

Weiss RA, Weiss MA. Continuous wave venous Doppler examination for pretreatment diagnosis of varicose and telangiectatic veins. *Dermatol Surg* 1995;20:58–62.

CHAPTER 4

Setting Up a Sclerotherapy Suite

Beginning a sclerotherapy practice is a relatively simple endeavor because there is no significant financial outlay for specialized equipment. However, as in the case of all other surgical procedures, a well-organized treatment locale with precise layout of instrumentation is of prime importance. A common question often asked by young physicians attempting to begin a sclerotherapy practice is "What type of equipment do I need to get started?" The goal of this chapter is to answer this question by instructing the sclerotherapist on how to set up an efficient, functional sclerotherapy suite. A list of materials necessary to begin sclerotherapy practice is given in Table 4-1.

Lighting

As sclerotherapy involves the treatment of small-diameter vessels in many instances, the accuracy of venous cannulation is of great relevance in the procedure; thus adequate side lighting is of prime importance. Many types of overhead lighting sources are available: however, a sclerotherapy light source should have the characteristic of being mobile on either a tract or pivot mechanism, so that the light can be adjusted to illuminate the area being treated. Two examples of light sources found to be helpful in the sclerotherapy suite are:

1. The Burton Fleximont Model 1004 Single ceiling-mount halogen lamp 115 V 50/60 Hz (Burton Medical Products, Van Nuys, CA, U.S.A.) (Fig. 4-1).
2. The Magnifying Flowlamp (Burton Medical Products) Van Nuys, CA, U.S.A.) (Fig. 4-2).

TABLE 4-1. MATERIALS NECESSARY FOR BEGINNING A SCLEROTHERAPY PRACTICE

Sterile gauze
Disposable 3-mL Becton Dickinson or 1-mL tuberculin syringes
Fine needles (#30, #32, #33)
Sclerosant
Normal saline
1% Lidocaine
Alcohol—$\frac{1}{2}$% acetic acid solution
Cotton balls
Compression pads (foam rubber)
Adhesive or elastic bandages (4 and 6 inches wide)
Support hose
Hyaluronidase
Nitroglycerin paste
Magnifying source (2× to 3×)
Clear light source
Hand-held Doppler (5- and 8-MHz)
Bard Parker surgical blade #11 or Beaver surgical blades #65 and handle
Emergency resuscitation kit
Consent form
Macro-lens photography system
Doppler examination treatment flow sheet
Anatomic region diagrammatic flow sheet

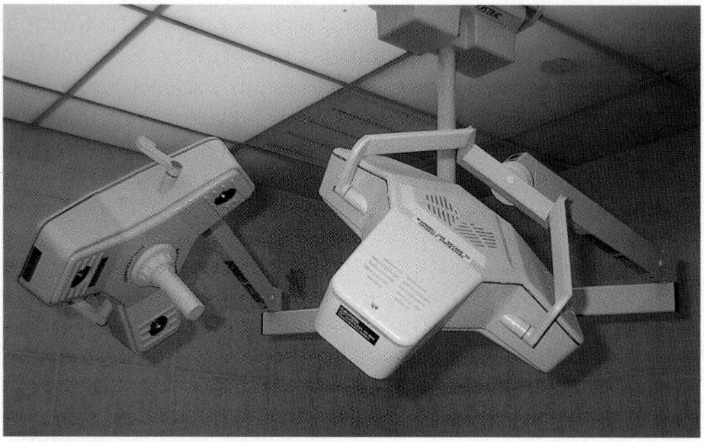

Figure 4-1

Burton overhead lamp. Provides excellent side lighting for improved vessel identification and cannulation sites.

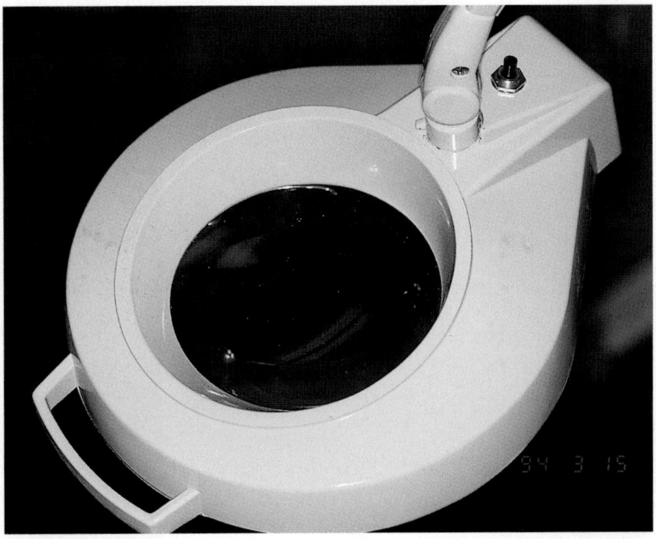

Figure 4-2
Burton floor magnifier (magnifying flow lamp). Provides simultaneous illumination and magnification, allowing the sclerotherapist improved optical visualization.

The Magnifying Flowlamp light source, although not as strong in terms of illumination as the Burton Fleximont, has the advantage of illuminated optical magnification. This light source may be used concomitantly to give synergistic illumination and magnification.

Tables

In performing sclerotherapy, positions varying from supine to Trendelenburg or reverse Trendelenburg are required. It is thus essential to have a power-assisted table (Fig. 4-3). More specifically, it is important to have a table with adjustable head and leg options so that appropriate positioning may be carried out in treating various problems. It is also efficacious to have motorized foot pedals, so that the physician can make adjustments without having to move.

For example, in treating telangiectasis or venulectasis, most sclerotherapists treat the patient in a supine position. In the case of large class IV truncal varicosities, many sclerotherapists prefer to treat the patient in a more vertical, dependent position. For ambulatory phlebectomy procedures, patients are initially placed in a reverse Trendelenburg position.

Examples of power-assisted tables with adjustable head and leg segments include:

1. The Midmark Model #111 or #119 power medical table (Midmark Corporation, Versailles, OH, U.S.A.).
2. The Ritter Model #119 power medical table (Ritter Corporation, Versailles, OH, U.S.A.).

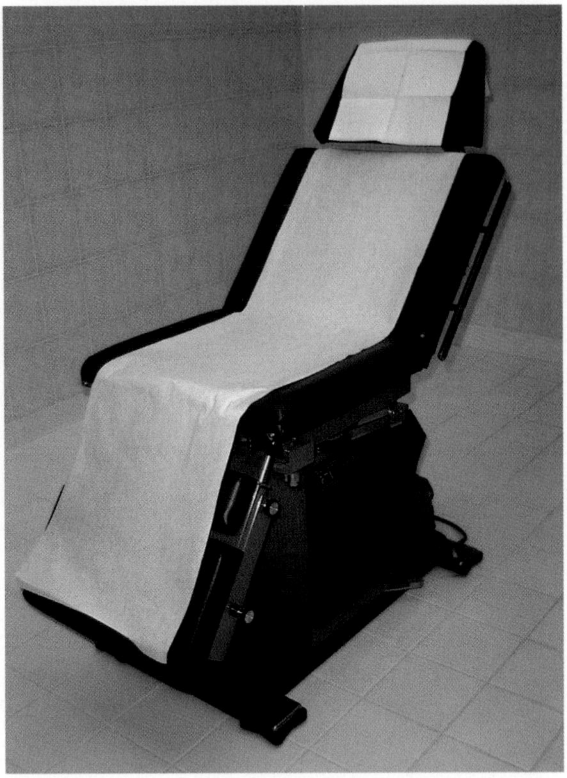

Figure 4-3
Power-assisted table.

Operator Stools

Adjustable stools (Fig. 4-4), either manual or hydraulically assisted, also are helpful in achieving proper physician-patient positioning in order to perform accurate and precise sclerotherapy. The addition of a back support is helpful in preventing low back strain in the operator who performs these procedures repetitively over long periods of time. Stools are available from most manufacturers, including those noted above.

Patient Examination Step Stools

As demonstrated in Chapter 3, for appropriate physical examination, Doppler evaluation, and in selected instances for the treatment of axial (class V: greater saphenous vein, lesser saphenous vein) and truncal class IV varicosities, it is often necessary to have a two-step stool (Fig. 4-5). Such a stool may be purchased commercially (E.F. Brewar, Bay Medical, Farmingdale, NY, U.S.A.), or it may be constructed by a carpenter with a custom-carpeted exterior.

The tables and stools described above will allow the sclerotherapist flexibility in treating all types of venous problems.

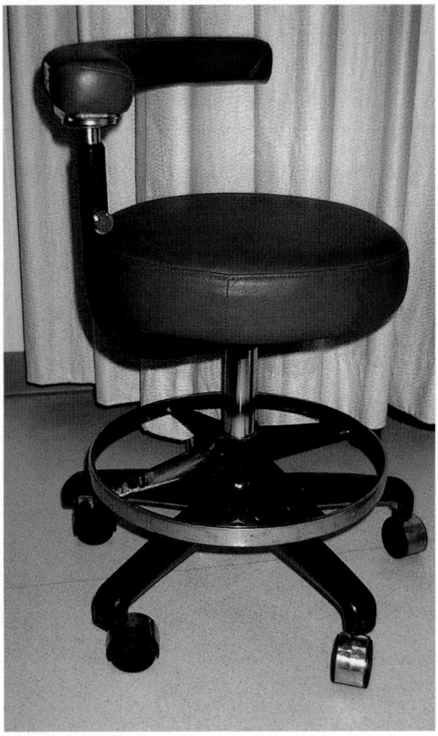

Figure 4-4

Sclerotherapy stool with back support. Helps prevent lower back fatigue in the sclerotherapy practice, where hours of injection and therapy are performed each day.

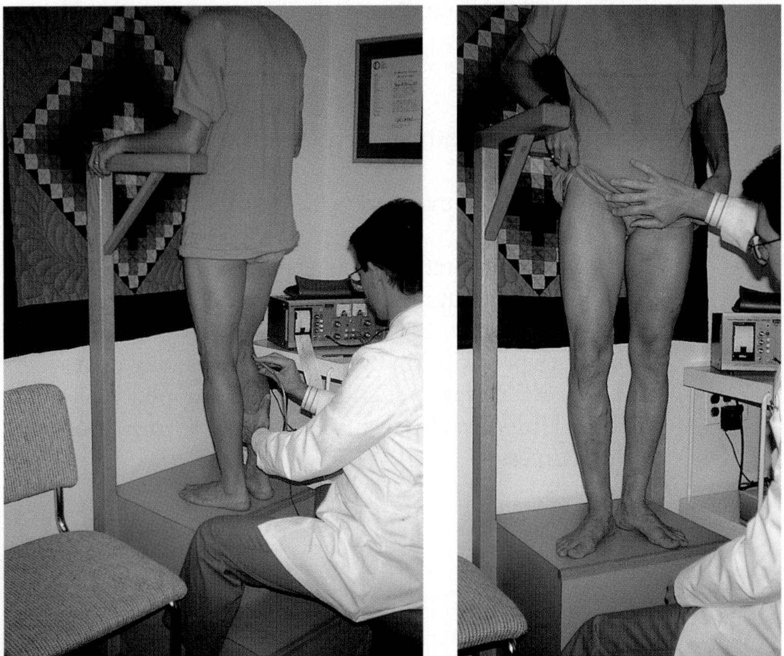

Figure 4-5

Custom-made two-step examination stool. Helps in the appropriate physical examination, Doppler analysis, and presclerotherapy marking of the patient presenting with venous problems.

Protective Eyewear

In the present environment of concern about HIV and hepatitis, and in order to meet the current standard of the Occupational Safety and Health Administration, it is important for the sclerotherapist to use protective eyewear (Fig. 4-6) in order to minimize contact with splashing blood and subsequent exposure to various viral and bacterial pathogens.

Examples of such eyewear include the Micron Wrap Around Glasses (Henry Schein Inc., Farmingdale, NY, U.S.A.).

Magnification Sources

Although magnification may not be necessary for treating large-diameter varicose veins, it is certainly helpful in treating smaller telangiectasias and venulectasias, where precise cannulation is important in attempting to minimize such postsclerotherapy complications as extravasation necrosis.

Five major factors must be considered in choosing the appropriate magnifying source:

1. Magnification
2. Lens-to-object distance
3. Eye-to-object distance
4. Field of view
5. Depth of view

Most magnifying sources employed in sclerotherapy have magnification sources of 2× to 3×.

Three basic types of magnifiers have been found useful in this setting:

1. Headband-mounted binocular magnifiers (Fig. 4-7A). Examples include the Optivisor, Magnivisor, and Mark II Magnifocuser (PSS Medical Supply, Plainview, NY, U.S.A.). These commonly utilized units may be worn over prescription eyewear. They usually provide magnification of 1.5× to 3.5× (many such units are equipped with interchangeable lens plates). Units are also available with superiorly mounted illuminating light sources.

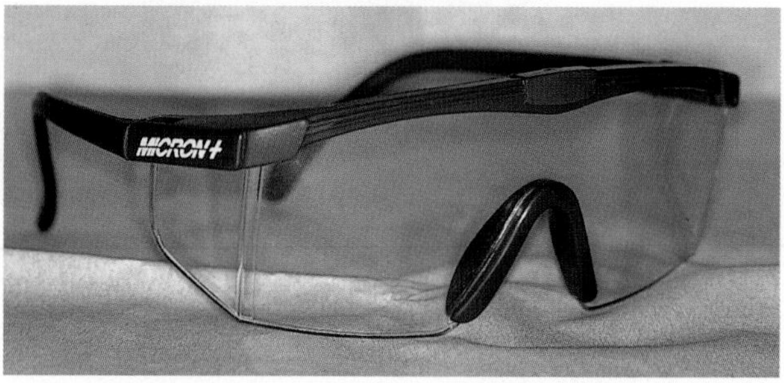

Figure 4-6
Protective eyewear helps protect against blood splatter and provides an ophthalmologic barrier against HIV and hepatitis viral exposure.

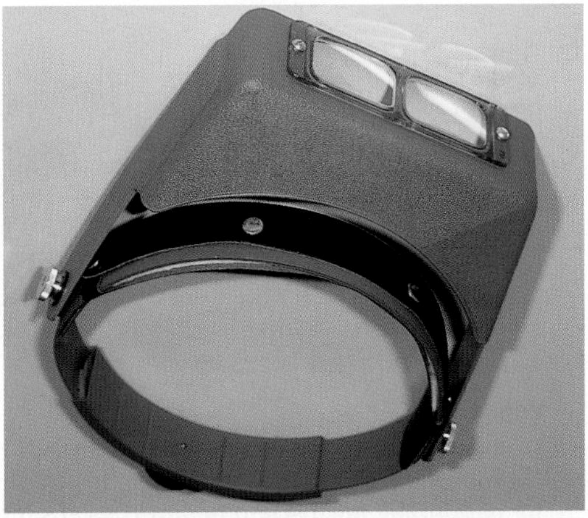

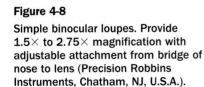

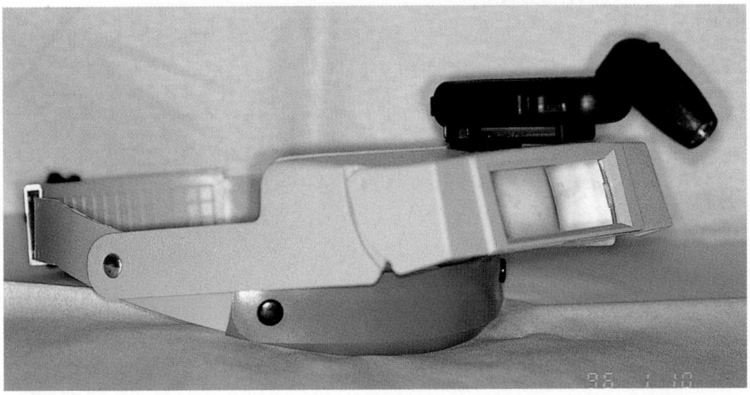

Figure 4-7

Headband-mounted binocular magnifier. **A:** Optivisor—available in 2.5× to 3.5× magnification. **B:** Units are also available with superiorly mounted illuminating light sources (PSS Medical Supply, Plainview, NY, U.S.A.).

2. Simple binocular loupes (Figs. 4-7B and 4-8). Examples are the Precision and Elsenbeck loupes (Robbins Instruments, Chatham, NJ, U.S.A.). Loupes of varying diopter are fitted on either a frame mount or double-hinged telescoping rod. These units come with an adjustable bridge-of-nose-to-lens and provide magnification of 1.5× to 2.75×. Both headband-mounted binocular magnifiers and binocular lamps are relatively inexpensive.

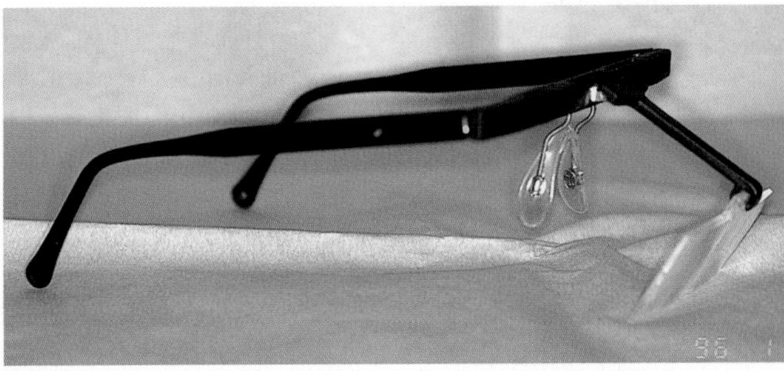

Figure 4-8

Simple binocular loupes. Provide 1.5× to 2.75× magnification with adjustable attachment from bridge of nose to lens (Precision Robbins Instruments, Chatham, NJ, U.S.A.).

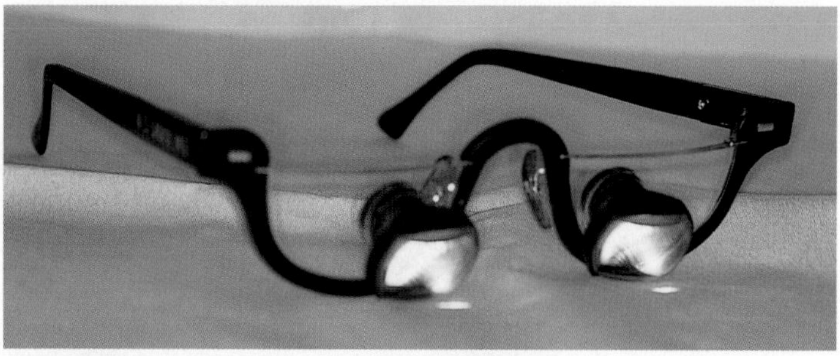

Figure 4-9

Multilens binocular magnifiers. These devices have greater magnification of 2× to 8× providing the clearest undistorted fields for performing microsclerotherapy (Designs for Vision, Ronkonkoma, NY, U.S.A.).

3. Multilens binocular magnifiers (binocular loupes, telescopic magnifiers, surgical telescopes) (Fig. 4-9). Examples include Designs for Vision (Ronkonkoma, NY, U.S.A.), Orascoptics (St. Louis, MO, U.S.A.), Surgitel (Los Angeles, CA, U.S.A.), and See Better loupes (Chatham, NJ, U.S.A.).

These devices have a greater magnification potential of 2× to 8×. The increased magnification is associated with a diminished optical field. These optical instruments provide the clearest undistorted field of any of the previously mentioned types of magnification, making this class of magnifiers clearly the one of choice for performing precise microsclerotherapy. However, such optical units are more expensive than the previously mentioned types.

Photography

As with all surgical procedures, photographic documentation is important in the sclerotherapy setting, allowing patients to see improvement in their legs, particularly when cosmetic small-diameter vessels are treated.

Basic parameters to be considered in choosing a photographic system are as follows:

1. Focus. Autofocus provides a great advantage at very close range, where depth of field is critically limited.
2. Flash. Autoexposure flash is essential at very close range, where the exposure varies greatly with a change of only inches in focus, demanding an accuracy that only electronic through-the-lens (TTL) exposure can provide.
3. Lens. A macro lens (60 to 105 mm, F2.8) is necessary for closeup imaging.

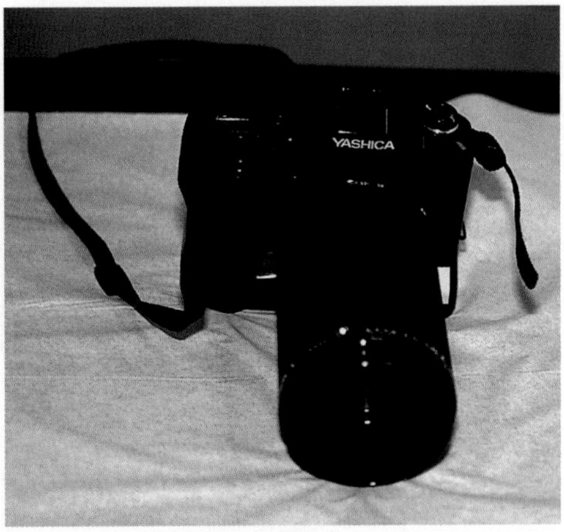

Figure 4-10
Yashica Dental Eye Camera. Built-in 100-mm macro lens offers a wide range of magnification ratios and working distances with an automatic programmed mode.

Photographic systems may be integrated separately; they are also available in "unibody" fully automatic modes.

Photographic units include the following:

1. Among automated units is the Yashica Dental-Eye II (Yashica Inc., Somerset, NJ, U.S.A.) (Fig. 4-10). Its built-in 100-mm macro lens offers a wide range of magnification ratios and working distances. It also has a quickly selectable ready flash with no flash exposure compensation necessary.
2. Integrated systems. Camera bodies, lenses, and flashes are available through a number of manufacturers. Two companies that offer such systems include Canfield Clinical Systems (Cedar Grove, NJ, U.S.A.) and Lester Dine (Palm Beach Gardens, FL, U.S.A.).

   An excellent unit producing high-quality closeup photography is the 35-mm camera (Nikon dual F4 with 50-mm F2 macro lens, TTL macro dual-speed light flash, and choice of manual focus or autofocus settings.

   Other cameras that can be used in the manual-focus mode include the Autofocus Nikon 2020, 4004, 5005, 6006 and 8008 cameras, equipped with Nikon speedlight 58-24 flashes.

Digital photography has evolved with systems such as the updated Sony Mavica showing promise for imaging microvascular lesion. Similar systems are available from Canfield Clinical Systems and Lester Dine.

Sclerotherapy Tray

The sclerotherapy suite should be a professional, well-equipped room that suggests relaxation and assurance to the patient. Within it there should be a distinct tray, cart, or Mayo stand apparatus equipped with appropriately labeled sclerosants, needles, syringes, compression pads, and gauze pads (Fig. 4-11). A solution of alcohol with ½% acetic acid should be on the sclerotherapy tray. Application of this solution prior to treating vascular areas increases the index of refraction and thus improves visualization of vessels, as previously stated.

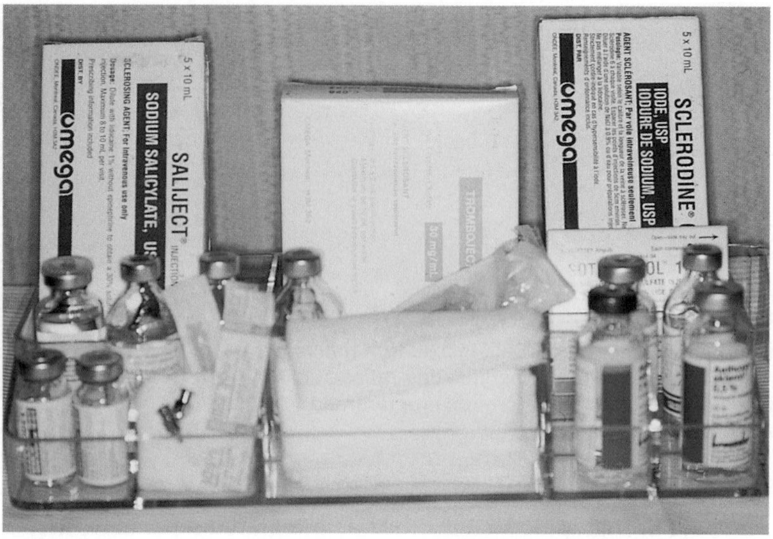

Figure 4-11

Sclerotherapy tray. Shows neatly laid out, labeled sclerosants and pads for local spot compression, which are easily accessible to the sclerotherapist.

Syringes

Although 2-mL autoclavable glass syringes have been used in the past, most sclerotherapists employ disposable 1- to 3-mL syringes (non-Luer-Lok) (Figure 4-12) as their mainline depots for microsclerotherapy (Becton Dickinson and Company, Franklin Lakes, NJ, U.S.A.). Insulin syringes, ½ mL, with 32-gauge ½-inch microfine needles (Becton Dickinson and Company) may be particularly helpful in treating areas of new angiogenesis "micromatting," where diminished injection pressures are preferable (Fig. 4-13).

Needles

The appropriate choice of needles is among the most important aspects of sclerotherapy instrumentation because brisk and accurate cannulation of veins will lead to improved results and a low sclerotherapy complication profile. Needles

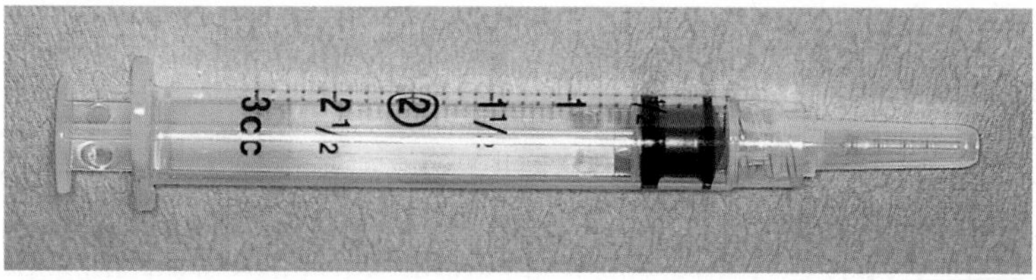

Figure 4-12

Disposable 3-mL syringe. These are the main sclerosant depots utilized in the daily sclerotherapy practice (Becton Dickinson and Company, Franklin Lakes, NJ, U.S.A.).

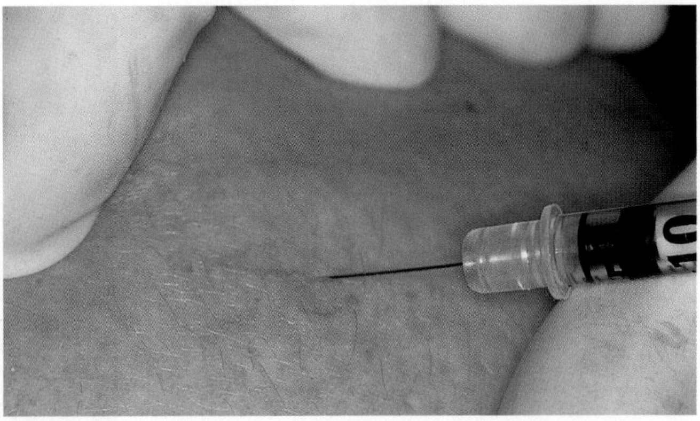

Figure 4-13
Microfine insulin syringe (½ mL with 28-gauge ½-inch microfine needle). This is helpful in treating areas of microvasculature where conventional 30-gauge needles do not allow vascular access.

should have a clear plastic hub to ensure visualization of blood with aspiration. There are three basic choices of needles that have been found by the author to be efficacious in treating patients with microsclerotherapy techniques.

I. Needle options for intermediate-size vessels
   A. Metal hub needles. Becton Dickinson (B-P) Precision Glide needle (Becton Dickinson and Company). This ½-inch needle has an elongated bevel on with a 45-degree angle at the tip.
   B. Silicone-coated tribeveled-point needles. An example is the Poly-Kote metal-bulb needle with a silicone-coated tribeveled point (Acuderm, Inc., Fort Lauderdale, FL, U.S.A.; Dermatology Lab and Supply Corp., Council Bluffs, IA, U.S.A.).
   C. Delasco tribeveled-point needles. These are perhaps the best and most durable needles for sclerotherapy. They are 30-gauge, ½-inch hypodermic needles. The tribeveled points add durability and improved skin transection with decreased pain upon injection.
   D. Air-Tite 30-gauge ½-inch needle (Air-Tite of Virginia Inc., Virginia Beach, VA, U.S.A.).

For improved results, it is often helpful to change needles after every 10 to 15 injections, particularly in areas of thickened skin (for example, inner thighs, popliteal fossae, feet, knees, or ankles). In addition, there are three options for needles that are used to treat class I vessels 1 to 2 mm in diameter and difficult-to-treat areas of neoangiogenesis.

II. Needle options for microvessels
   A. Nondisposable autoclavable needles. Multiple disposable 31- to 33-gauge needles have become available (Figure 4-14).
      1. 32-gauge: ¼, ⅜, and ½ inch
      2. 33-gauge ¼, ⅜, ½, and ⅝ inch

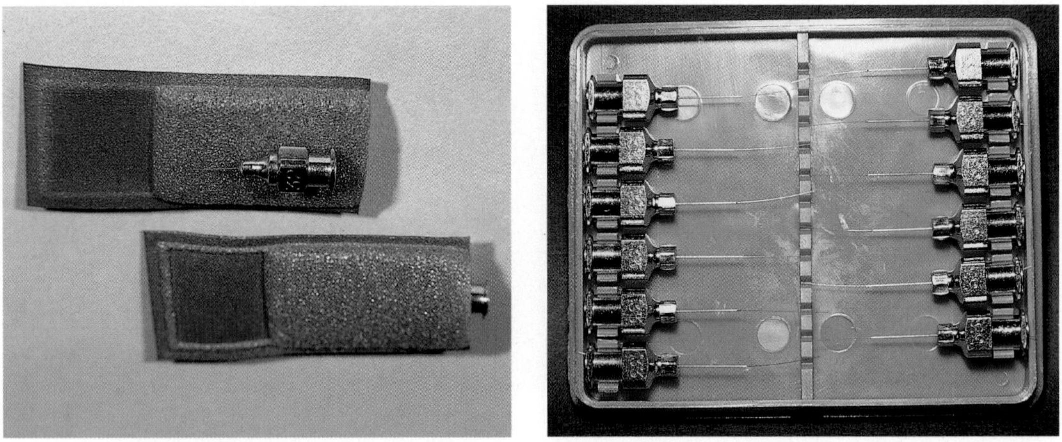

Figure 4-14

Autoclavable microneedles. These are now disposable and reusable and come in gauges 31 to 33 (Delasco Dermatologic Lab and Supply, Council Bluffs, IA, U.S.A.).

(Delasco, Dermatologic Lab and Supply, Corp.). These needles unfortunately have several drawbacks that have limited their usefulness:

1. They are more expensive than traditional 30-gauge needles.
2. They must be autoclaved after each use.
3. They often dull after several treatment sessions as they require sterilization after each use.
4. Their thin diameter makes them easily bendable; thus it is often difficult to obtain precise microdissection of small-diameter vessels, the very indication for which they are being employed.

B. Cannulas for small-vein infusion.

Two basic devices are presently available: a 33-gauge small-vein infusion system (Kawasumi, Labs America Inc., Tampa, FL, U.S.A) (Fig. 4-15), and a 30-gauge STD needle with microsclerotherapy infusion

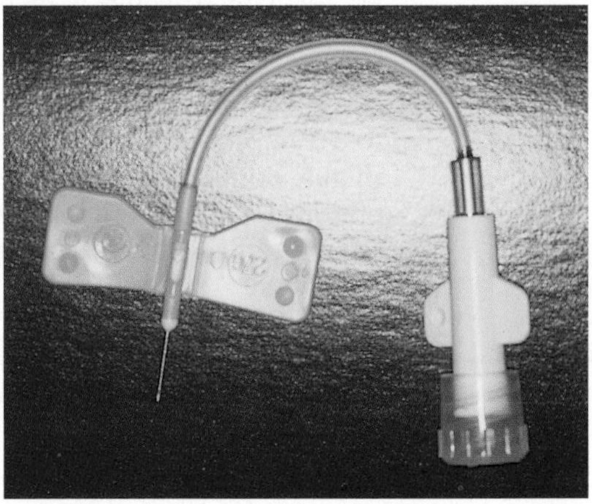

Figure 4-15

Small infusion cannula system, 33 gauge. This allows cannulation of small-diameter microtelangiectasia (Kawasumi Labs America Inc., Tampa, FL, U.S.A.).

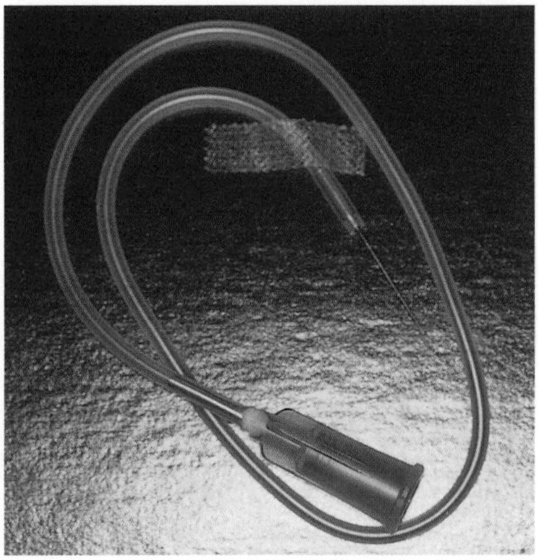

Figure 4-16

Microsclerotherapy infusion system, 30 gauge. Microneedle apparatus attached to infusion tubing allows microcannulation of small-diameter vessels (STD, Hereford, England).

system (STD/Hereford HR-OEL, England) (Fig. 4-16). These are microneedles attached to infusion tubing. Although these needles are more rigid than those previously described, their main drawback is that, because they have a tubing system that must be attached to a syringe, they require a second operator to accurately cannulate small diameter vessels. This becomes somewhat clumsy, considering the small size of the vessels and their relation to the cumbersome injection delivery system. Adhesive anchoring pads are currently being developed in order to counteract this deficiency.

C. Disposable microneedles (Fig. 4-17)

Commercially available insulin syringes include ½-mL, 28-gauge, ½-inch microfine needles and 1-mL, 25-gauge, ⅝-inch tuberculin syringes (Becton Dickinson and Company, Franklin Lakes, NJ, U.S.A.). These have been the best options in the author's experience. They are firm and easy for a single operator to use, they cannulate small-diameter vessels briskly, and they are both inexpensive and disposable.

III. Needle options for large vessels When injecting larger truncal and axial varicosities, one may choose to employ a larger-diameter needle. In these situations, the sclerotherapist is utilizing highly concentrated solutions with

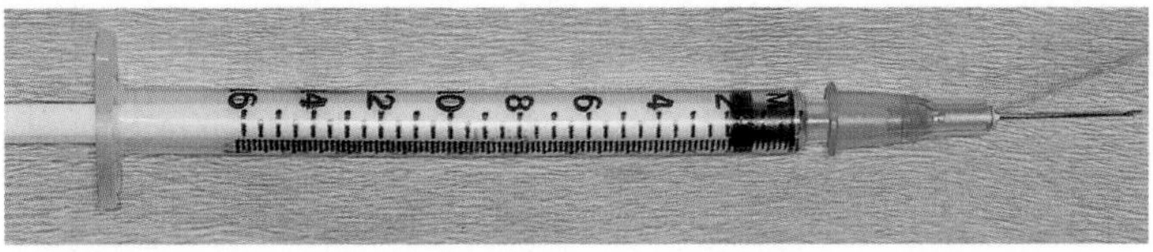

Figure 4-17

Disposable microneedle/tuberculin syringe, 1 mL, 25 gauge, ⅝ inch. These have been the best option in the author's experience for cannulation of microtelangiectasia (Becton Dickinson and Company, Franklin Lakes, NJ, U.S.A.).

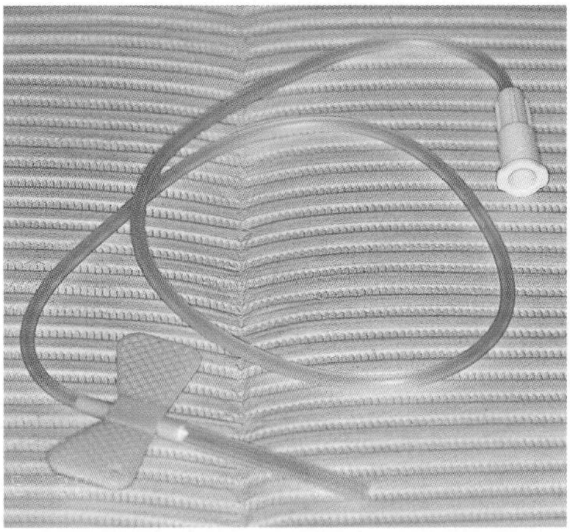

Figure 4-18
Large-bore 23-gauge needle angiocath system. Used for injecting larger truncal and axial varicosities (Becton Dickinson and Company, Franklin Lakes, NJ, U.S.A.).

a greater potential for adverse complications, including an increased risk of arterial injection.

Usually a 23- to 25-gauge needle is employed in this setting (Becton Dickinson and Company).

The author prefers utilization of an angiocath system to ensure adequate needle placement (Fig. 4-18) and visualization of venous return after performing venous cannulation. This system also allows for more mobility of needle angulation during injection of sclerosing agents.

Sclerosing Solutions

Of greatest import is having the necessary types and concentrations of sclerosing agents adequately drawn up and labeled prior to beginning the sclerotherapy procedure.

Since most sclerotherapists utilize sodium tetradecyl sulfate (Sotradecol, Wyeth-Ayerst Laboratories, Philadelphia, PA, U.S.A.; STD injection, S.T.D. Pharmaceuticals, Hereford, United Kingdom; Thrombojet, Omega Laboratories, Montreal, Canada) or hypertonic saline (American Regent Laboratory, Shirley, NY, U.S.A.), the two above agents may be easily labeled. As other agents—such as Polidocanol (Aethoxysklerol, Aeteoxisclerol, Sclerovein) and Polyiodide iodine (Varigloban, Variglobin)—reach FDA approval status and our sclerotherapy armentarium increases in size, labeling of sclerosants will gain increased importance. In addition, many sclerotherapists are compounding solutions such as hypertonic saline and dextrose, which also increases the importance of sclerosant labeling. Sclerosants should be laid out in a systematic fashion. The author uses colored labels for each sclerosant, which he sticks on the plunger base, then marking the concentration on the label (Fig. 4-19). Sclerosants are then laid out in order of increasing concentration.

Any labeling system the sclerotherapist chooses is adequate as long as it is well known to both physician and staff.

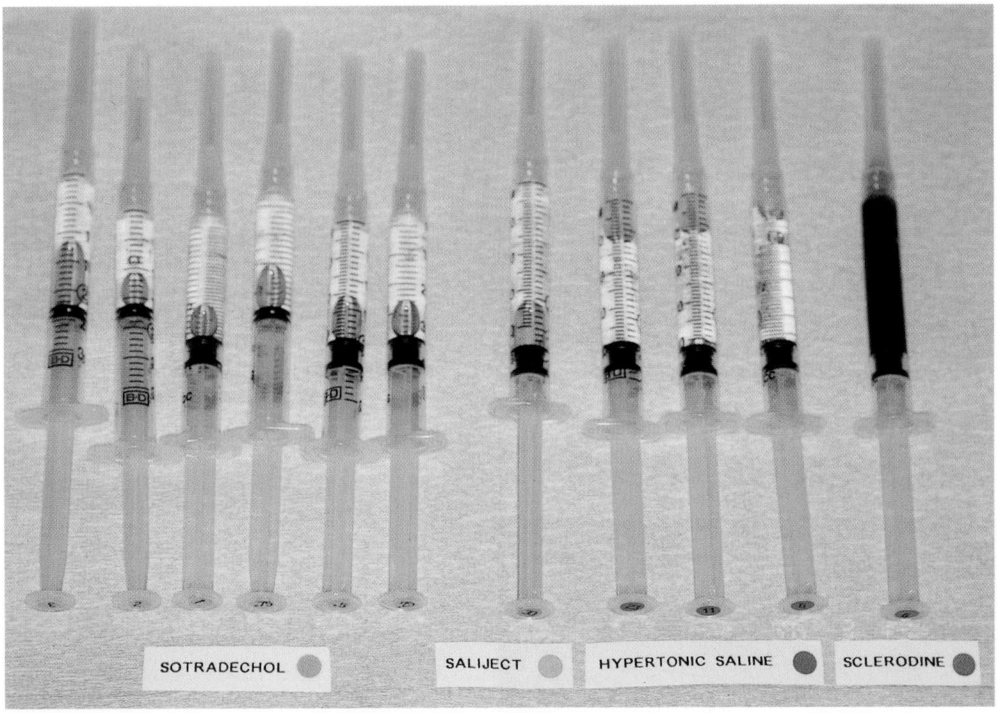

Figure 4-19

Sclerosant labeling. Colored labels for each sclerosant are located on the plunger base; these identify each sclerosant in a systematic fashion. Sclerosant concentrations are then marked on the labels.

▷ Compression Considerations

As previously stated, the most important supplementary measure after sclerotherapy remains the compression dressing. Having a well-stocked supply of compression garments available for patients is helpful for assuring patient compliance.

Compression materials may be divided into three basic categories:

1. Compression pads and tape

   Several alternatives exist, as listed below. Compression pads are more expensive and may be utilized in treating larger-diameter vessels. Pressure pads are also helpful in treating varicosities around the medial and lateral malleoli, where compression stockings are often poorly tolerated. Such pads are not necessary in treating small-diameter telangiectasias.

   Compression pad options:

   a. Gauze pads (4 × 4 inch)

   b. Cotton balls

   c. STD-E pads (STD Pharmaceuticals, Hereford, England) (Fig. 4-20)

   d. Jobst Stasis-Pads (Jobst-Baersdorf Company, Charlotte, NC, U.S.A.)

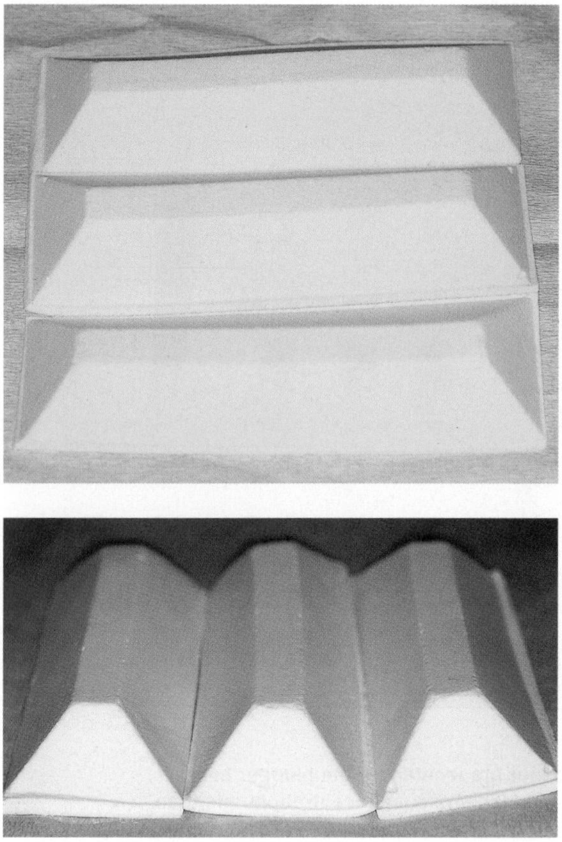

A

B

Figure 4-20

STD compression pads. These are an excellent option for treating larger-diameter varicosities. (STD Pharmaceuticals, Hereford, England).

Tape options:

e. Micropore tape (5 mm, ½ inch) (3M Medical Surgical Division, St. Paul, MN, U.S.A.) (Fig. 4-21)

f. Microfoam (3M Medical Surgical Division)

2. Compression bandages

Compression bandages are classified into three categories: short-stretch, long-stretch, and inelastic bandages. Most commonly employed in sclerotherapy practice are short-stretch bandages, which are utilized to supplement compression with graduated support stockings when patients with varicose veins are treated.

Short-stretch bandages:

a. Medi-Rip (Conco Medical Company, Bridgeport, CT, U.S.A.) (Figure 4-22)

b. Tubigrip (Pro Health Care Inc., Montgomery, PA, U.S.A.)

Inelastic bandages:

a. Circaid (Circaid Medical Products, Inc., Coronado, California, CA, U.S.A.)

3. Compression hosiery

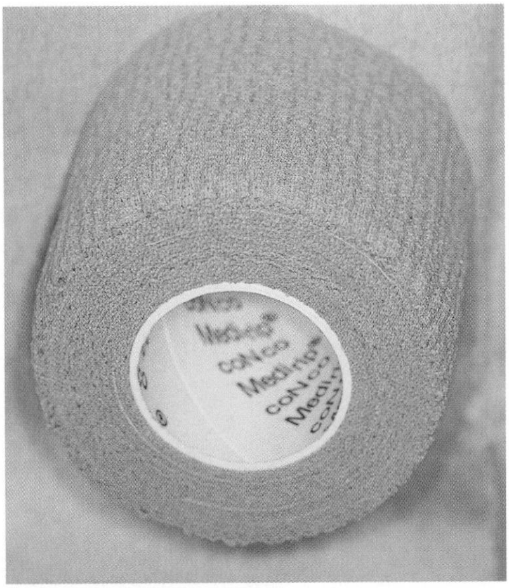

Figure 4-21
Micropore tape (5 mm, ½ inch) (3 M Medical Surgical Division, St. Paul, MN, U.S.A.).

In order to develop controlled levels of graduated support, compression hose are classified into four major classes, depending on the degree of compression, from class I (20 to 30 mm Hg) to class IV (50 to 60 mm Hg) (Fig. 4-23). This is covered in greater detail in Chapter 12. A listing of major compression hosiery products is given below. The reader is referred to Table 4-2 for a listing of each company's product lines. In setting up a sclerotherapy suite, the sclerotherapist may choose to sample one or two lines that he or she feels will be most beneficial. Dispensing of support hose within the office assures that such hose will be applied with appropriate instruction at the time of the sclerotherapy procedure.

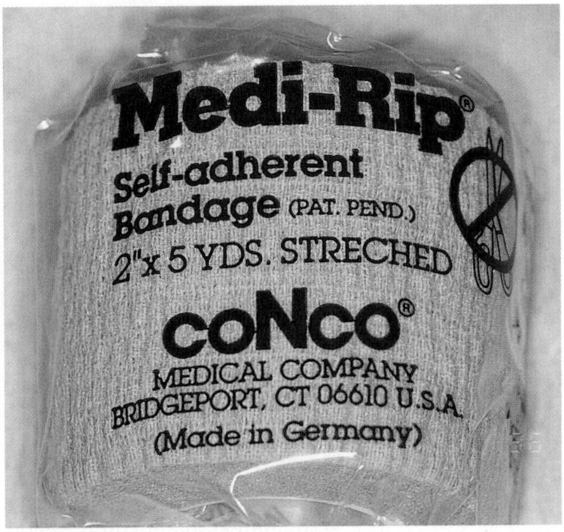

Figure 4-22
Short-stretch compression—Medi-Rip. This provides excellent compression locally following sclerotherapy of truncal or axial varicosities (Conco Medical Company, Bridgeport, CT, U.S.A.).

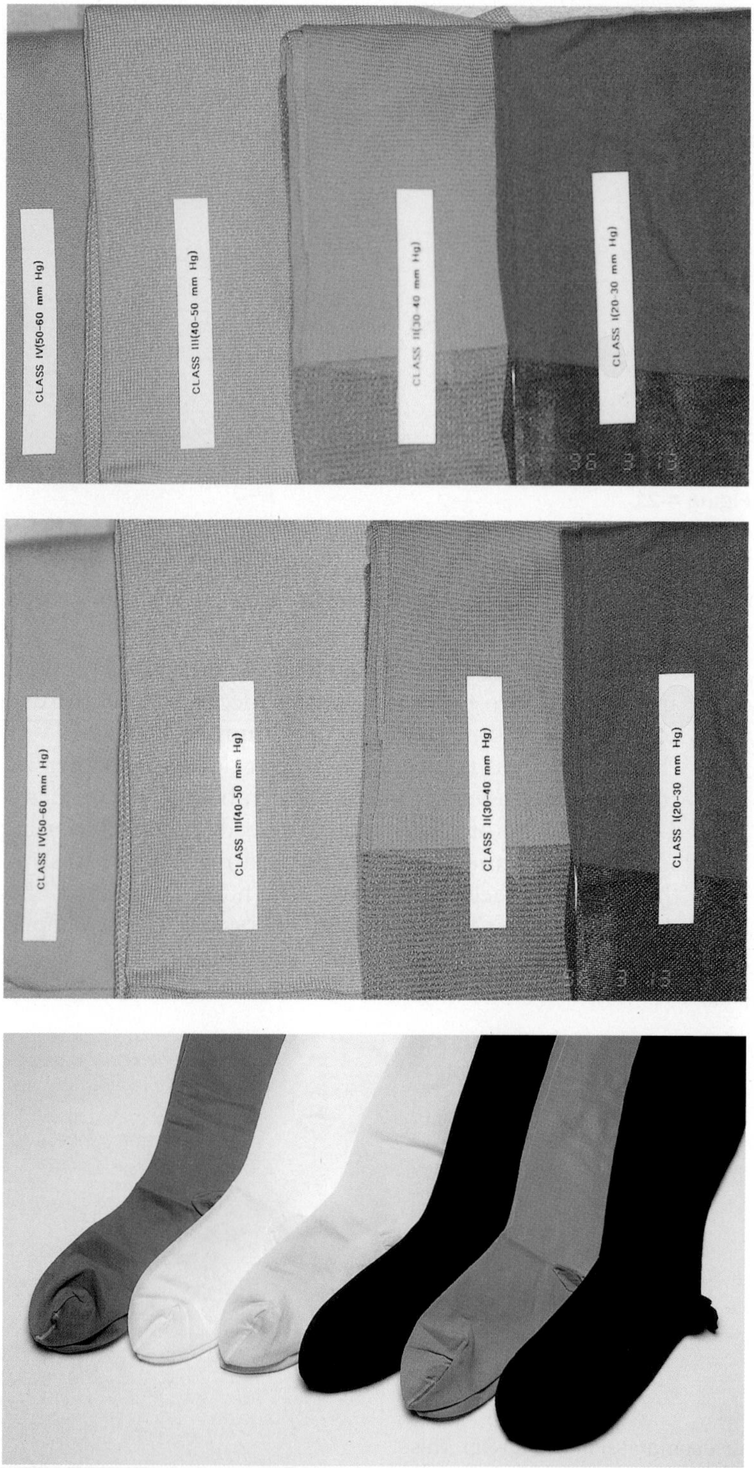

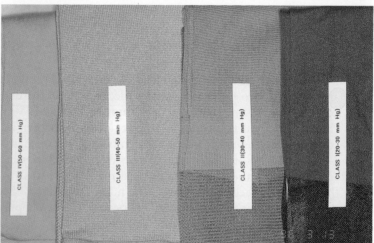

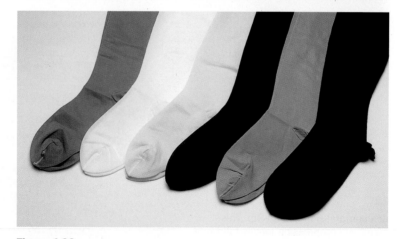

Figure 4-23

Graduated compression hosiery (classes I to IV). This provides excellent graduated-gradient compression after sclerotherapy.

Major manufacturers of compression hose are listed below:

a. Jobst (Jobst-Baersdorf Company)
b. Sigvaris (Branford, CT, U.S.A.)
c. Medi (Medi USA, Arlington Heights, IL, U.S.A.)
d. Juzo (Julius Zorn Inc., Cuyahoga Falls, OH, U.S.A.)
e. International Medi-Surgical (International Medi-Surgical, Houston, TX, U.S.A.)
f. Venosan (BioCompression, Asheville, NC, U.S.A.)
g. Camp (Camp International Inc., Jackson, MI, U.S.A.)
h. Elastic Therapy Inc. (Elastic Therapy Inc., Asheboro, NC, U.S.A.)
i. Hanes Alive (Hanes Inc., Winston-Salem, NC, U.S.A.)

TABLE 4-2. COMPRESSION GARMENTS AVAILABLE FOLLOWING SCLEROTHERAPY TREATMENTS

Compression Class	Manufacturer	Compression Stocking Styles
Fashion hose	Hanes	Hanes Alive
10–20 mm Hg	International Medi-Surgical	Cotton 70
	Sigvaris	Delilah
	Jobst	Men's:
		Lightweight dress
		Lightweight casual
		Women's:
		Sheer pantyhose
		Sheer maternity
		Ultrasheer
		Casual
		Relief
	Juzo	Lite Line 5000
Class I	Camp International, Inc.	Camp Model 01606
20–30 mm Hg		Camp Model N1606
		Camp Model 01608
		Camp Model N1608
		Camp Model 01681
		Camp Model 01683
	International Medi-Surgical	IMS SS
		Maternity 140
	Jobst	Jobst Custom
		Compriform
		Relief
		Fast Fit
	Juzo	Juzo Hostess 2501
		Juzo Hostess 2581
		Juzo Varin Super 3531
	Medi U.S.A.	Mediven
		Medi 15
		Medi Plus
		Medi Custom
		Medi Plus Custom
	Sigvaris	801, 901
	Venosan U.S.A.	Venosan U.S.A. 2030

(continued)

TABLE 4-2. (Continued)

Compression Class	Manufacturer	Compression Stocking Styles
Class II 30–40 mm Hg	Camp International, Inc.	Camp Model 01626 Camp Model 01628 Camp Model 01634 Camp Model 01640 Camp Model 01686 Camp Model 01648 Camp Model 01650L Camp Model 01650R Camp Model 01660L Camp Model 01660R Camp Model 01826 Camp Model 01828 Camp Model N1828 Camp Model 01846 Camp Model 01848 Camp Model 01885 Camp Model 01887 Camp Model 01926 Camp Model 01934
	International Medi-Surgical	Segreta Plus
	Jobst	Ultimate
	Juzo	Juzo Hostess 2502 Juzo Hostess 2582 Juzo Varin Soft 3512 Juzo Varin Cotton 3512 Juzo Varin Soft-in 3512 Juzo Varin Super 3532
	Medi U.S.A.	Medi 75 Medi Man Medi 32 Medi Lastex Mediven Custom
	Sigvaris	202, 503, 702, 802, 902
	Venosan U.S.A.	Venosan U.S.A. 3040
Class III 40–50 mm Hg	Camp International, Inc.	Camp Model 01627 Camp Model 01629
	Jobst	Varox
	Juzo	Juzo Varin Super 3533 Juzo Varin Soft 3513 Juzo Varin Soft-in 3513 Juzo Varin Soft-in Silk 3513 Juzo Helastic 3023 Juzo Helastic Cotton 3023
	Medi U.S.A.	Medi Plus Custom Medi Plus
	Sigvaris	504
Class IV 50–60 mm Hg	Medi U.S.A.	Thrombexin
	Juzo	Helastic 3024
	Sigvaris	505

CPR Cart

Emergency equipment is a must in every sclerotherapy office. A crash cart is ideal (Fig. 4-24) and must be regularly inspected and restocked. This cart should be clearly marked, mobile, and easily accessible throughout the sclerotherapy suite. The sclerotherapist should be trained and certified in basic cardiac life support at least but preferably in advanced cardiac life support (ACLS). All medical person-

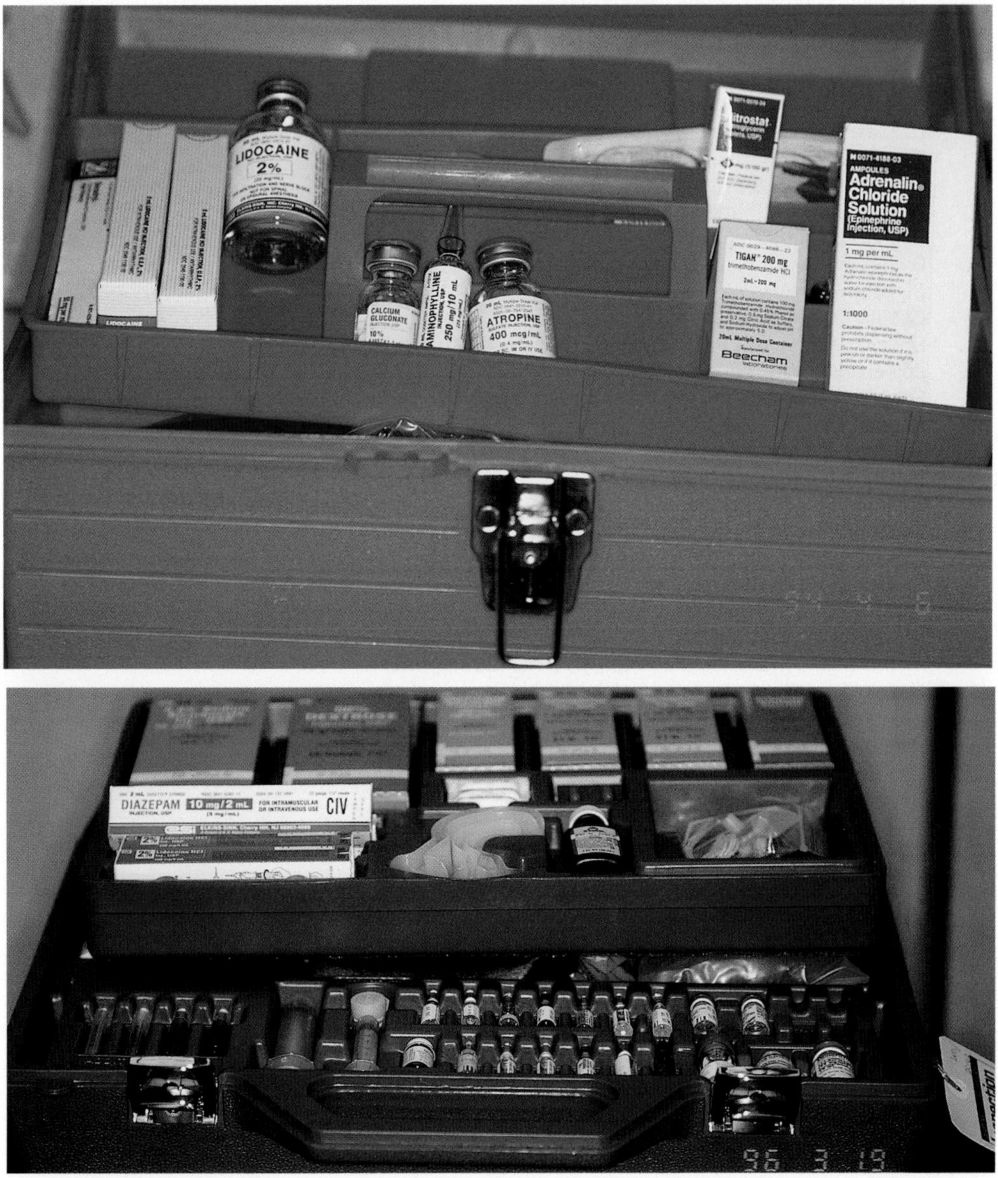

Figure 4-24

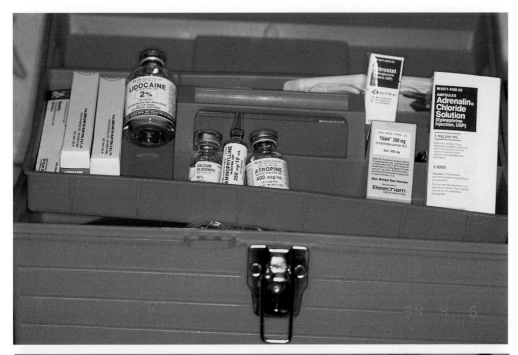

Emergency cardiopulmonary resuscitation cart. This should be clearly marked, mobile, easily accessible, and regularly inspected in the event of a sclerotherapy-induced medical emergency.

TABLE 4-3. SUGGESTED DRUGS FOR THE CPR CART IN A SCLEROTHERAPY PRACTICE

Atropine sulfate 10 mL (0.1 mg/ mL)
Abuterol (Ventolin inhaler) mg
Aminophylline 10 mL (25 mg/ mL ampule)
Amyl nitrate (Aerosol) 0.3 mL
Aromatic spirits of ammonia (Aerosol) 0.3 mL
Antrilium 2 mL (1 mg/ mL ampule)
Bretylium (Bretylol) 10 mL (50 mg/ mL)
Bumetanide (Bumex) 4 mL (1-mg vial)
Calan (Verapamil) 2 mL (2.5 mg/ mL)
Calcium chloride 10% (10 mL, 100 mg/ mL)
Calcium gluconate 10% (10 mL, 100 mg/ mL)
Dexamethasone sodium phosphate 5-mL vial
Dextrose 25% (10 mL, 250 mg/ mL)
Diazepam 2 mL (5 mg/ mL)
Digoxin 1 mL (0.25 mg/ mL)
Dilantin 2 mL (50 mg/ mL)
Diltiazem (Cardizem) IV 10 mg (5 mg/ mL)
Diphenhydramine (Benadryl) 1 mL (50 mg/ mL)
Dobutamine hydrochloride (Dobutrex) 20 mL (250-mg vial)
Dopamine 5 mL (40 mg/ mL)
Epinephrine 1 mL (1:1000)
Ephedrine sulfate 1 mL (50 mg/ mL)
Heparin 10,000 U/mL
Inderal 1 mL (1 mg/ mL)
Isuprel 1 mL (0.2 mg/ mL)
Lactated Ringer's solution with 5% dextrose
Lanoxin 2 mg (0.25 mg/ mL)
Lidocaine 2%, 5 mL (20 mg/ mL)
Lanoxin 2 mL (0.025 mg/ mL)
Levophed 4 mL (1 mg/ mL)
Lopressor 5 mL (1 mg/ mL)
Methoxamine hydrochloride (Vasoxyl) 1 mL (20 mg/ mL)
Nalbuphine HCl (Nubain) 1 mL (10 mg/ mL)
Naloxone (Narcan) 1 mL (0.4 mg/ mL)
Nifedipine (Procardia) 10 mg
Nitroglycerine (Nitrostat) 0.4 mg (1/150 g)
Nitrolingual spray 14.49 g
Normal saline 0.9%
Phenothiazine (Phenergan) 25 mg/ mL
Procainamide 500 mg/ mL
Regitine 5 mg/ mL
Ramazicon 5 mL (0.1 mg/ mL)
Solu-Medrol 40 mg (40 mg/ mL)
Sodium bicarbonate 8.4%, 10 mL (10 mEq)
Trimethobenzamide HCl (Tigan) 2 mL (100 mg/ mL)
Wyamine sulfate 10 mL (15 mg/ mL)
Xylocaine hydrochloride 2%, 5 mL (20 mg/ mL)

nel should be familiar with the cart and its contents. Suggested contents of a well-supplied sclerotherapy cardiopulmonary resuscitation (CPR) cart are listed in Table 4-3. Such a preequipped cart is available from Banyan International Corp. (Abilene, TX, U.S.A.).

Patient Information Brochures

Patient information brochures are an excellent way to educate patients about sclerotherapy and related procedures such as ambulatory phlebectomy and laser/pulsed-light-source modalities. Such brochures may carefully describe these procedures, outline indications for diagnostic vascular testing, and discuss insurance reimbursement issues, fee schedules, and compression considerations. They may also outline varicose vein risk factors as well as posttreatment activity modifications. Finally, they may include a brief outline of the sclerotherapist's experience and expertise in performing each of the procedures mentioned above. Fig. 4-25 shows such a brochure utilized in the author's practice.

How to Build a Sclerotherapy Practice

There are key elements that may help the physician to gain expertise in the treatment of varicose vein disease and to enlarge his or her patient population base in developing a successful sclerotherapy practice.

1. Attend a American College of Phlebology Regional Symposium. These hands-on educational workshops are held twice a year throughout the United States. They give the novice sclerotherapist a chance to learn up-to-date techniques of physical examination, vascular testing, and sclerotherapeutic modalities.
2. Preceptorship in the office of an experienced sclerotherapist. Obtaining in-office training from a physician well versed in sclerotherapy can provide invaluable experience to the beginning sclerotherapist.
3. Educational pamphlets. As stated, in-office educational pamphlets tell patients that the physician is serious about treating venous disorders. They are often distributed to friends and family members as well.
4. Physician announcement letters. Professional letters announcing to community physicians that you are interested in treating varicose vein disease and that you have developed expertise in the areas of sclerotherapy, ambulatory phlebectomy, and/or laser pulsed-light-source modalities will often lead to increased physician referrals. Often physicians of unrelated subspecialities are unaware of which physicians in the community are actively involved in phlebology patient care.
5. American College of Phlebology (ACP) membership. Membership in the ACP carries, along with its other educational benefits, inclusion in a regionally based referral service where physicians' addresses and phone numbers are distributed to patients who call in for referrals. These are

Dr. Sadick has a special interest in varicose veins. He is a member of the Board of Directors of the North American Society of Phlebology and has numerous publications in the field. Dr. Sadick is the recipient of the Conrad Jobst Award for his extensive research in phlebology and has treated thousands of patients with venous disorders.

Initial Consultation

Upon your initial consultation with Dr. Sadick, a complete medical history will be taken and physical examination will be completed to determine whether you are a candidate for treatment. Pre-sclerotherapy photographs will be taken to document your progress and long term improvement.

Testing Requirements

If you have symptoms of deep varicose veins (pain), you will be scheduled for an examination of the venous blood system using a non-invasive technique called "Light Reflective Rheology" or Doppler.

The Sclerotherapy Procedure

During the actual treatment, a solution of saline (salt water) or sotradechol (detergent sclerosant) will be injected directly into the veins with a tiny needle. A few areas on each leg can be treated during a session. The initial treatment is usually light so that you can get used to the therapy and so that we can observe your healing pattern. The entire treatment will take no longer than fifteen minutes. A small square bandage will be placed on each injection site for compression and healing. You will walk out with minimal to no discomfort.

Number of Treatments Required

Usually, a few treatments will be necessary to treat all the existing veins. Then, a yearly or twice yearly session of small sclerotherapy treatments may be needed for any new vein formation.

What the Procedure Feels Like

You can expect to feel a tiny pin-prick, then a slight burning and/or cramping sensation which will dissipate completely within five minutes.

After Care

The small square bandage that was placed on each injection site can be removed the night of the treatment. You may wish to wear a long skirt or pants to cover these bandages when you leave the office.

Please be prepared to wear support stockings for at least three consecutive days following your treatment while you are up and about. If you like, we have medical support hose available in the office by special order. Please call a few days in advance with your height, weight, and color preference. The available colors in women's hose are black and nude.

Daily Activities Post Procedure

We ask that you refrain from any high impact exercise, such as jogging or aerobics, for three days following your treatment.

Appearance of Legs During Healing Process

Over a period of weeks the veins undergo resolution and fade from view. Within a month you will no longer feel self-conscious of your bare legs -- and if you had painful veins, you will feel at ease standing and walking.

Figure 4-25

Sclerotherapy brochure. Describes procedures, insurance reimbursement issues, fee schedules, and postsclerotherapy compression/activity considerations. Such a brochure helps educate patients concerning the breadth of modalities now available to treat telangiectasias and varicose veins.

provided in the patients' home regions to physicians who have a special interest in the treatment of venous diseases.

6. Media contacts. Correspondence with local newspapers and radio and television stations may lead to published and network appearances once the sclerotherapist has gained experience and expertise in the treatment of various diseases. Particularly new techniques such as echosclerotherapy, duplex-guided sclerotherapy, ambulatory phlebectomy, endoscopic

fulgration and valvuloplasty, laser/pulsed-light-source techniques, and radiofrequency vein obliteration procedures often elicit public interest and are publicly aired. These communications benefit the participating physician as well as the subspecialty as a whole.

Conclusion

As in all surgical procedures, adequate instrumentation and a well-equipped, up-to-date medical facility—that is, the development of a properly functioning sclerotherapy suite—are of paramount importance in performing optimal sclerotherapy and related treatment of venous disorders.

BIBLIOGRAPHY

Duffy DM. Setting up a vein treatment center—incorporating sclerotherapy into the dermatologic practice. *Semin Dermatol* 1993;12:150–158.

Geisse JK. The dermatologic surgical suite. *Semin Dermatol* 1994;13:2–9.

Marley WM, Marley NF. Sclerotherapy treatment of varicose veins. *Semin Dermatol* 1993;12:98–101.

Ramelet AA. Primer of phlebology. *Int J Dermatol* 1992;31:833–839.

Widmer LK. The time has come for vascular medicine angiology: a subspecialty of internal medicine and dermatology in Switzerland. *Int Angiol* 1995;27:162–166.

CHAPTER 5

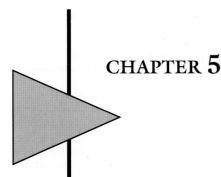

PATIENT INFORMATION

The present chapter deals with patient-related information issues, which are helpful in providing well-consented, well-documented, and thoughtful treatment to patients who will benefit from sclerotherapy.

Photographs

As it is difficult for both the patient and physician to recollect the exact amount of improvement after sclerotherapy treatment—as well as any pretreatment imperfections, such as regions of pigmentation that may have been present prior to institution of therapy—it is important to have excellent presclerotherapy photographic documentation. In addition, it is often difficult to recollect areas of class I telangiectatic vessels that may have been present prior to treatment and may become more apparent after treatment of larger-diameter vessels; such vessels may thus be incorrectly interpreted as a minor postsclerotherapy sequelae, i.e., telangiectatic matting. It is helpful at defined intervals to review pre- and postsclerotherapy photographs with patients in order to document therapeutic progress. Photographs can also help the sclerotherapist to make decisions concerning sclerosant concentrations, the use of compression, and frequency of treatment sessions. A summary of the use of photographic documentation in sclerotherapy is presented in Table 5-1.

A summary of specific camera types is presented in Chapter 4. Specific photographic approaches are outlined below.

1. Patients should initially be photographed both at distant and close ranges in order to demonstrate the nature and extent of vessels before treatment.
2. A natural landmark should be chosen for photographic documentation, and one must have sufficient landmarks to take precise follow-up pictures. Three landmarks the author has found to be important in this regard include (Fig. 5-1):

TABLE 5-1. INDICATIONS FOR PHOTOGRAPHIC DOCUMENTATION IN SCLEROTHERAPY

1. Pretreatment consultation—discuss plan with patient.
2. Document any presclerotherapy cutaneous imperfections (i.e., scars, pigmentation, etc.).
3. Monitor results of pretreatment.
4. Sclerotherapist decision making concerning sclerosant concentrations, grade of compression, and frequency of treatments.
5. Distinguish presclerotherapy landmarks (i.e., class I–II telangiectasia/venulectasia) after larger-diameter vessels are treated from postsclerotherapy complications (i.e., telangiectatic matting).

a. The inguinal crease

b. The prepatellar notch

c. The lateral/medial malleoli

The author prefers photographs taken with the knee bent at a 135-degree angle for references purposes.

3. Utilization of a clear light source. Fluorescent lighting tends to provide shadow-free illumination overhead. Adjustable surgical spotlights are helpful in converging a concentrated light source on anatomic areas to be treated.
4. It is helpful to show both slides as well as standard 5- by 7-inch photographs. The photographs are easier to review with patients, can be conveniently left in chart records, and can be used to construct a sclerotherapy album, which can be used as a future consultative tool.
5. Finally, insurance companies often ask for presclerotherapy photographs as part of their medical review. Such pictures often play an integral role in the determination of decisions concerning medical necessity.

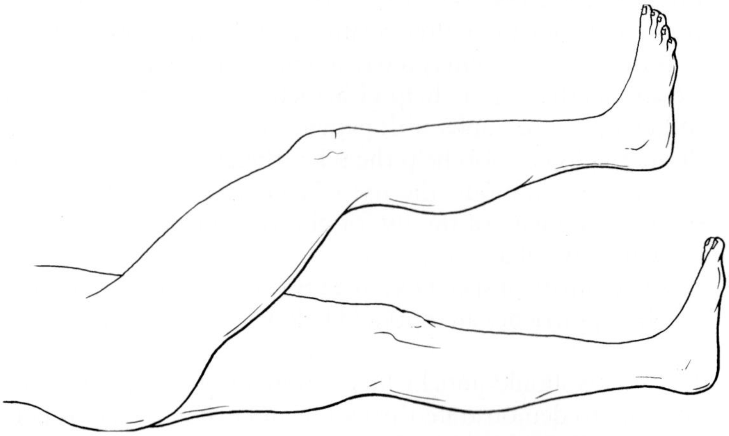

Figure 5-1

Photographic landmarks for sclerotherapy: The inguinal crease, prepatellar notch, and lateral malleolus are major photographic reference points in sclerotherapy documentation

Checklists

The sclerotherapist may keep for him or herself a useful checklist before instituting treatment in order to make sure that all pretreatment diagnostic, consent-related, and treatment considerations have been adequately addressed. The following is a suggested format:

I. Sclerotherapy consultation
  A. History
    1. Drug/hormone history
    2. Drug allergies
    3. Coagulation considerations
    4. Risk factors—varicose vein disease
  B. Patient brochure/video
  C. Photographic documentation
  D. Medical/surgical history
  E. Discussion of fee considerations (The fee schedule should be signed prior to beginning sclerotherapy and should include a signed statement as to whether the treatments are being performed for medical or cosmetic indications and thus whether they are submittable for insurance reimbursement considerations.)
II. Diagnostic evaluation
  A. Physical examination
    1. Trendelenburg test
    2. Perthes test
    3. Documentation of cutaneous sequelae of varicose vein disease
    4. Doppler
  B. Photoplesythmography (PPG)/light-reflective rheography (LRR)[a]
  C. Duplex ultrasound[a]
  D. Venoscopy[a]
III. Informed consent
IV. Treatment considerations
  A. Primary source of reflux
    1. Deep venous system
    2. Saphenofemoral/saphenopopliteal junction
    3. Axial veins (greater and lesser saphenous veins)
    4. Truncal (branch) varicosities
    5. Perforators
    6. Reticular veins
    7. Telangiectasia/venulectasia

[a]As indicated.

FEE FORM FOR PERFORMING SCLEROTHERAPY (TO BE DISCUSSED DURING THE INITIAL SCLEROTHERAPY CONSULTATION)

Name: ______________________ Date: ______________________

I understand and have fully discussed by Dr. ______________________ the following fee schedule for treatment of my spider/varicose veins. All fees are payable at the time of administration of services.

Spider/telangiectatic veins

$ ________ /injection session/per leg

An estimate of ______________ injection sessions are needed in order to attempt to provide adequate improvement

Varicose/reticular veins

$ ________ /injection session/per leg

An estimate of ______________ injection sessions are needed in order to attempt to provide adequate improvement

Treatment sessions are carried out at 1- to 6-week intervals depending upon the individual patient. It is recommended that patients be seen for routine follow-up at 1 to 2 weeks

- Ambulatory phlebectomy

  $________per procedure includes cost of operating and all instrumentation

- Laser/flash-lamp

  $________/treatment session

  An estimate of ______________treatment sessions are needed in order to provide adequate improvement

Additional fees have been fully explained and are charged according to the following schedule:

_______ Doppler ultrasound evaluation
_______ Photoplethysmography (PPG)
_______ Light-reflective rheography (LRR)
_______ Duplex ultrasound evaluation
_______ Spider/varicose vein tray per session
_______ Vigilon dressing (for Sclerolase treatments)
_______ Compression garment below knee, midthigh stockings or pantyhose

I understand that some medical implications are associated with the treatment of my varicose veins; however, I have been advised that there is no guarantee of insurance reimbursement.

I understand that my spider veins/varicose veins are being treated for cosmetic purposes only and as such may not be submitted for insurance reimbursement.

I have received full explanation of and duly understand the above fee schedule and agree to these terms.

Date: ______________ Time: ______________

______________________ ______________________

Patient's Signature Witness

B. Treatment options (Pending vessel type and primary source of reflux as determined by diagnostic investigations listed above.)
   1. Surgery (junction ligation and short stripping)
   2. Ambulatory phlebectomy (stab avulsion procedure)
   3. Sclerotherapy
   4. Laser, filtered flash-lamp light therapy
C. Sclerosant options
D. Compression considerations

Once the sclerotherapist has gone through the preceding sequence of diagnostic and thought-related processes, he or she is assured that the presclerotherapy evaluation is complete and that appropriate therapeutic intervention may commence.

▶ Consent Forms

Of course, of greater importance in the age of modern risk-containment medicine is the consent form for sclerotherapy of varicose and spider veins. Any consent form employed in this setting should include the following elements:

1. Nature and purpose of sclerotherapy.
2. Treatment alternatives. In this case—i.e., surgical ligation and stripping/ambulatory phlebectomy and laser-filtered flash-lamp therapeutic approaches—all the alternatives must be discussed as well as why sclerotherapy has been shown to be the optimal therapeutic approach in the given clinical setting.
3. Risks. Discussion of risks should include common and infrequent adverse sequelae. The patient should also be given a rough estimate of the relative incidence of each of the aforementioned complications.
4. Proposed treatment. This statement should include a description of the type of sclerosing agent being employed, including its concentration, U.S. Food and Drug Administration FDA status, and the estimated number of injections. The patient should also be given an approximation of the number of treatment sessions necessary in order to attempt to achieve a significant improvement in the patient's condition.
5. Cooperation. This statement will share responsibility with the patient to immediately inform the physician if any unexpected adverse sequelae occur.
6. Photography. The consent should emphasize that photographs are part of the permanent patient record and should indicate the potential for viewing by outside individuals for educational or publication purposes if so intended.
7. Informed consent. A final statement should summarize that the patient has received and understands all of the previously described information and that he or she accepts full responsibility for any complications that may arise as a result of the procedure as performed at the patient's request according to the aforementioned principles. A sample consent form employed in the author's practice embellishing these issues is presented.

SCLEROTHERAPY INFORMED CONSENT FORM

This form is designed to provide you with the information you need to make an informed decision about whether to have sclerotherapy performed. If you have any questions or do not understand any potential risks, please do not hesitate to ask us.

What is sclerotherapy?
Sclerotherapy is a popular method of eliminating varicose veins and superficial telangiectasias ("spider veins") in which a solution, called a *sclerosing agent*, is injected into the veins. The injection causes sclerosis or the formation of fibrous tissue in the vessel subsequent to an inflammatory reaction. This process causes a gradual fading of the treated vessel over a period of several weeks to several months.

Does sclerotherapy work for everyone?
The majority of persons who have sclerotherapy performed will be cleared of their varicosities or at least see good improvement. Unfortunately, however, there is no guarantee that sclerotherapy will be effective in every case. Approximately 10% of patients who undergo sclerotherapy have poor to fair results. ("Poor results" means that the veins have not totally disappeared after six treatments.) In very rare instances, the patient's condition may become worse after sclerotherapy treatment. I also understand the sclerosing solution being used, its dosage, and its present FDA status.

How many treatments will I need?
The number of treatments needed to clear or improve the condition differs from patient to patient, depending on the extent of varicose and spider veins present. One to six or more treatments may be needed; the average is three to four. Individual veins usually require one to three treatments.

What are the most common side effects?
The most common side effects experienced with sclerotherapy treatment are as follows:

1. *Bruising*: Occurs in treated areas and lasts from one to several weeks. It may occur in association with tenderness and firmness of the treated vein. Use of prescribed support hose and the utilization of Vitamin K cream for 72 hours before and after each treatment session along with avoidance of alcohol and anticoagulant medications for 72 hours prior to each treatment session may minimize this effect.
2. *Transient hyperpigmentation*: Approximately 30% of patients who undergo sclerotherapy notice a discoloration of light brown streaks after treatment. In almost every patient, the veins become darker immediately after the procedure. In rare instances, this darkening of the vein may persist for four to twelve months.
3. *Sloughing*: Sloughing occurs in less than 3% of patients who receive sclerotherapy. Sloughing consists of a small ulceration at the injection site that heals slowly. A blister may form, open, and become ulcerated. The scar that follows should return to a normal color.
4. *Allergic reactions*: Very rarely, a patient may have an allergic reaction to the sclerosing agent used. The risk of an allergic reaction is greater in patients who have a history of allergies.

continued

SCLEROTHERAPY INFORMED CONSENT FORM—*Continued*

5. *Pain*: A few patients may experience moderate to severe pain and some bruising, usually at the site of the injection. The veins may be tender to the touch after treatment, and an uncomfortable sensation may run along the vein route. This pain is usually temporary, in most cases lasting from 1 to 7 days at most.
6. *Blood accumulation in the treated vessel*: May present as a tender bump at a treatment site. If this develops it can be simply drained by notifying the physician. The use of prescribed compression hosiery will minimize this possibility.

What are the other side effects?
Other side effects include a burning sensation during injection of some solutions and neovascularization (the development, usually temporary, of new tiny blood vessels); transient, phlebitic-type reactions (swelling of the vein might cause the ankles to swell); temporary superficial blebs or wheals (similar to hives); and, very rarely, wound infection, poor healing, or scarring.

Phlebitis is a very rare complication, seen in approximately 1 of every 1,000 patients treated for varicose veins greater than 3 to 4 mm in diameter. The dangers of phlebitis include the possibility of pulmonary embolus (a blood clot to the lungs) and postphlebitis syndrome, in which the blood clot is not carried out of the legs, resulting in permanent swelling of the legs.

What are the possible complications if I do not have sclerotherapy?
In cases of large varicose veins (greater than 3 to 4 mm in diameter), spontaneous phlebitis and/or thrombosis may occur, with the associated risk of possible pulmonary emboli. Additionally, large skin ulcerations may develop in the ankle region of patients with long-standing varicose veins with underlying venous insufficiency. Rarely, these ulcers may hemorrhage or become cancerous.

Are there other types of procedure to treat varicose veins and telangiectasias?

1. Vein stripping and/or ligation may also be used to treat large varicose veins.
2. Ambulatory phlebectomy is a surgical alternative for removing diseased varicose veins. It is performed under local anesthesia.
3. Laser and filtered flash-lamp therapies can be utilized to treat small spider veins less than 1 mm in size, which are difficult to treat with conventional sclerotherapy injections.

Patients with significant coagulation, circulatory problems, or diabetes should not undergo the procedure.

Photographs

I consent to be photographed before, during, and after the treatment. These photographs shall be the property of Dr. ______________________________ and may be published in scientific journals and/or shown for scientific reasons.

By my initials, I acknowledge that I have received a copy of this sclerotherapy informed consent form. ______________________________

continued

SCLEROTHERAPY INFORMED CONSENT FORM—*Continued*

By signing below, I acknowledge that I have read the foregoing informed consent form and that the doctor had adequately informed me of the risks of sclerotherapy treatment, alternative methods of treatment, and the risks of not treating my condition, and I hereby consent to sclerotherapy treatment performed by Dr. ______________________.

Date: ______________________, 19____ Time: ______________________ AM/PM

______________________	______________________
Patient's signature	Patient's representative (If patient is a minor or is mentally incompetent, signature of parent or legal guardian is required.)
______________________	______________________
Witness	Relationship to patient

Instructions

Sclerotherapy instruction sheets should include pretreatment as well as postprocedural instructions, so that the patient is well prepared prior to arrival at the sclerotherapist's office on the day of treatment. Such informational forms should emphasize the points listed below.

Presclerotherapy Care

1. Cleanse the legs with an antibacterial soap such as Dove or Lever 2000 (Unilever, Greenwich, CT, U.S.A.) on the day of the procedure.
2. Bring prescribed support hose to the office on the day of the procedure.
3. Apply vitamin K cream twice a day 3 days before and after the procedure to indicated areas (optional).
4. Discontinue alcohol and anticoagulant medications 48 hours before the procedure.
5. Eat a light meal before coming to the physician's office.
6. Be prepared to remain in the physician's office for at least 15 minutes after the first procedure when a sclerosing agent with theoretical anaphylactic potential is used.
7. A sclerotherapy disposable garment will be provided to you at the time of the procedure.

Postoperative Care

1. Taped compression pads are to be gently removed the day after the sclerotherapy procedure.

2. Immediately after the injection session, you will be asked to put on your previously prescribed compression hose.
3. You will then be asked to walk around the office for 10 to 15 minutes.
4. Bring loose-fitting clothing and comfortable shoes to be worn immediately after the procedure.
5. Maintain normal activities immediately after the procedure. You are encouraged to walk as much as possible and avoid standing in a single position for prolonged periods of time.
6. Avoid strenuous activity such as running, high-impact aerobics, and weight lifting for 72 hours after the sclerotherapy procedure.
7. Compression hosiery should be worn for __ days after the procedure. The hosiery should be worn for __ nights, while sleeping, as well.
8. A plastic shower bag may be used to protect the leg while bathing during the prescribed compression interval.
9. If any unusual postprocedure symptoms occur—such as persistent pain, unusual diffuse bruising, or skin breakdown—call the office immediately.
10. Avoid blood-thinning medications such as aspirin and other nonsteroidal antiinflammatory drugs, dipyridamole, warfarin, and heparin for 24 hours after the sclerotherapy procedure. Consult your internist prior to this change in medications if you have been placed on them for medical indications.

All patients should have a customized informational instruction sheet such as the above prior to returning to the office for their sclerotherapy procedure and after the initial consultation.

Flow Sheets

It is important to use a sclerotherapy flow sheet to document which anatomic areas are treated during each treatment session, since this is often difficult for the busy sclerotherapist to remember treatment locations for each patient on a regular basis despite adequate written documentation in the chart.

As previously stated, the sclerotherapist does not want to treat a given anatomic area a second time for at least 4 to 6 weeks in order to assure maximal endofibrosis of treated vessels. Re-treatment within shorter periods of time can lead to further inflammation and a resultant increase in the incidence of adverse sequelae.

Such a flow sheet may include the following parameters:
Diagnosis—vessel class treated
cosmetic/medical indications
Sclerosant solution
Postsclerotherapy instruction documentation
Numerically labeled anatomic flow sheet
Treatment date flow sheet
Resolution scale

−1 Blue—increased
0 No change
+1 Mild fade
+2 Moderate fade
+3 Total fade

Side-effect profile
E Edema
P Pigmentation
M Mottling
U Ulcer
B Bruising
O Other

Such a well-devised flow sheet will enable the sclerotherapist to carefully monitor the progress of each individual patient, along with precise photographic documentation. It will also avoid overtreatment of various areas and give a precise record of the therapeutic/complication index of each individual patient at a glance.

A sample sclerotherapy flow sheet is presented.

Insurance Reimbursement

Confusion has arisen in the insurance industry over "cosmetic" leg veins as opposed to normal veins. This, in addition to the cost-cutting approach of managed care, has left the issue of insurance reimbursement for the treatment of varicose vein disease in a state of confusion.

The term *cosmetic varicosity* should be reserved to describe a slight dilatation of a normal vein, usually no greater than 1 to 2 mm in diameter, without symptoms and without physiologic reflux (leaky valves) detected at its source. This definition fits within the American Medical Association (AMA) criteria for a cosmetic procedure, "taking a normal feature and improving it by means of a medical or surgical procedure." Symptomatic varicose veins are diseased, abnormal veins; therefore their treatment is not cosmetic.

The American College of Phlebology (ACP) has taken a rational approach as to reasonable guidelines for reimbursement of sclerotherapy for the treatment of varicose vein disease in the form of an Insurance Advisory Committee Report (published in *Dermatologic Surgery* 1992; 18:609–616).

In this report, medical necessity (for which sclerotherapy reimbursement is deemed reasonable by the insurance carrier) includes the following criteria:

1. Abnormally enlarged veins that cause pain, usually over 4 mm in diameter
2. Demonstrable reflux or reverse flow, causing increased venous pressure documented by a noninvasive diagnostic technique such as Doppler ultrasound
3. Evidence of adverse sequelae of venous disease, i.e., ulceration, stasis dermatitis, lipodermatosclerosis

SAMPLE LETTER TO INSURANCE COMPANY FOR DETERMINATION OF REIMBURSEMENT FOR MEDICAL NECESSITY OF SCLEROTHERAPY

Date:

Insurance Company
Street Address
City, State, Zip Code

Claims Reimbursement Supervisor:

My patient, ______________________ requires sclerotherapy in order to treat medically significant varicose veins. Her veins have been present for ________ years. Her venous disease is accompanied by the following symptoms ________________. The patient has the following risk factors for progression of venous disease: ____________. In addition there is a family history of ________________ with varicose vein disease.

Previous conservative therapies prior to sclerotherapy attempting to treat the patient's venous disease include ________________. The patient has undergone the following pre-sclerotherapy vascular examinations ________________ which reveal ________________.

The treatment plan for this patient includes approximately ________________ sclerotherapy treatments of vessels up to ________ mm. in diameter.

This is to be accompanied by long-term class _____ _____ mmHg graduated compression. This treatment program will require approximately ______ treatments at a cost of _______ /leg per treatment for a total cost of $ ________ over ________ months.

Pre- and postsclerotherapy documentation is available upon request.

In the present setting the patient is being treated solely for medical indications, as previously stated.

The sclerotherapy technique employed is a combination of the Swiss (Sigg) and Irish (Fegan) schools. Over the past decade in the United States it has provided favorable results in treating varicose vein disease.

The technique of compression sclerotherapy will enable the patient to be treated without surgical removal of the diseased veins, (i.e., ligation, vein stripping). This will give effective symptomatic treatment while minimizing cost (i.e., hospitalization, operating room fee, anesthesiologist). This technique will also help the patient to minimize absence from work as patients are able to return to work on the same or the next day.

Each treatment session requires 30 to 45 minutes. Our sclerotherapy suite is well equipped with CPR equipment in case an allergic reaction or other adverse sequela occurs. Each injection session is followed by a special bandaging and compression protocol. Patients are instructed to walk for 10 to 15 minutes in the office following each treatment and then reassessed prior to discharge from the office.

Compression sclerotherapy is a cost-effective treatment modality for treating symptomatic varicose/telangiectatic venous disease.

Sincerely,

Doctor's signature

SCLEROTHERAPY OPERATIVE REPORT

Patient ______________________________

Date / Time ______________________________

Physician ______________________________

Treated vessel	Location	___________
	Class	___________
	Diameter	___________
Sclerosing agent	Type	___________
	Concentration	___________
	Quantity	___________
	Number of injections	___________

Procedure

After signing informed consent, the patient was placed on the operating table in a reverse-Trendelenburg position. The area to be treated was prepped with alcohol utilizing Doppler-assisted guidance; 23- to 30-gauge needles were inserted into the entire varicosity beginning with areas of proximal reflux. The leg was elevated 180 degrees and the limb emptied of blood. The entire vein segment was treated with sclerosant (0.5 mL per injection site at 3- to 5-cm intervals) followed by immediate compression employing cotton/foam rubber pads under a 3- to 4-inch microfoam-type dressing. The sequela of treated vessels was varicose veins followed by reticular veins and finally, residual telangiectatic veins. A 3-mL syringe containing 2 mL of sclerosant was employed utilizing the ____________________ technique.

After the vessels were injected along their entire length, a Class ____ ____ mmHg graduated support stocking was applied with the patient still on the operating table. The stocking will be worn for ________ weeks.

The patient was given a follow-up appointment in 7 days to assess any complications such as microthrombus which might occur and was instructed to contact the office immediately if any symptoms indicating adverse sequela such as bleeding, thrombophlebitis, or signs of infection occur sooner.

____

Physician's signature

Conclusion

The patient information issues outlined above allow the practicing sclerotherapist to prepare the patient in a well-defined, systematic fashion for the treatment programs discussed in the remainder of this text. Adherence to the rational approach mentioned above will help the physician to achieve optimal results in his or her sclerotherapeutic management of the individual patient.

BIBLIOGRAPHY

DeGroot WP. Practical phlebology—sclerotherapy of large veins. *Dermatol Surg* 1991; 17:589–595.

Goldman MP, Weiss RA, Bergan JJ. Diagnosis and treatment of varicose veins: a review. *J Am Acad Dermatol* 1994; 31:393–413.

Pordes JB, Nemeth AJ. Adverse sequelae of venous hypertension. *Semin Dermatol* 1993; 12:66–71.

Weiss MA, Weiss RA. Sclerotherapy in the U.S. *Dermatol Surg* 1995; 21:293–396.

Weiss RA, Heagle CR, Raymond-Martimbeau DM. Insurance Advisory Report: The Bulletin of the North American Society of Phlebology. *Dermatol Surg* 1992; 18:609–616.

CHAPTER 6

CHOOSING THE RIGHT SCLEROSING AGENT

Once the patient has undergone comprehensive physical examination and appropriate laboratory testing and subsequently has been deemed to be a good candidate for sclerotherapy, the initial approach to treatment is to determine the choice of sclerosing agent and the optimal concentration that will accomplish the desired clinical effect. Although many phlebologists will utilize only a single sclerosant (that is, the one that he or she feels most comfortable with), a more flexible attitude and experience with several agents will allow a more directed, diversified approach for a given clinical situation. What are the parameters upon which the clinician must decide in choosing a given sclerosing agent?
These include:

1. Vessel diameter
2. Reflux considerations
3. Approval by the U.S. Food and Drug Administration (FDA)
4. Patient allergy profile
5. Pain tolerance
6. Previous treatment response to a given agent
7. Minimal sclerosant concentration
8. Sclerosant complication profile

It is with these factors in mind that one may begin to make a rational decision about which sclerosing agent should be employed in a given clinical setting.

Sclerosant Considerations

Sclerosing agents have been employed since the mid-1800s for the treatment of many diverse conditions, including recurrent pleural effusions, ganglions, hernias, esophageal varices, and hemorrhoids in addition to varicose veins and spider veins.

Regardless of which class of sclerosing agents one employs, the final goal is the same—that is, injury to endothelial surfaces (endosclerosis) resulting in obliteration of damaged surfaces and leading to reabsorption of the damaged vessel wall and subsequent fibrosis, which is the last stage of sclerosant action, assuring lack of reappearance of treated vessels (Fig. 6-1).

There are several important points to remember when choosing a given sclerosant and determining the appropriate sclerosant concentration.

1. If the sclerosant is too weak, insufficient endothelial damage will occur, leading to thrombosis secondary to varicose vessel damage. However, there will be no fibrosis and thus recanalization of the vessel often occurs, with persistence of an incompetent pathway for retrograde blood flow.
2. Too strong a solution leads to uncontrolled destruction of vascular endothelium. In addition, the sclerosant may flow into adjacent normal vessels and perivascular tissues, causing damage to them as well. Such uncontrolled inflammatory stimulation may lead to an increased incidence of hyperpigmentation, neoangiogenesis (telangiectatic matting), and even ulceration subsequent to vessel wall damage and associated sclerosant extravasation.
3. Choose the minimum sclerosant concentration. The key goal in sclerotherapy regardless of the sclerosant concentration employed is to deliver the minimum volume and concentration of sclerosant that will cause irreversible damage to the endothelium of the abnormal vessel wall while leaving adjacent normal vessels intact.
4. Correct patient positioning. Regardless of the sclerosant agent employed, elevation of a treated extremity with emptying of a given vessel by hand kneading (Fig. 6-2) will allow maximum sclerosant contact with the vascular endothelium so that the lowest concentration of sclerosant will achieve adequate endothelial injury, thus maximizing results while minimizing inflammation and the potential side effects in a given patient.

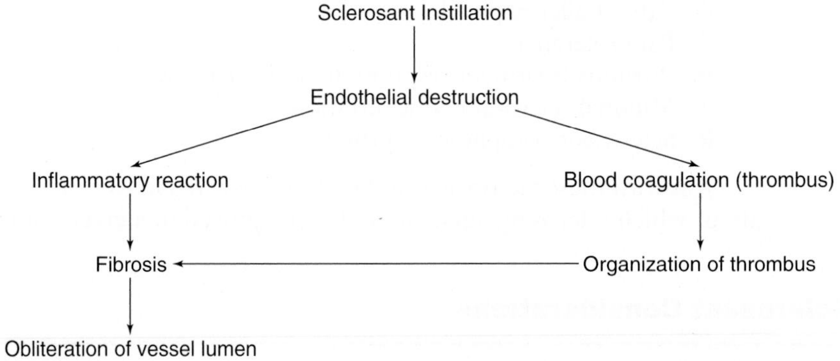

Figure 6-1

Diagrammatic illustration of the mechanism of action of desired sclerosing agents leading to the common desired endpoint of fibrotic obliteration of treated vessels.

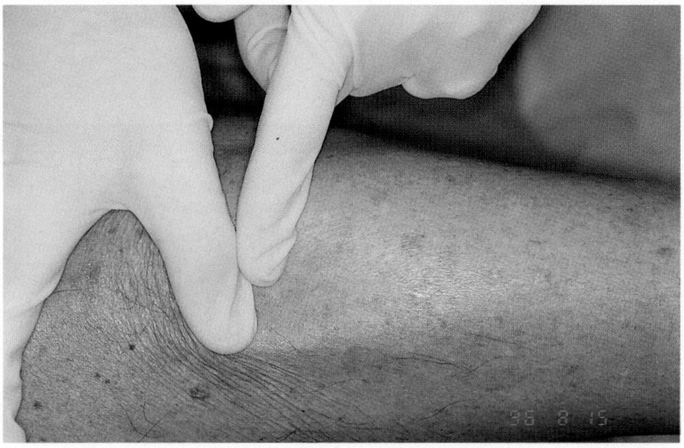

Figure 6-2
Elevation of a treated extremity with emptying of vessel by hand kneading will allow maximal sclerosant-endothelial contact, yielding the greatest potential intravascular effects.

Classification of Sclerosing Agents by Mechanism of Action

Sclerosing agents are classified into three groups, based on the mechanism whereby they cause injury to the endothelium (Table 6-1).

1. *Detergent agents.* The detergent agents include polidocanol, sodium tetradecyl sulfate, and sodium morrhuate. This group of agents causes vascular injury by altering the surface tension around endothelial cells. These agents contain one pole that is hydrophilic and one pole that is hydrophobic. They cause endothelial cell wall damage as the hydrophobic portion of the detergent molecule attaches to cells on the vein wall while the hydrophilic portion attracts and draws water into the cell, resulting in rapid overhydration (maceration) (Fig. 6-3).
2. *Osmotic agents.* The osmotic sclerosants include hypertonic saline and hypertonic saline-dextrose. Their primary mechanism of action involves endothelial cell damage through dehydration (Fig. 6-4).

TABLE 6-1. MECHANISMS OF ACTION OF SCLEROSING AGENTS

Detergents
Polidocanol (Aethoxysklerol)
Sodium tetradecyl sulfate (Sotradecol)[a]
Sodium morrhuate (fatty acids in cod liver oil)[a]
Ethanolamine oleate
Osmotic agents
Hypertonic saline (18%–30%)[a]
Hypertonic saline/dextrose (10% saline, 5% dextrose)
Chemical irritants
Chromated glycerin[a]
Polyiodide iodide

[a] FDA-approved.

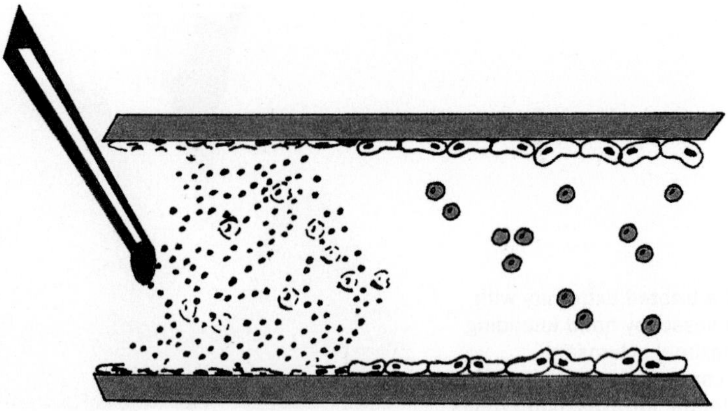

Figure 6-3

Mechanism of action of detergent sclerosant. The hydrophobic portion of the detergent molecule attaches to the endothelial cell wall while the hydrophilic portion draws water into the cell, leading to an overhydrated maceration effect.

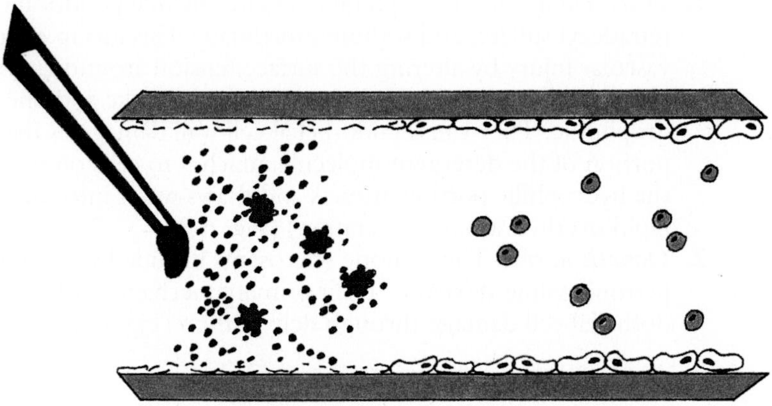

Figure 6-4

Mechanism of action of osmotic sclerosant. Endothelial damage is produced by a gradient dehydration effect.

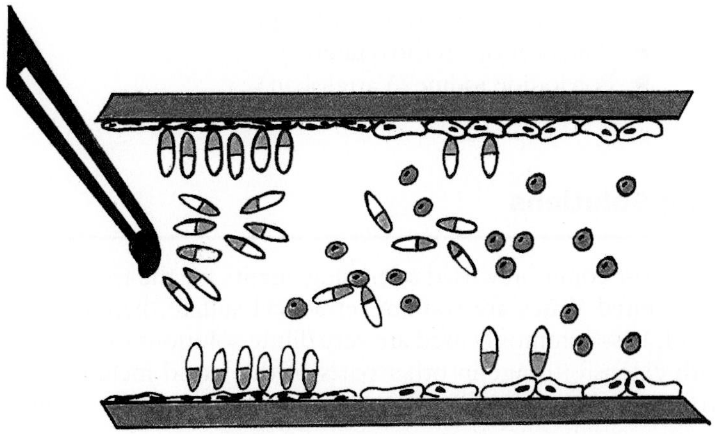

Figure 6-5

Mechanism of action of chemical irritant sclerosant. A cauterizing corrosive effect directly damages treated vascular endothelium.

3. *Chemical irritants.* The chemical irritants include chromated glycerin and polyiodide iodine. They act as corrosives by producing a cauterizing action, which injures cells by means of a heavy metal effect (Fig. 6-5).

▶ FDA-Approved Sclerosants

The detergent sclerosants are the only agents currently approved for use in sclerotherapy by the FDA. These agents include sodium tetradecyl sulfate and sodium morrhuate. Sodium morrhuate is appropriate for use in varicose veins but is "highly caustic" and is not recommended for use in the treatment of class I telangiectasis and class II venulectasis.

Although polidocanol is not yet approved by the FDA for treatment of varicose veins, it is hoped that it will soon be cleared for this indication.

Of the osmotic agents, hypertonic saline has been approved by the FDA for indications other than the treatment of varicose vein disease (that is, as an abortifacient).

Finally, of the chemical irritants, polyiodinated iodide is used in Europe and Canada for treatment of large varicose veins, including the saphenofemoral and saphenopopliteal junctions. Clinical dosing studies are now under way in the United States, and hopefully this agent will be incorporated into the sclerotherapeutic armentarium in the near future.

Sclerosing agents approved by the FDA (1996)

- Sodium tetradecyl sulfate (Sotradecol)
- Sodium morrhuate (fatty acids in cod liver oil)
- Hypertonic saline (18% to 30% saline) approved as an abortifacient rather than for treatment of varicose veins

Sclerosing agents awaiting FDA approval
- Polidocanol (Aethoxysklerol)
- Polyiodide iodine (Varigloban)

Sclerosing Solutions

The most commonly used sclerosing agents for the treatment of varicose veins in the United States are sodium tetradecyl sulfate, hypertonic saline, and polidocanol. Less commonly used are very dilute solutions of sodium morrhuate. Agents with extensive usage in other parts of the world include hypertonic saline/dextrose (widely used in Canada) and chromated glycerin (widely used in Europe).

Detergents

Polidocanol (Aethoxysklerol, Chemische Fabrik Kreussler and Company Wiesbaden, Biebrich, Germany) (Fig. 6-6) is a urethane anesthetic agent. It differs from the more classic ester and amide anesthetics by lacking an aromatic ring. It may be employed in 0.5% to 3% concentrations. It is classified as a relatively weak sclerosant for the treatment of smaller-diameter vessels. The unique characteristics of this sclerosing agent are that it is relatively painless to inject and poses minimal risk of extravasation necrosis as compared with other agents such as hypertonic saline. Concentrations of 0.25% to 1.0% may be utilized to treat telangiectasis and reticular veins less than 4 mm in diameter. Polidocanol is available from Europe in 30-mL vials and 2-mL ampules of 0.5%, 1%, 2%, and 3% solutions. A daily dose of 2 mg per kilogram of body weight should not be exceeded. It is presently in Phase III clinical trials by the FDA and hopefully will soon be approved for clinical use. Its FDA clearance will make it an integral part of the sclerotherapeutic armentarium for the treatment of diseased small and intermediate-size vessels.

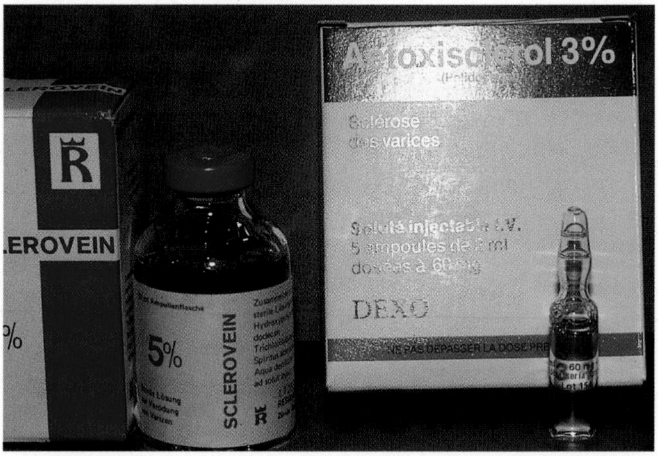

Figure 6-6
Polidocanol (Aethoxysklerol, Sclerovein), available in 0.05% to 3% concentrations. Phase III FDA trials are presently in progress.

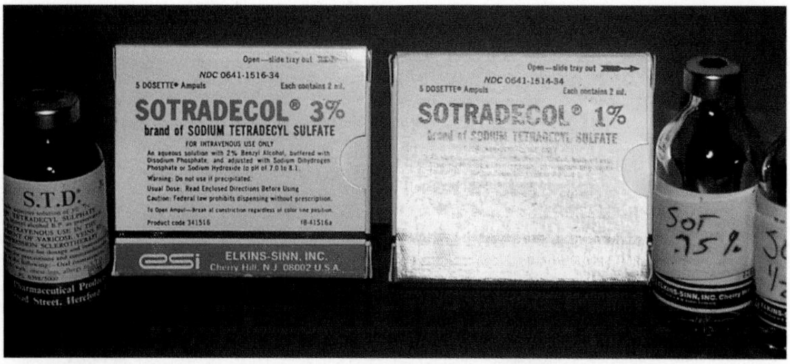

Figure 6-7

Sodium tetradecyl sulfate (Sotradecol). Major efficacy is in the treatment of small and intermediate-size vessels. The most commonly used detergent sclerosant available in the United States is available in 1% or 3% ampules which may be diluted to desired concentrations for the treatment of small-to larger-diameter vessels.

Sodium tetradecyl sulfate (Sotradecol, Elkin-Sinn, Inc., Cherry Hill, NJ, U.S.A.) (Fig. 6-7) (STS, Wyeth-Ayerst Laboratories, Philadelphia, PA, U.S.A.; STD Pharmaceuticals, Hereford, United Kingdom; Throm-boject, Omega Labs, Montreal, Canada) is available in 1% or 3% ampules. It is the most frequently employed agent in the United States for the treatment of larger varicose veins. It is also gaining increasing popularity for the treatment of telangiectasia and reticular vein disease as well. STS is a long-chain fatty acid salt with significant detergent properties. Classified as a medium-potency sclerosing agent, it is relatively painless to inject and is thus well tolerated. However, it must thus be injected fastidiously in order to prevent extravasation necrosis.

Current recommendations for usage include 0.1% to 0.25% for treatment of class I to class II telangiectasis/venulectasis up to 2 mm in diameter, 0.25% to 0.5% for treatment of reticular veins, 0.5% to 1% for treatment of small varicosities less than 4 mm in diameter, and 1% to 3% for treatment of large varicosities and incompetent saphenofemoral and saphenopopliteal junctions.

The maximum recommended dosage per treatment session is 10 mL of 3% solution. Sotradecol is photosensitive and thus must be stored away from light.

Sodium morrhuate (Scleromate, Glenwood, Tenafly, NJ, U.S.A.) (Fig. 6-8), a 5% solution of a complex mixture of fatty acids, is essentially a cod liver oil extract. Approximately 10% of its fatty acid composition is unknown. The major usage of this agent has been in the treatment of esophageal varices. It has been used in the past for treatment of both varicose veins and telangiectasis. It has been used in dilute concentrations of 0.25% to 0.5%.

Although this agent is FDA approved for the treatment of varicose veins, it is not commonly employed for treatment of varicose veins or telangiectasia in this country because of its caustic qualities and its high side-effect profile, to be discussed in the next section.

Ethanolamine oleate (Cypros, Carlsbad, CA, U.S.A.) is a synthetic mixture of oleic acid and ethanolamine. It has weak detergent properties, making high concentrations necessary for effective treatment. Its relative lack of sclerosant strength as well as its highly viscous quality, making it difficult to inject, have made this agent an unpopular choice for treating varicose veins in the United

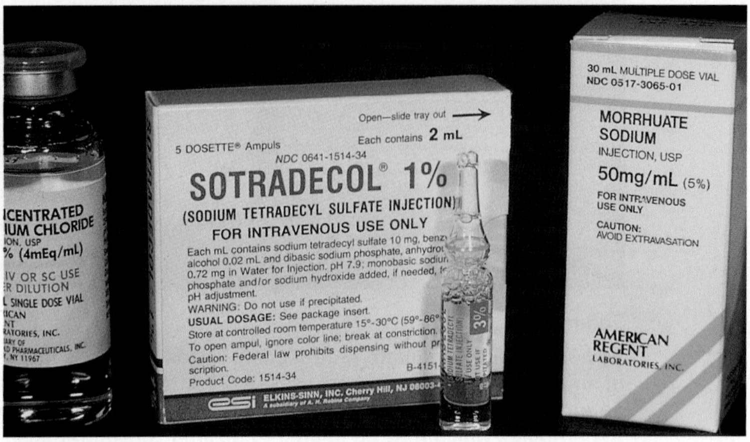

Figure 6-8

Sodium morrhuate, a detergent sclerosant, has been employed in dilute concentrations of 0.25% to 0.5%; however, its highly caustic nature and increased anaphylactic risk has limited its usefulness in daily sclerotherapy practice.

States, although it is more commonly used for this purpose in Australia and New Zealand. In the United States, ethanolamine oleate is used mainly for sclerosis of esophageal varices.

Osmotic Agents

Hypertonic saline (Fig. 6-9) has been utilized for treatment of small-vein disease for four decades in the United States. It has been used in concentrations of 10% to 30% for the treatment of class I to III telangiectasia, venulectasia, and reticular

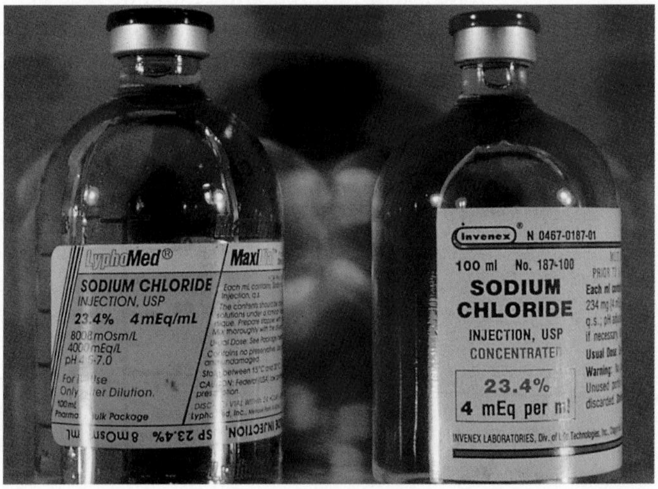

Figure 6-9

Hypertonic saline, utilized in concentrates of 6% to 30%, is a commonly employed minor sclerosant. Desired concentrations may be achieved utilizing procaine, lidocaine, or bacteriostatic water. Pain upon injection and high ulcerogenic potential are limiting factors to its widespread usage.

veins. It is available commercially in a concentration of 23.4% in 30-mL vials. In the past, this agent had been diluted with heparin (Heparsal) in an attempt to prevent embolization; however, in studies carried out by the author, this has not been shown to change the complication profile of hypertonic saline. More commonly, hypertonic saline may be diluted with procaine, lidocaine, or bacteriostatic water. The author routinely utilizes concentrations of 6% to 7% for treating vessels 1 mm or less in diameter, 11.7% for treating vessels 1 to 2 mm in diameter, and 23.4% for the treatment of vessels 2 to 4 mm in diameter.

In previous studies, the author has shown that such diluted agents may be left for periods of up to 12 weeks without risk of bacterial contamination. The author has also shown that selected sclerosing agents such as hypertonic saline and sodium sotradecol sulfate have intrinsic antimicrobial properties, also contributing to the lack of vascular infections noted in patients treated with sclerotherapy techniques.

The major benefit of treating patients with hypertonic saline derivatives is the relative lack of allergenicity associated with these agents. However, when they are diluted with agents such as lidocaine, which may contain preservatives such as methylparabens, there is a minor risk of secondary allergic reactions.

The major disadvantages of this agent include its weak sclerosing potential as well as the cramping pain that occurs after the injection of 23% hypertonic saline (HS) and to a lesser extent when 11.7% or 6.7% HS is employed.

Sclerodex (Hypertonic dextrose/hypertonic saline Sclerodex, Omega Laboratories, Ltd., Montreal, Canada) (Fig. 6-10) is a mixture of 25% dextrose and 10% sodium chloride with a small quantity of phenethyl alcohol.

This relatively weak sclerosant is utilized predominantly in Canada. It has two particular advantages over straight HS. First, it presents a reduced salt load and, second, the nonionic dextrose moiety causes hypertonic injury without stimulating the nerve endings, thus inducing less burning than would occur with straight HS. Finally, the combined glucose-saline moieties produce a higher viscosity, allowing increased endothelial vascular contact time and producing improved synergistic results as compared with each of these agents alone.

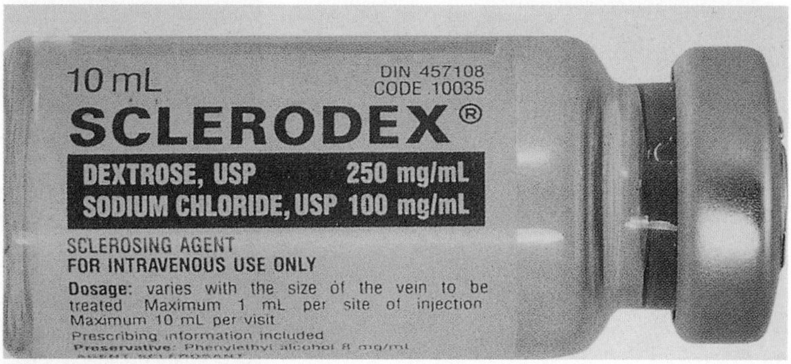

Figure 6-10

Hypertonic dextrose/hypertonic saline (Sclerodex) is a mixture of 25% dextrose and 10% sodium chloride. Decreased pain, reduced salt load, and a synergistic effect of glucose/saline moieties makes this is useful hypoallergenic minor sclerosant.

This agent is utilized for the treatment of class I to II telangiectasia/venulectasia, with a total volume of injection not to exceed 10 mL per visit and 1.0 mL per injection site.

Chemical Irritants

Chromated glycerin 71% (Scleremo, Chromex, Omega Laboratories, Montreal, Canada; Laboratories E, Bauteille, Paris, France) (Fig. 6-11), polyalcohol agent, is a mild sclerosing agent popular in Europe for the treatment of small-vessel disease. It is a highly viscous agent and thus is usually diluted 1:1 to 4:1 with normal saline or 1% lidocaine. The addition of the chromium salt potentiates the corrosive activity of glycerin.

Chromated glycerin may cause local pain on injection as well as cramping in remote areas. This effect may be minimized with the use of lidocaine as a diluent.

Chromated glycerin is painful on extravasation. Finally, because of its weak sclerosing potential, it may be necessary to switch to another agent of medium potency when expected results are not achieved in a reasonable number of treatment sessions.

Polyiodide iodine (Varigloban, Chemische Fabrik, Kreussler and Company, Wiesbaden–Biebrich, West Germany; Sclerodine, Omega, Montreal, Canada) (Fig. 6-12) is a mixture of elemental iodine with sodium iodide and a small amount of benzyl alcohol. The active ingredient is iodine. This agent is the strongest presently available for the treatment of large-diameter veins and associated points of axial reflux. This agent produces rapid and localized corrosive endothelial destruction. Blood neutralization of PII occurs within seconds, so that its sclerosant effect is highly localized.

Polyiodide iodine is highly painful when inadvertent extravascular injection occurs. Finally, its sclerosing power is strengthened by increasing the concentra-

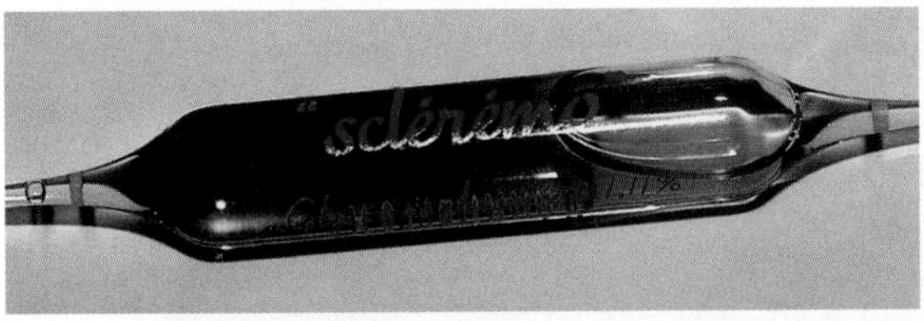

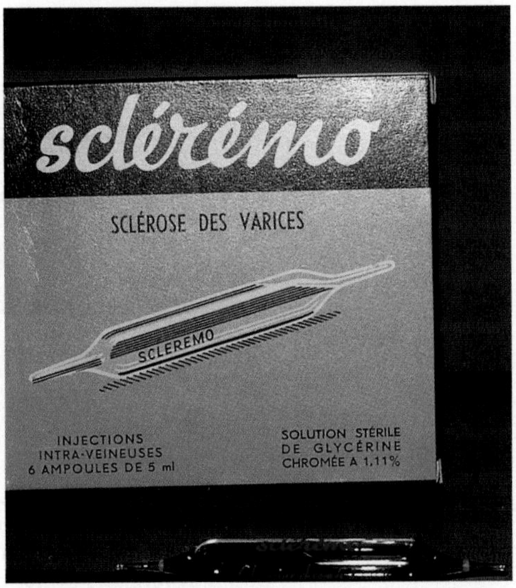

Figure 6-11

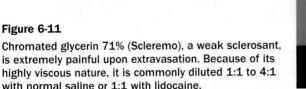

Chromated glycerin 71% (Scleremo), a weak sclerosant, is extremely painful upon extravasation. Because of its highly viscous nature, it is commonly diluted 1:1 to 4:1 with normal saline or 1:1 with lidocaine.

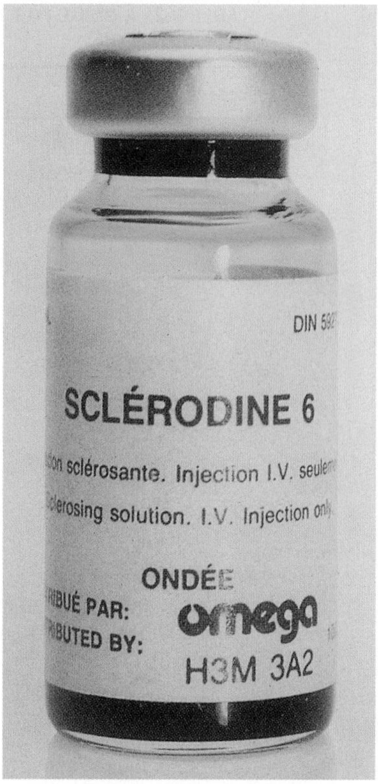

Figure 6-12

Polyiodide iodine (Sclerodine, Varigloban), a mixture of elemental iodine with sodium iodide and a small amount of benzyl alcohol, is the strongest sclerosant presently available. A broad concentration profile of 0.1% to 12% makes this agent useful for the treatment of vessels of varying diameters.

tion of the agent rather than making incremental increases in volume. This agent has a broad spectrum of sclerosing power. Suggested concentrations are as follows: for vessels less than 2 mm in diameter 0.1% to 1%; for vessels 3 to 5 mm in diameter, 2%; for vessels greater than 5 mm in diameter, perforators, and saphenofemoral and saphenopopliteal junctional incompetence, 3% to 12%.

Determining the Appropriate Sclerosing Concentration for a Given Vessel Diameter

Determining the minimum volume and minimal concentration of the most appropriate sclerosing agent is the major goal consideration in producing effective sclerotherapy results. This concept, termed the *minimal sclerosant concentration* (MSC) by the author, will enable the sclerotherapist to achieve maximal results while minimizing his or her complication profile.

A guide to suggested sclerosing agents and initial choices of sclerosant concentrations and volume instillation as related to vessel type and diameter is presented in Table 6-2. Suggested ways to dilute to these appropriate concentrations are presented in Table 6-3.

TABLE 6-2. A GUIDE FOR THE SELECTION OF SCLEROSING SOLUTION AND VOLUME INSTILLATIONS BY VESSEL TYPE[a]

Vessel	Solution Concentration	Volume (per region)
Telangiectatic matting (after previous treatment)	Chromated glycerin, diluted by 50%	0.1–0.2 mL
Telangiectasia (up to 1 mm)	Hypertonic saline, 11.7% Sodium tetradecyl sulfate, 0.1% Hypertonic saline and dextrose, Chromated glycerin, 50% Polidocanol, 0.25% Polyiodide iodine 0.1%	0.1–0.3 mL
Venulectasis (1–2 mm)	Hypertonic saline, 11.7%–23.4% Sodium tetradecyl sulfate, 0.2–0.25% Hypertonic saline 10% and dextrose, 25% (Sclerodex) Chromated glycerin, 100% Polidocanol, 0.5% Ethanolamine oleate 5% Sodium morrhuate 2.5%	0.2–0.5 mL
Reticular veins (2- to 4-mm subcutaneous blue veins)	Hypertonic saline, 23.4% Sodium tetradecyl sulfate, 0.33%–0.5% Sodium morrhuate, 2.5% Polidocanol, 1.0% Polyiodide iodide, 0.3%–1.0%	0.5 mL (may increase to 1 mL if filling of reticular vein is observed)
Nonsaphenous varicose veins (3–8 mm)	Sodium tetradecyl sulfate, 0.5%–1.0% Sodium morrhuate, 5% Polidocanol, 1.0%–3.0% Polyiodide iodine, 1.0%–2.0%	0.5 mL (may increase to 1 ml per injection site in large capacity vein, except for polyiodide)
Saphenous varicose trunks (usually >5 mm)	Sodium tetradecyl sulfate, 1.0%–3.0% Polidocanol, 3.0%–5.0% Polyiodide iodide, 2.0–6.0% (rarely to 12%)	0.5 mL (low-volume injection critical at high concentrations)

[a] FDA-approved solutions shown in italics.

Complication Profiles

Understanding major risk profiles for each of the sclerosing agents is an important factor in attempting to determine which agent to employ in a given clinical setting. Presented below is a major summary of important complication issues as related to each of the previously discussed sclerosing agents.

Detergents

Polidocanol (Aethoxysklerol)

- Allergic and anaphylactic reactions are rare: 0.01% to 0.02%.

  Recent data indicate that its hypersensitivity potential is similar to that of sodium tetradecyl sulfate. The manufacturer warns against use in patients with a history of bronchial asthma. This is a relative contraindication.

TABLE 6-3. COMMON DILUTIONS USED FOR SCLEROTHERAPY SOLUTIONS

Aethoxysklerol (available in 0.5%, 1%, 2%, and 3% in 30-mL vials and 2-mL ampules) (usually diluted in 30-mL vial of 0.9% NaCl for injection)

1. 0.5% Aethoxysklerol[a]
   5 mL 3% Aethoxysklerol
   25 mL 0.9% NaCl for injection or in bacteriostatic water
2. 0.75% Aethoxysklerol
   7.5 mL 3% Aethoxysklerol
   22.5 mL 0.9% NaCl for injection or bacteriostatic water

Hypertonic saline (available in 23.4% in a 30 mL vial) (usually diluted in 3-mL syringes for injection)

1. 18.7% hypertonic saline with 0.4% lidocaine
   2 mL hypertonic saline 23.4%
   0.5 lidocaine 2% plain or in bacteriostatic water

Sotradecol[b] (available in 1% or 3% in 2-mL ampules) (usually diluted in 30-mL vial of 0.9% NaCl for injection)

1. 0.5% Sotradecol
   5 mL 3% Sotradecol
   25 mL 0.9% NaCl for injection or in bacteriostatic water
2. 0.33% Sotradecol
   3.3 mL 3% Sotradecol
   26.7 mL 0.9% NaCl for injection or in bacteriostatic water

[a] Polidocanol.
[b] Sodium tetradecyl sulfate.

- ▶ The extravasation necrosis potential is minimal as compared with that of agents such as hypertonic saline, but it still exists and extravascular injection, which was advocated in the past for treatment of noncanulizable veins, is absolutely contraindicated.
- ▶ A secondary related contraindication is the utilization of polidocanol in patients receiving disulfiram after alcohol withdrawal treatment because a small amount of absolute ethyl alcohol is added to polidocanol to furnish heat stability, which may lead to a "flushing reaction" in susceptible individuals.

Sodium Tetradecyl Sulfate (Sotradecol)

- ▶ Various allergic reactions—from urticaria to anaphylaxis—have been reported; however, their incidence is extremely low and is estimated to be at 0.2% to 0.3%. In-office observation for 20 to 30 minutes after an initial injection session will give both the patient and physician assurance that no such reaction has occurred. With increasing usage it is now felt that the incidence of severe type I anaphylactic reactions is minimal.
- ▶ Hyperpigmentation has been mentioned in 5% to 30% of case reports. However, in the author's experience, its true incidence parallels that of other sclerosing agents of similar potency and is more related to concentration as well as to host skin type, vessel type, and other vascular fragility factors.

- Extravasation necrosis has been reported and probably has an incidence falling between the polidocanol and hypertonic saline spectrum.

Sodium Morrhuate

- In the past, allergic reactions, varying from urticaria to anaphylaxis, have been reported with incidences as high as 48%. However, there have been no reports of severe allergic reactions in the recent medical literature.
- An increased incidence of extravasation necrosis reactions has been reported with this agent.

Ethanolamine Oleate

- Urticarial and anaphylactic reactions have been reported in up to 0.25% of treated individuals.
- A hemolytic reaction has been reported in one patient.
- Acute renal failure with spontaneous recovery has been reported in two patients.

Osmotic Agents

Hypertonic Saline

- Stinging and cramping occur uniformly after treatment with 23.4% HS. These effects are minimized when the agent is diluted to a 11.7% or 6.7% concentration. Immediate kneading of the involved area will minimize this discomfort.
- This agent causes reproducible extravasation neurons when it is injected extravascularly.
- Because intravascular hemolysis occurs immediately and there is rapid disruption of vascular endothelial continuity, there is an increased incidence of postsclerotherapy hyperpigmentation secondary to hemosiderin staining.

Hypertonic Saline/Dextrose

- Allergenicity of the phenethyl alcohol component of this agent is possible, with a reported incidence of allergic reactions being 0.2%.
- Burning and cramping on injection is minimal as compared with HS.
- Extravasation necrosis and hyperpigmentation profiles are similar to that reported with HS.

Chemical Irritants

Chromated Glycerin

- This agent is extremely viscous and thus often difficult to inject.
- Pain and cramping may occur with injection; however, dilution with 1% lidocaine without epinephrine may minimize these side effects.

- The chromate moiety has been associated with rare hypersensitivity reactions, including anaphylaxis.
- Ureteral colic and hematuria have rarely been reported with this agent.
- Because of its weak sclerosing power, a correspondingly low incidence of pigmentary abnormalities and ulcerative necrosis has been reported.

Polyiodide Iodine

- There is an increased incidence of extravasation necrosis with this agent.
- This agent has limited effectiveness at a short distance from the injection site.
- There have been reported cases of anaphylaxis, although minimal considering the nature of the ionic iodinated moiety.
- Rare cases of renal toxicity have been reported.

The Perfect Sclerosant

The ideal sclerosant remains to be elucidated. It would be an agent that produced greatest clinical efficacy with minimal side effects. It should produce irreversible endothelial injury in the desired location while minimizing damage to normal vessels.

Conclusion

When choosing a given sclerosant for treating a particular vascular problem, the practicing sclerotherapist must be aware that different sclerosing agents have varying sclerosing potentials and side-effect profiles. Also, the relative strength of a sclerosant as it related to a given vessel diameter must be understood.

By choosing the MSC for a given situation, it is possible to minimize side effects by producing less vascular irritability with subsequent decreased diapedesis of erythrocytes and cytokine release, leading to a diminished incidence of postsclerotherapy adverse sequelae, including hyperpigmentation, edema, thrombophlebitis, and bruising.

The ultimate goal of sclerotherapy is to deliver the minimum volume and minimum concentration of the most appropriate sclerosant and to inject it under conditions that will achieve the maximal effective endothelial exposure. Sclerosant concentration, volume, temperature, mixing, and patient positioning are important factors in attempting to achieve optimal results when performing sclerotherapy.

A summary of important characteristics of sclerosing solutions is presented in Table 6-4.

TABLE 6-4. IMPORTANT CHARACTERISTICS OF SCLEROSING SOLUTIONS

Sclerosing Solution (Brand Name)	Class	Allergenicity	Risks	FDA Approval	Dose Limitation[a]
Hypertonic saline (HS)	Hyperosmotic	None	Necrosis of skin Pain and cramping Hyperpigmentation	Yes, as abortifacient	6–10 mL (estimate based on author's experience)
Hypertonic saline and dextrose (HSD) (Sclerodex)	Hyperosmotic	Low (due only to added phenethyl alcohol	Pain (much less than HS)	No (sold in Canada)	10 mL of undiluted solution
Sodium tetradecyl sulfate (STS) (Sotradecol, S.T.D., Injection, Thrombojet)	Detergent	Rare anaphylaxis	Pigmentation Necrosis of skin (higher concentrations) Pain with perivascular injection	Yes	10 mL of 3%
Polidocanol (POL) (Aethoxysklerol, Aetoxisclerol, Sclerovein)	Detergent	Rare anaphylaxis	Lowest risks of necrosis Lowest risks of pain Pigmentation at higher concentrations Disulfarim like reaction	No	10 mL of 3%
Sodium morrhuate (SM) (Scleromate)	Detergent	Anaphylaxis, highest risk	Pigmentation Necrosis of skin Pain	Yes	10 mL
Ethanolamine oleate (EO) (Ethamolin)	Detergent	Urticaria Anaphylaxis	Pigmentation Necrosis of skin Pain Viscous, difficult to inject Acute renal failure Hemolytic reactions	Yes (used primarily for esophageal varices)	10 mL

Polyiodide iodine (PII) (Varigloban, Variglobin, Sclerodine)	Chemical irritant	Anaphylaxis, iodine hypersensitivity reactions	Pain on injection Necrosis of skin Dark brown color makes intravascular placement more difficult to confirm Renal insufficiency	No	5 mL of 3%
72% glycerin with 8% chromium potassium alum (Chromex, (Scleremo)	Chemical irritant	Extremely rare anaphylaxis	Ineffective sclerosis (weak agent) Very low risk of pigmentation Viscous—difficult to inject Pain and cramping Ureteral colic/hematuria	No	5 mL (estimate)

[a] Increased volume per session associated with increased risks of allergenicity.

BIBLIOGRAPHY

Carlin MC, Ratz JL. Treatment of telangiectasia: comparison of sclerosing agents. *J Dermatol Surg Oncol* 1987;13:1181–1184.

Conrad P, Malouf GM, Stacey MC. The Australian Polidocanol (Aethoxysklerol) Study: results at 1 year. *Phlebology* 1994;9:17–20.

Conrad P, Malouf GM, Stacey MC. The Australian Polidocanol (Aethoxysklerol) Study—results of 2 years. *Dermatol Surg* 1995;21:334–336.

Feied CF, Jackson JJ, Bren TS, Bond OB, Fernando CE, Young VCY, Hashemiydon RB. Allergic reactions to Polidocanol for vein sclerosis. *J Dermatol Surg Oncol* 1994;20:466–468.

Goldman MP. A comparison of sclerosing agents—clinical and histologic effects of intravascular sodium morrhuate ethanolamine oleate, hypertonic saline 11.7% and Sclerodex in the dorsal rabbit ear vein. *J Dermatol Surg Oncol* 1991;17:354–362.

Guex JJ. Indications for the sclerosing agent Polidocanol. *J Dermatol Surg Oncol* 1993;19:959–961.

Martin EE, Goldman MP. A comparison of sclerosing agents—Clinical and histologic effects of intravascular sodium tetradecyl sulfate and chromated glycerin in the dorsal rabbit ear vein. *J Dermatol Surg Oncol* 1990;16:18–22.

Norris MJ, Carlin ML, Raiz JL. Treatment of essential telangiectasia: effects of increasing concentrations of Polidocanol. *J Am Acad Dermatol* 1989;20:643–649.

Rotter SM, Weiss RA. Human saphenous vein in vitro model for studying the action of sclerosing solutions. *J Dermatol Surg Oncol* 1993;19:59–62.

Sadick NS. Advances in sclerosing solutions. Cosmet Dermatol 1996;9:9–13.

Sadick NS. Hyperosmolar versus detergent sclerosing agents in sclerotherapy: Effect on distal vessel obliteration. *J Dermatol Surg Oncol* 1994;20:313–316.

Sadick NS. Treatment of varicose and telangiectatic leg veins with hypertonic saline: A comparative study of Heparin and saline. *J Dermatol Surg Oncol* 1995;16:24–28.

Sadick NS. Sclerotherapy of varicose and telangiectatic leg veins: minimal sclerosant concentration of hypertonic saline and its relationship to vessel diameter. *J Dermatol Surg Oncol* 1991;20:65–70.

Sadick NS, Farber B. A microbiological study of diluted sclerotherapy solutions. *J Dermatol Surg Oncol* 1993;19:450–454.

CHAPTER 7

TREATMENT OF TELANGIECTATIC LEG VEINS

In previous chapters, the history, physical examination, and vascular laboratory evaluation of the patient with venous disease have been discussed. The present chapter begins with the technical approach to treating telangiectatic and varicose veins.

The Right Approach

Sclerotherapy of telangiectasia and venulectasia (spider veins) involves treatment of vessels less than 1 to 2 mm in diameter (class I to II vessels). Treatment of such small-diameter vessels should only ensue after treatment of areas of reflux and associated larger-diameter vessels have been addressed. In practical terms, telangiectatic vessels are the last to be considered in the treatment cascade. Table 7-1 emphasizes this point and portrays a rational approach to the treatment of venous pathology.

The first question the sclerotherapist must ask is: What are the absolute and relative contraindications to performing sclerotherapy?

Absolute Contraindications

1. Pregnancy
2. Advanced collagen vascular disease
3. Osteoarthritis or other diseases that interfere with the patient's mobility
4. Acute deep venous thrombophlebitis
5. Acute febrile illness
6. Anticoagulant therapy

TABLE 7-1. A CLINICAL APPROACH TO THE TREATMENT OF VENOUS PATHOLOGY

Axial reflux—greater and lesser saphenous veins and associated junctional incompetence (surgical ligation/stripping procedures/ duplex-guided sclerotherapy, echosclerotherapy) Radiofrequency ablation

↓

Truncal varicosities (sclerotherapy, ambulatory phlebectomy) Radiofrequency ablation

↓

Perforating veins (sclerotherapy, ambulatory phlebectomy)

↓

Reticular veins (sclerotherapy, ambulatory phlebectomy)

↓

Telangiectasia (microsclerotherapy, laser, noncoherent light-source therapy)

Relative Contraindications

1. Acute superficial thrombophlebitis
2. "Needle phobia"
3. Hypercoagulable states (protein S or protein C deficiency, circulating antiphospholipid antibody syndrome, factor V Leyden mutation)
4. Severe obesity
5. Elderly debilitated individuals

Once the above issues have been addressed, the physician is ready to begin treating the patient with telangiectasia.

Patient Instructions

Patients may be treated on the day of the initial consultation and evaluation. However, more commonly, patients are treated on separate days after they have been well instructed and counseled on what to do to prepare for the injection procedure and how to proceed with postsclerotherapy compression.

Patient Preparation Instructions for Sclerotherapy Treatments

1. If telangiectasias are symptomatic or associated with symptomatic reticular or perforator veins, contact your insurance company for advice on extent of benefits coverage.

2. Shave with an antibacterial soap such as Lever 2000 (Unilever, Greenwich, CT, U.S.A.) on the morning of the procedure.
3. Bring prescribed compression stockings to the office on the day of the procedure.
4. Minimize the use of emollients on the legs the evening prior and on the day of injection therapy.
5. Dress in loose-fitting clothing and comfortable loose shoes in order to accommodate postsclerotherapy dressings.
6. Be prepared to ambulate for several hours following your sclerotherapy procedure.
7. Be prepared to sit in the office for at least 15 minutes after your initial treatment session in order to rule out any potential postsclerotherapy allergic reactions.
8. If you have a history of easy bruisability, consult your physician about the topical application of vitamin K cream prior to your treatment.

Appropriate Sclerosant Concentrations for Treating Telangiectasias

In treating all venous ectasias, one should also employ the minimal sclerosant concentration (MSC). This concept is particularly important in treating small-diameter vessels, where the risks of extravasation necrosis, hyperpigmentation, and telangiectatic matting are maximized.

Suggested choices of sclerosing agents and suggested initial concentrations for treating telangiectasias are presented below and fully outlined in Chapter 6.

Vessel Diameter	Sclerosant Concentration
Less than 1 mm	Hypertonic saline 11.7%[a]
	Sodium tetradecyl sulfate 0.1%
	Polidocanol 0.25%
	Scleremo 100%
	Polyiodide iodine 1%
	Sclerodex
	Ethanolamine oleate 2%
	Sodium morrhuate 1%[a]
1 to 3 mm	Hypertonic saline 23.4%[a]
	Sodium tetradecyl sulfate 0.25%[a]
	Polidocanol 0.75%
	Polyiodide iodine 1%
	Ethanolamine oleate 5%
	Sodium morrhuate 2.5%[a]

In principle, if resolution of treated veins does not occur as expected, the sclerotherapist can increase the concentration of sclerosant at subsequent treat-

[a] Approved by the U.S. Food and Drug Administration (FDA).

ment sessions. Alternatively, a different sclerosing agent can be chosen if vessels do not respond to a sclerosant at suggested concentrations for given vessel diameters.

Technique Modifications

Regardless of the sclerosant used, microsclerotherapy utilizes a standard technique. The patient who has been dressed in the previously discussed sclerotherapy garment (Chapter 4), is placed in a supine position on the treatment table. Proper visualization of the treatment sites requires bright shadow-free lighting and is aided by the use of a lighted high-intensity magnifying head lamp, magnifying glasses, or loupes (2× to 5× magnification). The skin is then cleansed with either an alcohol swab or a 1:1 compound of 70% alcohol compound with 1% acetic acid solution. The glistening effect of alcohol may be synergistically augmented with the addition of acetic acid, rendering the skin more transparent. This changes the refraction coefficient of the skin, allowing improved visualization of surface telangiectasia.

Injections are performed in most cases with 30-gauge ½-inch disposable needles (Becton Dickinson and Company, Franklin Lakes, NJ, U.S.A.; Air-Tite, Newport News, VA, U.S.A.). In addition 31-, 32-, and 33-gauge needles are available (Chapter 4); however, these needles are nondisposable (steam autoclaved), clog easily upon repeated usage, and lose their sharpness upon repeated puncture of telangiectasias. Regardless of the needle employed it is inserted at a 30- to 45-degree angle with the bevel side up; allowing the vascular lumen will be transected at an acute angle, thus minimizing the possibility of transecting the vessel (Fig. 7-1).

A 3-mm syringe is of adequate size yet allows for slow, low-pressure injection of the sclerosant (gentle pressure is desirable to prevent "blowout" of telangiectatic vessels and consequent extravasation of the sclerosant and venous blood). The routine utilization of smaller 1-mL tuberculin or insulin syringes is commonly associated with leakage of sclerosant and high injection pressures, which may lead to suboptimal results.

For treatment of vessels less than 1 mm in diameter, noncannulizable with the needle-syringe apparatus mentioned above, or for extensive telangiectatic matting, alternative approaches include injection with either a 31-gauge 1-mL insulin or tuberculin syringe or utilization of one of the previously described 33-gauge angiocath apparatuses (STD, Hereford, England; Kawasumi Laboratories, Tampa, FL, U.S.A.). These smaller-diameter systems are not practical for the treatment of large surface areas of telangiectasia; however, they are helpful in selected situations where microvessels cannot be appropriately cannulized utilizing the conventional 30-gauge needle, 3-mL syringe apparatus.

Appropriate surgical gloves are part of universal precautions in this blood contact procedure. These should be particularly snug-fitting in order to minimize interference with palpation, which becomes of paramount importance as larger-diameter vessels are treated. Regardless of vessel type or an individual physician's approach to treating telangiectasias and varicose veins, a definite set of principles

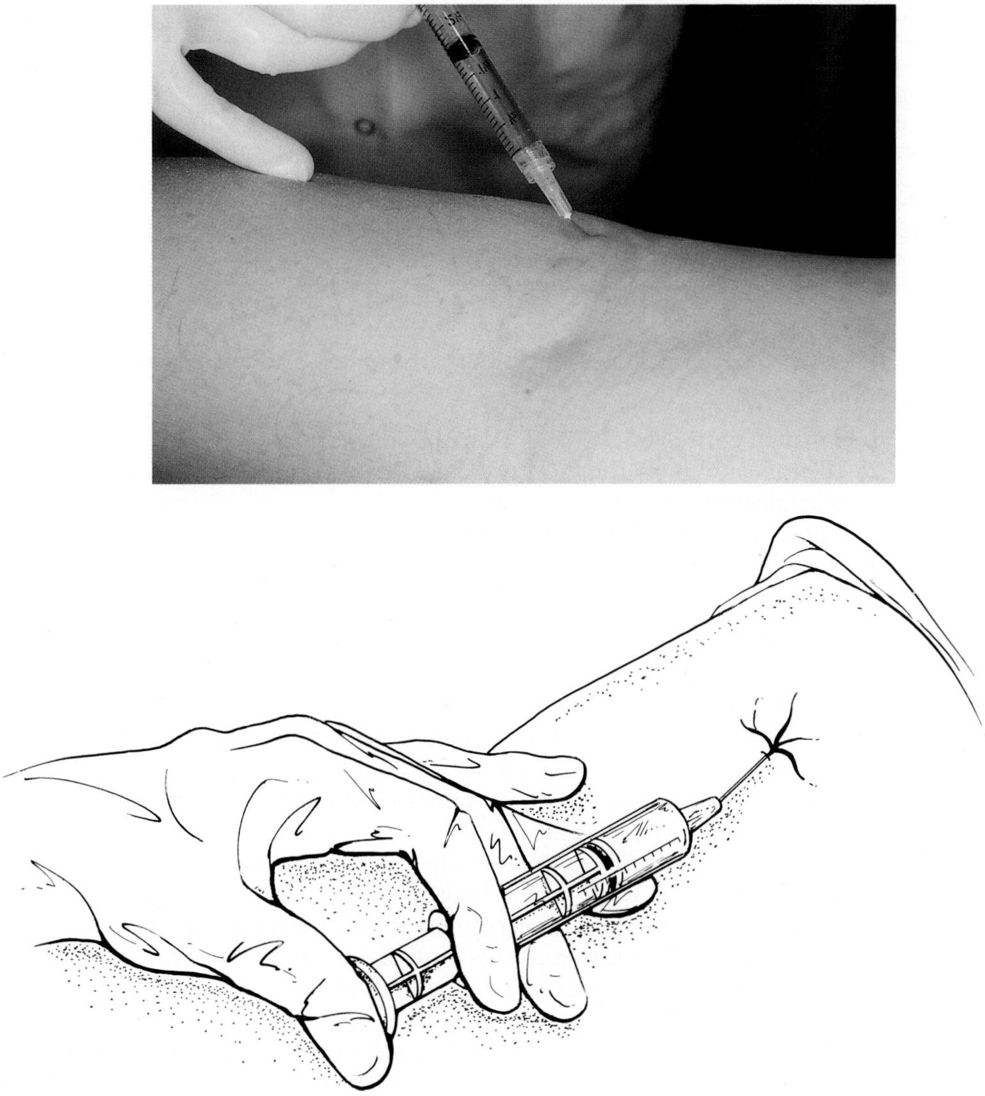

Figure 7-1

A 30- to 40-degree injection angle, bevel up, produces optimal results in sclerotherapy by minimizing vascular transection.

must be adhered to and is universally accepted within the sclerotherapy community. These guidelines are presented in Table 7-2.

Whether sclerotherapy should proceed from the top of the leg downward (French school), whether the clinician should start distally and work proximally (Swiss school), or whether random-site injection is acceptable are questions of discussion and individual preference. At this time insufficient data are available to establish whether efficacy, safety, or other factors are significantly affected by the choice of injection pattern. The author prefers a proximal-to-distal approach in treating both small- and medium-to large-diameter vessels.

TABLE 7-2. PRINCIPLES OF VARICOSE VEIN/TELANGIECTASIA SCLEROTHERAPY

Proximal-to-distal treatment is the rule
Largest veins are treated before smaller veins
Veins must be emptied of blood by various maneuvers
Distal finger pressure in a spreading and compressing motion is applied after injection
The entire varicosity is treated at one time
Reflux points are determined initially and treated specifically
Immediate and adequate compression is applied
Adequate ambulation immediately after treatment

There are, however, four principles that should be adhered to in all cases of injection therapy:

1. Treat an entire vessel at a given treatment session.
2. Identify and inject the most proximal "arborizing feeder" vessel in a telangiectatic cluster.
3. Empty the vein prior to injection (Fig. 7-2).
4. Knead the sclerosant immediately postinstillation into the surrounding periinjection vessel area (Fig. 7-3).

Treatment of an entire vessel at a given treatment session will minimize incomplete vessel dissolution and also minimize the probability of recanalization and thus suboptimal therapeutic results.

Treat feeding arborizing foci of telangiectasia, which will minimize the number of puncture sites necessary to achieve desired results. This will lead to a decreased complication profile in terms of postsclerotherapy hyperpigmentation and extravasation necrosis (Fig. 7-4).

Emptying of vessels prior to injection increases sclerosant-endothelial contact, and thus, theoretically at least, should improve endosclerosis, the ultimate goal of the sclerotherapy procedure. The persistence of telangiectasia and varicose veins after treatment is usually due to recanalization of the intramural thrombus that develops. Proper vein emptying prior to treatment may help minimize this occurrence.

Finally, local kneading or distribution of sclerosant should theoretically lead to diminished "pooling of sclerosant" and thus produce more uniform results; it should also minimize the potential for sclerosant "sludging," which could lead to an increased incidence of superficial thrombophlebitis and postsclerotherapy hyperpigmentation.

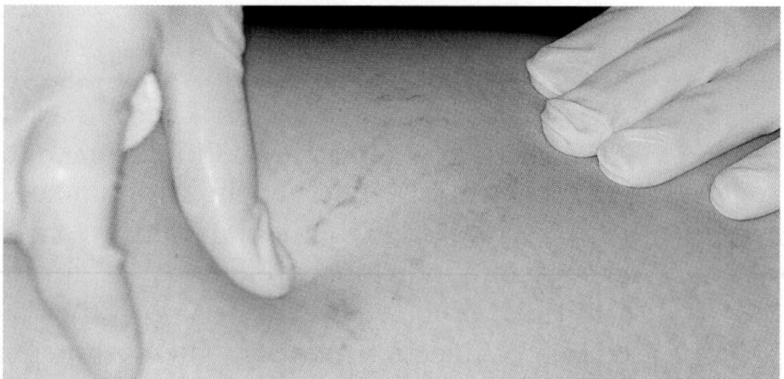

Figure 7-2

Emptying of the full vein prior to injection improves results in sclerotherapy by improving sclerosant-endothelial contact.

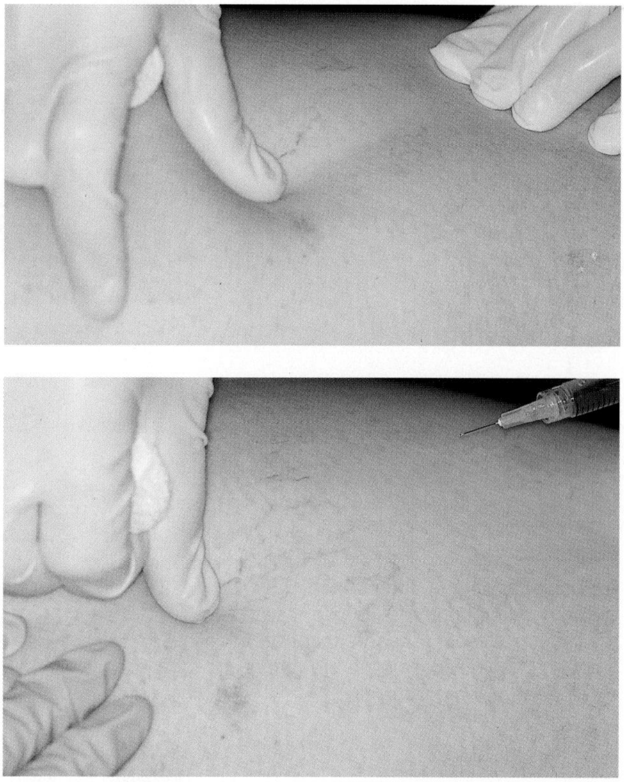

Figure 7-3

Kneading of sclerosant postsclerotherapy improves sclerosant-endothelium contact, optimizing potential sclerosant efficiency.

There are four basic techniques that may be employed when injecting telangiectasia:

1. Air bolus technique (Fig. 7-5)
2. Aspiration technique (Fig. 7-6)
3. Puncture "feel" technique (Fig. 7-7)
4. Empty vein technique (Fig. 7-8)

(text continues on page 28)

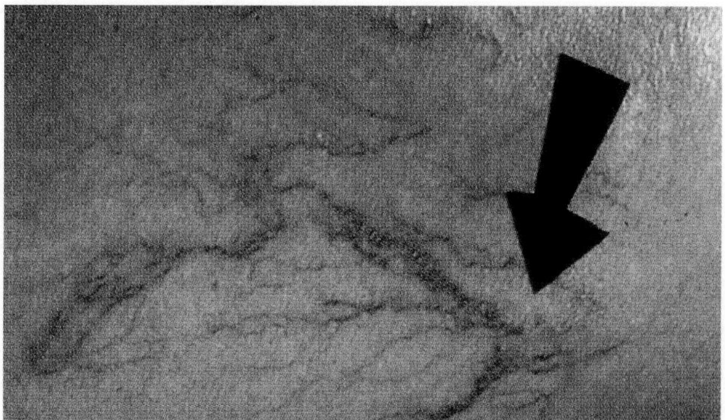

Figure 7-4

Treatment of arborizing feeder veins diminishes the number of injections required in a given sclerotherapy treatment session, thus minimizing potential side effects.

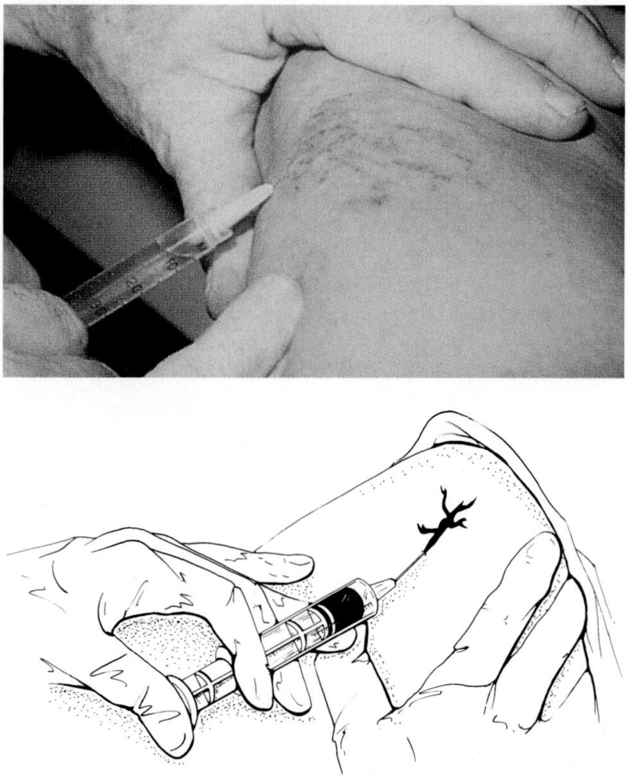

Figure 7-5

Air bolus technique. Injection of 0.5% of air prior to injection of sclerosant will ensure intravascular needle location by showing perivascular tissue blanching if extravasation has occurred.

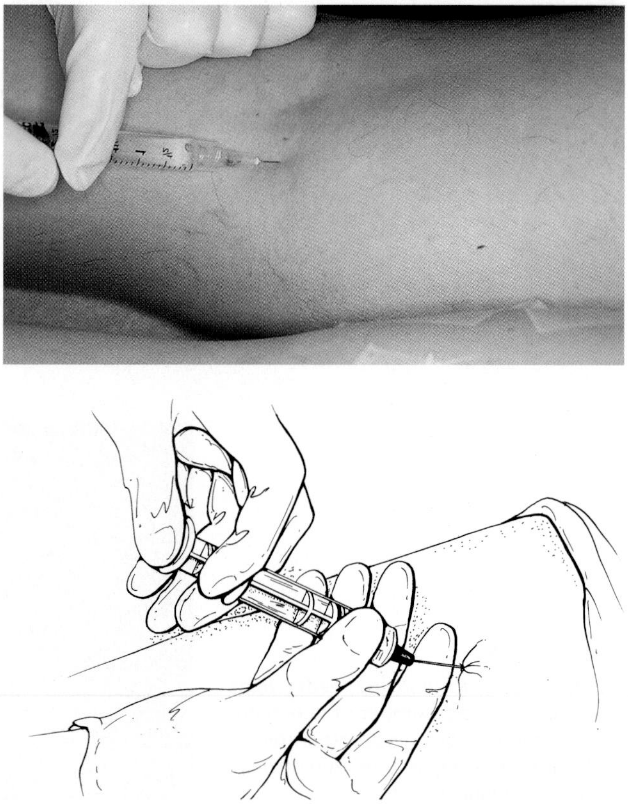

Figure 7-6

Aspiration technique. Aspiration of a small amount of blood ensures appropriate intravascular needle placement.

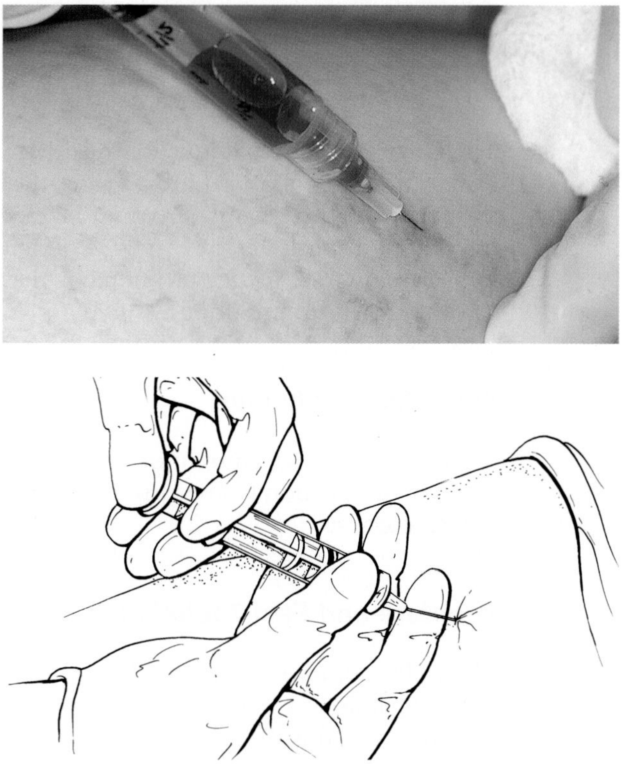

Figure 7-7

Puncture "feel" technique. Feel of entering the vein by means of endothelial wall perforation is employed in this technique modification and should be the ultimate technique mastered by the experienced sclerotherapist.

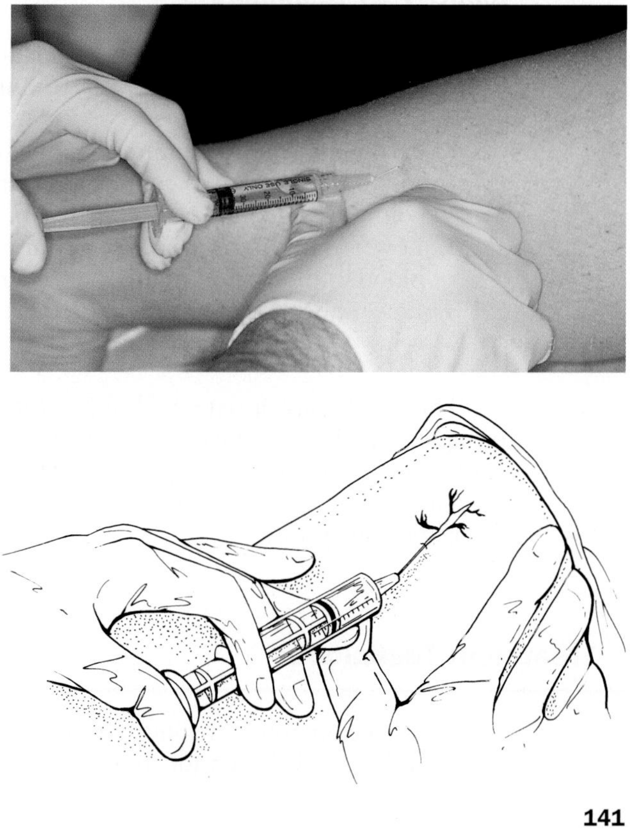

Figure 7-8

Empty vein technique. Vein emptying prior to vessel cannulation by kneading with gentle pressure improves sclerosant-endothelial interaction, thus optimizing the potential for effective endosclerosis.

Air Bolus Technique

This is an excellent technique for the novice beginning to treat leg veins. Injection of 0.5 mL of air prior to introducing the sclerosant will show air in soft tissue (blanching) rather than sclerosant. This helps to minimize the potential for extravasation necrosis.

The drawback to this technique is that too strong a push of air may lead to vascular spasm or distention.

Aspiration Technique

Aspiration of a small amount of blood into the hub of the syringe ensures that intact vein cannulation has occurred. However, aspiration that is too strong can lead to vein collapse.

Puncture and Feel Technique

The feeling of having entered the vein by perforating the endothelium is an excellent technique as there is no change in the pressure dynamics of the treated vessel. However, this modification is precarious for the beginner because of the increased risk of extravascular injection.

Empty Vein Technique

The vein is emptied prior to vessel cannulation by kneading the vessel with gentle hand pressure. The advantages of this technique are that:

1. An empty vein has minimal volume; therefore a smaller volume of sclerosant is necessary to contact the intraluminal surface, compared with the volume needed for a distended vein.
2. Lower concentrations of sclerosant may be employed, since there is less blood in the vein to dilute the solution.
3. Lower injection pressures are required to deliver the solution into the vein.

The most appropriate technique for performing microsclerotherapy on telangiectasias is that which produces the best results in the individual sclerotherapist's hands and results in the least complications. Finally, different techniques or combined techniques such as empty vein/puncture-fill may be employed in various clinical situations.

Treatment Techniques

A copy of the anatomic mapping diagram (see Chapter 5, page 109) should be placed at the patient's bedside in order to allow accurate charting of all injections.

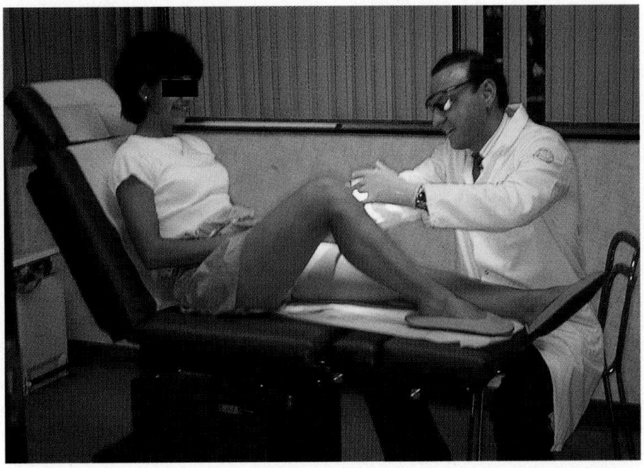

Figure 7-9
Patient positioned in recumbent position on a power-assisted table ready for the sclerotherapy procedure.

Patient Positioning

Patients are usually positioned in a recumbent position, as previously stated, on a power-assisted table with the sclerotherapist positioned at or below the level of the patient's knee (Fig. 7-9). Inaccessible vessels on the lateral posterior thigh may be treated with the patient in the prone position.

Physician/Assistant Positioning

Skin tension is an important factor in achieving accurate and precise vessel cannulation. While the sclerotherapist holds the syringe in his or her dominant hand between the index and middle fingers, an assistant can often help by stretching the patient's skin in two opposing directions. The physician can achieve appropriate three-point tension unaided, when necessary, by proper hand placement. The nondominant hand is used to stretch the skin adjacent to the treated vessels in two directions and then the fifth finger of the dominant hand exerts countertraction in a third direction (Fig. 7-10).

Sclerosant Quantity

Regardless of the technique employed, injections are begun after venous emptying of the projected treatment site. The author uses a maximum of 5 mL of sclerosant per treated extremity/patient treatment session. It should be noted that maximum recommended dosages vary among the sclerosants. The extent and duration of the treatment session is determined largely by the maximum dosage of the agent used. The quantity of solution to be injected should be enough to produce an obliteration 1 to 2 cm in diameter around the point of injection. Usually not more than 0.5 ml of sclerosant per injection site is employed in order to avoid the risk of initiating the formation of new telangiectasia around the edge of the treatment zone. One should not be overzealous at a given treatment session for several reasons. One is that sclerotherapy of telangiectasias requires concentration

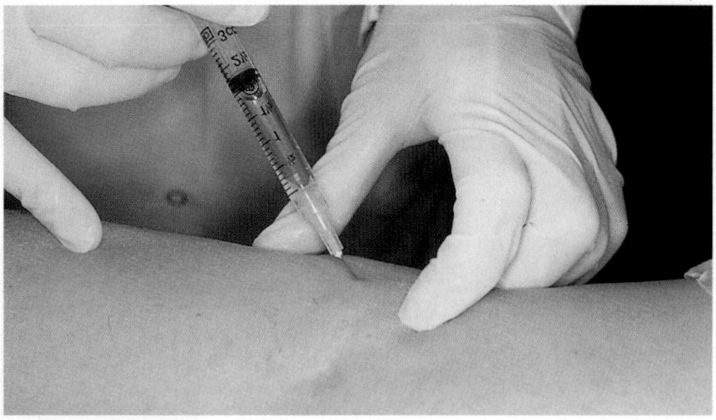

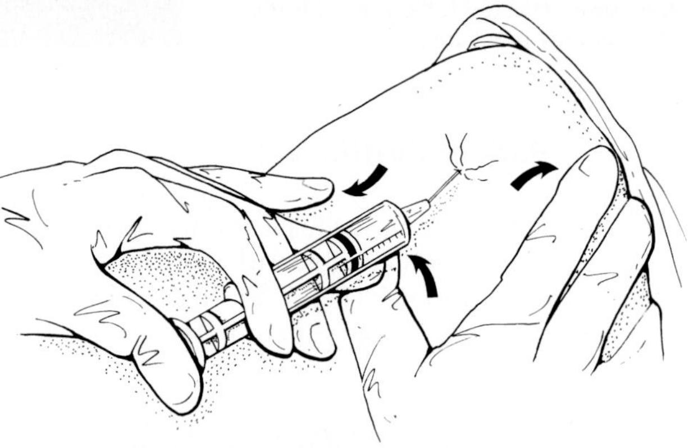

Figure 7-10

Proper hand placement. A nondominant hand stretches the skin adjacent to the treated vessels while the fifth finger of the dominant hand exerts countertraction during injection of sclerosant.

and a steady hand: Clinician fatigue may greatly reduce therapeutic efficiency. In addition, inducing large amounts of inflammation to the venous system at a single point in time may lead to an increased incidence of neoangiogenesis (telangiectatic matting) superficial thrombophlebitis, and postsclerotherapy hyperpigmentation.

Injection Technique

With continuous tissue tension applied, the sclerosant is slowly injected. Since most telangiectasias are located in the upper papillary dermis, a common problem in technique is to insert the needle too deeply, resulting in vascular transection. If the vessel is appropriately cannulated, immediate blanching will occur in the treated vessel and its adjacent tributaries. If the needle is not within the vessel, extravasation will occur and either a superficial tissue wheal will appear or the sclerosant will leak out onto the skin surface. Injection with the bevel of the needle facing the skin surface will minimize the possibility of vascular transection by decreasing the vacuum produced by the bevel and the skin surface. Entire vessels must be treated at each treatment session.

Finally, brisk cannulation and small volumes of sclerosant instilled at a given injection site regardless of the sclerosant employed will minimize patient discomfort, extravasation, and damage to the deep venous system.

Choosing the Optimal Sclerosant

The workhorse sclerosants in the author's practice for treating telangiectasias are sodium tetradecyl sulfate (Sotradecol) 0-1% to 0.25% and hypertonic saline 11.7% to 23.4%. With impending FDA approval of polidocanol (Aethoxysklerol) (0.25% to 1.0%) this agent will also play an important role in the treatment of telangiectasis in the near future.

Injection Pressures

Gentle injection of low volumes (less than 0.5 mL per injection site) of sclerosant that produces a small (less than 2-cm) blanch will improve sclerotherapy results while minimizing complications. This is accomplished by decreasing vascular trauma and increasing the duration of contact between sclerosant and the vascular endothelium. It should take between 5 and 10 seconds to fill a given vessel. Rapid pushes of large amounts of sclerosant can lead to sclerosant localization in deeper vessels, resulting in potential deep venous thrombosis and pulmonary emboli.

If the sclerosant appears to dissipate into the deeper venous system during the injection of superficial vessels, the sclerotherapist should immediately stop the injection and begin cannulation at an adjacent site, looking for blanching of superficial vessels.

Posttreatment Modifications

After sclerotherapy of telangiectasis, patients must recognize that burning, swelling, vein refilling, and urticaria can occur; these usually resolve rapidly.

After injection of hypertonic saline, cramping may occur; this can be alleviated with gentle massage of the treated area, although this effect usually resolves spontaneously within 5 to 10 minutes posttreatment.

Immediate postsclerotherapy urticaria does not portend systemic sclerosant allergy but rather is a local effect mediated by the release of histamine and other inflammatory cytokines. If this condition is symptomatic, it can be treated by medium-potency topical steroids such as fluocinonide 0.05% (Lidex E Cream, Roche Laboratories, Nutley, NJ U.S.A.) or fluorandrelone 0.05% (Cordran Cream, Oclassen, San Rafael, CA, U.S.A.). The patient should remain in the physician's office for 15 minutes following the first treatment session if any sclerosing agent with hypersensitivity potential is employed (all agents other than saline) to ensure that no hypersensitivity reaction ensues.

Posttreatment Compression of Telangiectasis

Immediately following injection, one assistant may apply either a cotton ball, gauze, and/or a foam-rubber compression pad (STD-E pad, Hereford, England) over the injected veins which is secured with a tape dressing (Duracil–3M, St. Paul, MN, U.S.A.) (Fig. 7-11). This provides local compression over the treated

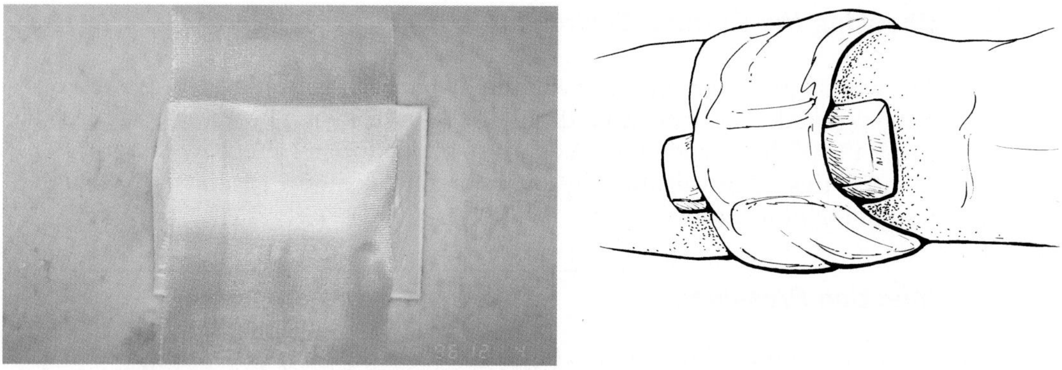

Figure 7-11
Foam rubber compression pad (STD-E pad, STD Pharmaceuticals) applied over injected vein and secured with a tape dressing (Duracil, 3M).

vein (the entire vein, not just the puncture site should be adequately compressed). These local compression dressings are removed the morning following treatment. More recently, the author has abandoned the use of spot local compression in treating small microtelangiectasias.

Full compression following the treatment of telangiectasis remains a point of controversy. How much compression is necessary and how long should it be worn are also points of contention.

Previous studies have stated that posttelangiectatic compression may decrease posttreatment hyperpigmentation, ankle edema, and telangiectatic matting. However, a cooperative recently published national study looking into these issues (Sadick, Weiss, Goldman, *Dermatologic Surgery*, 1999) has shown that 3 weeks of compression following treatment of telangiectasias and reticular veins produces optimal clinical results and that 3 days or 1 week of compression produce better clinical results than no compression at all. Compression appears to have its greatest effect in minimizing post-sclerotherapy hyperpigmentation as shown in this study as well.

On a more theoretical basis compression should improve clinical results by occluding the treated vascular lumen, decreasing recanalization, and finally by reducing the risk of vascular thrombosis.

It has been the author's experience that patients treated for telangiectasia will rarely wear class II 30- to 40-mm Hg graduate stockings and are much more compliant with class I 20- to 30-mm Hg support hose, which are lighter and are available in a number of fashionable colors (Fig. 7-12). Most companies—including Sigvaris, Jobst, and Medi-USA—manufacture such hose. This subject is covered in greater detail in Chapter 11.

As in all cases of sclerotherapy treatment, graduated support hose should be applied immediately posttherapy, before the patient has left the office.

Posttreatment Activity Regime

Patients are encouraged to ambulate following treatment. All activities other than high-impact exercise may be carried out. The latter is discouraged for a period of 48 hours posttreatment. Walking, riding bicycles, and low-impact aerobics are ideal exercises following sclerotherapy.

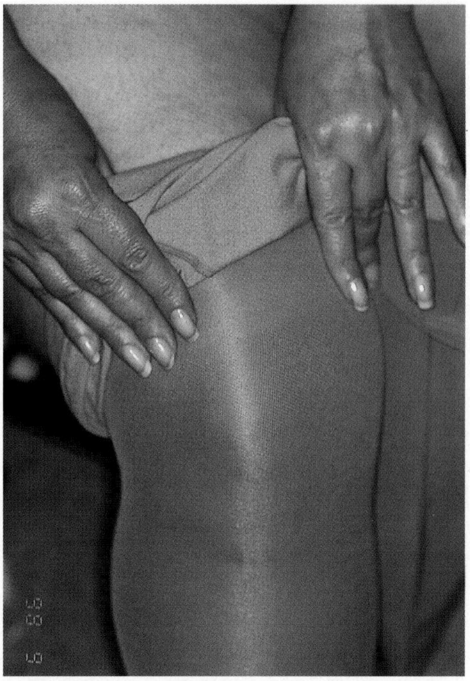

Figure 7-12
Class I 20- to 30-mm Hg support hose, light and fashionable in texture and color, may be applied immediately postsclerotherapy.

Repeat Treatment Sessions

A given anatomic area is usually not retreated for a period of 4 to 6 weeks in order to assess the response to the previous treatment session, since this is the duration of time for maximum sclerotherapy-induced endosclerosis to occur.

Anatomic treatment charts documenting the anatomic region treated at a given session, the size and number of vessels treated, and the amount of sclerosant employed are extremely useful (Chapter 5).

Resistant Telangiectasia

What does the clinician do when results are not as expected after a reasonable number (two to four) of treatment sessions in a given anatomic area utilizing an appropriate sclerosant concentration (MSC) is employed for a given vessel diameter?

1. Look for areas of larger feeding vessels such as reticular veins or perforators that might have been initially missed on physical and laboratory evaluation. Treatment of these feeder sources of reflux with Doppler guidance may be helpful in this clinical setting.
2. Use a stronger concentration of the same sclerosing agent.
3. Choose an alternative sclerosing agent.
4. Finally, there is an X factor, in that for some unknown reason, 1% to 2% of individuals do not respond to sclerotherapy treatments regardless of

which sclerosing agent is employed. These patients may be helped by alternative treatment approaches such as microambulatory phlebectomy or laser/noncoherent pulsed-light-source therapies.

Conclusion

By adhering to the basic principles stated in this chapter, the sclerotherapist may achieve gratifying results in treating telangiectasias of the lower extremities. Appropriate choice of sclerosant, utilization of the minimal sclerosant concentrations (MSC), and the practice of fastidious technique are the cornerstones of success.

BIBLIOGRAPHY

Bodian EL. Techniques for sclerotherapy for sunburst venous blemishes. *J Dermatol Surg Oncol* 1985;11:696–704.

Duffy DM. Small vessel sclerotherapy: an overview. *Adv Dermatol* 1988;13:221–242.

Duffy DM. Sclerotherapy. *Clin Dermatol* 1992;10:373–380.

Foley WT. The eradication of venous blemishes. *Cutis* 1975;15:665–668.

Goldman MP, Bennett RG. Treatment of telangiectasia: a review. *J Am Acad Dermatol* 1987;17:167–182.

Guex JJ. Microsclerotherapy. *Semin Dermatol* 1993;12:129–134.

Sadick NS. Sclerotherapy of varicose and telangiectatic leg veins: minimal sclerosant concentration of hypertonic saline and its relationship to vessel diameter. *J Dermatol Surg Oncol* 1991;17:65–70.

Weiss RA, Goldman MP. Advances in sclerotherapy *Dermatol Clin* 1995;13:431–443.

Weiss RA, Sadick NS, Goldman MP, Weiss MA. Post-sclerotherapy compression: controlled comparative study of duration and its effect on clinical outcome. *Dermatol Surg* 1999;25:106–108.

CHAPTER 8

TREATMENT OF RETICULAR VEINS

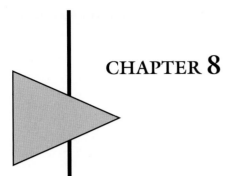

As stated in the previous chapter, the treatment of telangiectasias is not performed until larger feeding veins into which they drain are adequately addressed. This will prevent unsuccessful results and early recurrences. Thus, prior to microsclerotherapy of telangiectasia, one must consider treatment of the "connecting veins" or reticular veins. The evaluation and treatment of reticular veins is the focus of the present chapter.

The Right Approach

Reticular veins have also been called minor varicose veins or feeding veins. These veins are green or blue, usually 1 to 4 mm in diameter, and located parallel to the skin surface. They are most prominent over the posterolateral aspects of the thigh and the lateral aspects of the calf and tend to drain toward the popliteal fossa, with associated telangiectasia appearing in a centripetal fashion. As has been shown in numerous studies, these vessels are usually associated with telangiectasis in up to 80% to 90% of cases. This condition is particularly prominent along the outer aspect of the thigh, where a prominent interconnecting net of telangiectasia and reticular veins, known as the "Albanese complex," may be seen. It is speculated that this incompetent reticular venous network represents an embryonal vestige of the lesser saphenous vein, which is present within the calf and thigh during embryologic development and is connected at that time with the deep venous system. With later development, the lesser saphenous vein disappears above the knee, and it appears that the lateral subdermal venous complex of Albanese represents a vestigial remnant of this early developmental connection between the high developing lesser saphenous vein and the deep venous system. A summary of communication points or possible sources of reflux for reticular veins is presented in Table 1.

TABLE 8-1. REFLUX CONSIDERATIONS IN THE TREATMENT OF RETICULAR VEINS

1. Direct communication with high-pressure reflux from incompetent main truncal varicosities (long or short saphenous vein)
2. Communication with incompetent perforating veins
3. Association with arborizing foci of telangiectasia

Another point of importance when treating reticular veins is that, for some unknown reason, vein walls in this subset of vessels tend to be more fragile, so that injection technique (see below) becomes of paramount importance.

Examination

Several methods can be used to determine the presence, source, and intensity of reflux in reticular veins.

Physical Examination

A complete examination of the treatment site looking and palpating for reticular veins and their associated interconnections to feeding truncal and perforating varicosities as well as feeder sites or "telangiectatic flares" is the first step in establishing the sclerotherapist's treatment plan. The patient is initially examined in a standing position and subsequently placed supine to ensure that all incompetent reticular veins are clearly visualized. Vein marking is recommended once reticular veins are visualized; however, if a vein is not visible in the supine state, it may then be marked with the patient standing (Fig. 8-1). Finally, venoscopy is carried out on the limb in order to look for possibly hidden reticular veins, not visible to the human eye, that may be sites of occult hidden reflux. Veins such as those previ-

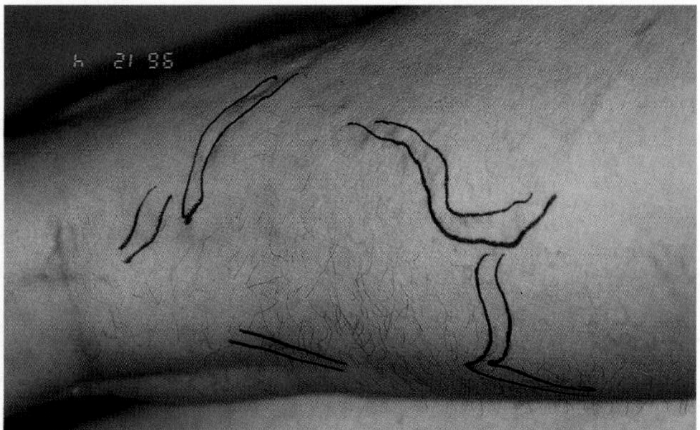

Figure 8-1
Marking of a reticular vein with the patient in standing position; this site was not visible in the recumbent state.

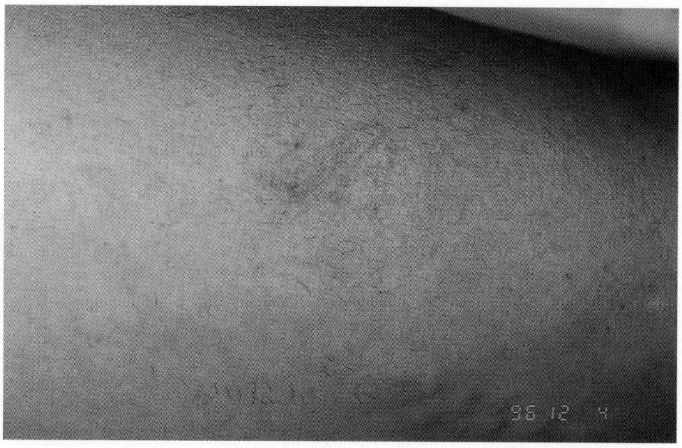

Figure 8-2
The lateral subdermal venous system of Albanese is noted, with reticular veins and overlying telangiectasia and feeding reference point at the distal lateral femoral condyle.

ously described, not visible in a supine position, may be picked up by this diagnostic maneuver.

Continuous-Wave Doppler

This will help to determine reflux in suspicious reticular veins as well as to determine the site of loudest reflux, which often corresponds to the site of an incompetent perforating vein.

As related to the lateral subdermal complex of Albanese, this site is most commonly noted immediately distal to the lateral femoral condyle, which would be the appropriate site for initial treatment of this unique drainage system (Fig. 8-2).

The examination is performed by repeatedly compressing the calf or veins distal to the Doppler probe, with the patient standing. In this fashion, reflux is easily heard at the site of an incompetent reticular vein (Fig. 8-3).

Duplex Ultrasound

Ultrasonography, although providing the most accurate anatomic localization as well as hemodynamic information concerning the reticular venous complex, in

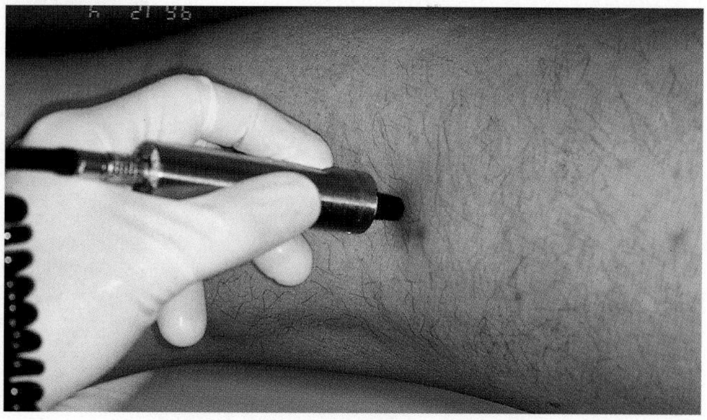

Figure 8-3
Localization of reflux in the reticular vein of the thigh by means of a distal compression maneuver employing the continuous-wave Doppler apparatus.

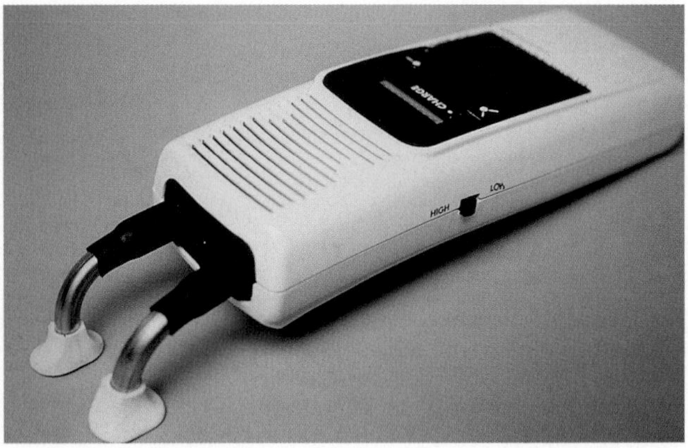

Figure 8-4

The venoscope operates on the principle of infrared transillumination. It is helpful in delineating subcutaneous veins such as reticular veins, which are not visible to the naked eye.

practicality is often necessary only when reflux sources cannot be adequately evaluated by physical examination and continuous-wave Doppler techniques. This set of circumstances is rare but may arise in situations where treatment failure or unexpectedly frequent recurrences manifest themselves.

Venoscopy

The venoscope (Applied Products, Biotech Inc., Lafayette, LA, U.S.A.) (Fig. 8-4) is a transilluminator with a dual encapsulated krypton lamp spotlight that is helpful in transilluminating abnormally dilated subcutaneous veins such as reticular veins, which may not be visible to the naked eye. It is particularly helpful in looking for possible points of reflux in association with cutaneous flares of telangiectasia, which may not be obvious upon routine examination (Fig. 8-5). The examination is conducted in a dark room so that transillumination may be adequately assessed.

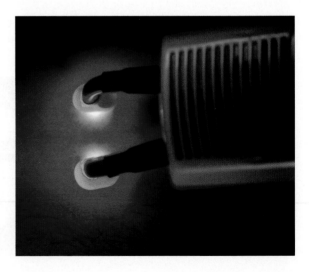

Figure 8-5

Utilization of the venoscope in order to isolate reticular veins associated with telangiectatic flares that are not obvious to the naked eye is performed in a "dark setting."

TABLE 8-2. SCLEROSANT CONCENTRATIONS FOR TREATING RETICULAR VEINS

Sodium tetradecyl sulfate[a]	0.3%–0.6%
Hypertonic saline[a,b]	23.4%
Polidocanol[c]	0.75%–1.5%
Polyiodide iodine	2%–3%

[a] FDA-approved.
[b] FDA-approved for nonsclerotherapy indications.
[c] non–FDA-approved.

Appropriate Sclerosant Concentrations for Treating Reticular Veins

Because of the previously described fragility of the reticular veins and, consequently, the inherently increased probability for sclerosant extravasation—leading to an increased risk of both hyperpigmentation and ulceration—the sclerotherapist should again choose the lowest concentration of sclerosant that will produce effective endosclerosis while minimizing inflammation and vascular spasm.

Suggested choices of sclerosants with concentrations appropriate for the injection of reticular veins are presented in Table 8-2.

Technique Modifications

After the vein has been completely emptied, the puncture feel or blood aspiration techniques (see Chapter 7) are the technique modifications that the author has found most helpful in treating reticular veins (Fig. 8-6).

As in the treatment of all types of varicose veins, the treatment should proceed in an orderly fashion. The following sequence is recommended in treatment of reticular veins:

1. Treatment proceeds from proximal to distal.
2. Areas of proximal reflux are to be treated first.

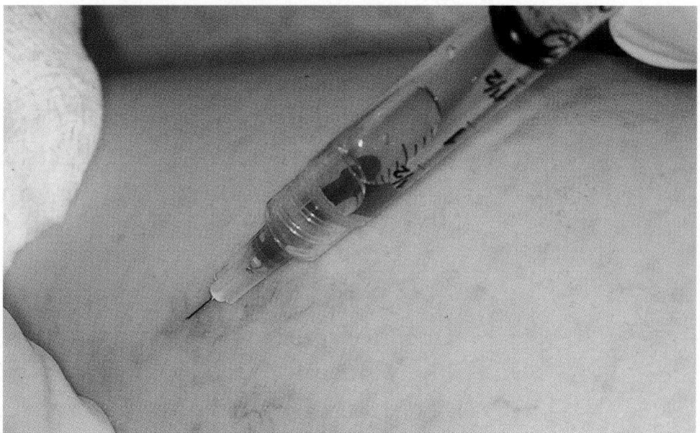

Figure 8-6
Blood aspiration technique of injecting reticular veins.

3. Larger-caliber veins are treated before smaller-caliber veins.
4. An entire reticular vein is treated at a given treatment session.
5. The author begins injections at the proximal posterior thigh with the patient lying prone.
6. Injections proceed distally towards the ankle.
7. The patient is then placed in a lateral position, where again injections are carried out in a proximal-to-distal sequence.

This systematic approach minimizes the chance of producing "skip zones" in treating desired vessel sites and assures maximal vessel obliteration.

Adequate side lighting and utilization of the Doppler to identify feeding reflux points are of paramount importance in achieving successful results in the treatment of reticular veins.

As previously stated, the venoscope may also be useful in identifying difficult-to-visualize reticular vein sites feeding clusters of telangiectasia.

Treatment Techniques

There are two basic modifications of techniques that may be employed in treating reticular veins.

Classic Supine Technique

1. The majority of reticular veins are treated in this fashion, with the patient lying in a supine position. The desired treatment vein is emptied by hand massage.
2. A 3-mL disposable syringe filled with appropriate sclerosant is connected to a 30-gauge needle (Becton Dickinson, Franklin Lakes, NJ, U.S.A.; Air-Tite of Virginia, Inc., Newport News, VA, U.S.A.).
3. The skin is cleansed with alcohol or a 1:1 mixture of alcohol and acetic acid.
4. The needle is bent to a 30-degree angle with the hub facing the skin surface.
5. Two-finger traction of skin to ensure tautness is accomplished with the opposite hand (Fig. 8-7).
6. The skin is pierced briskly and a second motion is employed to accurately cannulate the veins.
7. If the sclerotherapist is not sure that the vein has been cannulated, a small amount of blood may be aspirated into the hub of the syringe to ensure intravascular status (Fig. 8-8). (Caution: Too much negative pressure should not be employed because this may lead to intravascular spasm and subsequent compromise of results.)
8. Injection is subsequently carried out with a low injection pressure, utilizing not more than 0.5 mL of sclerosant at a given injection site.
9. If resistance is encountered or vascular spasm (vessel blanching) occurs, the needle is withdrawn and cannulation is repeated at a distal site.

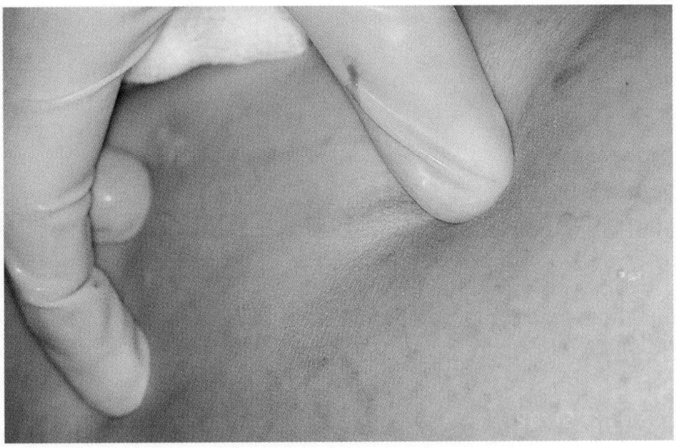

Figure 8-7
Traction on the skin directly over reticular veins with rapid biphasic cannulation of the skin surface and subsequent endothelium is the technique of choice in treating such vessels.

10. Injections are performed at intervals of 3 to 6 cm along the entire treated reticular varicosity.
11. The sclerosant is then spread along the treatment site by gentle hand kneading in order to ensure even distribution and uniform sclerosant-endothelial contact.

Butterfly Cannulation Technique

If large reticular veins are present, techniques similar to those employed in the treatment of large varicose veins may be utilized (Chapter 9).

1. Veins are mapped out, as previously stated, with the patient in a standing or supine position
2. Points of maximum reflux, as determined by physical examination and continuous-wave Doppler, are marked by a skin marker [the author's preference is the Sharpee (Sanford, Bellwood, IL, U.S.A.) or the Pilot Explorer (fine tip, Pilot Pen Corp., Trumbell, CT, U.S.A.)] at 5- to 7-cm intervals along the reticular vein to be treated (Fig. 8-9).
3. The patient is placed supine or sitting with the leg hanging over the

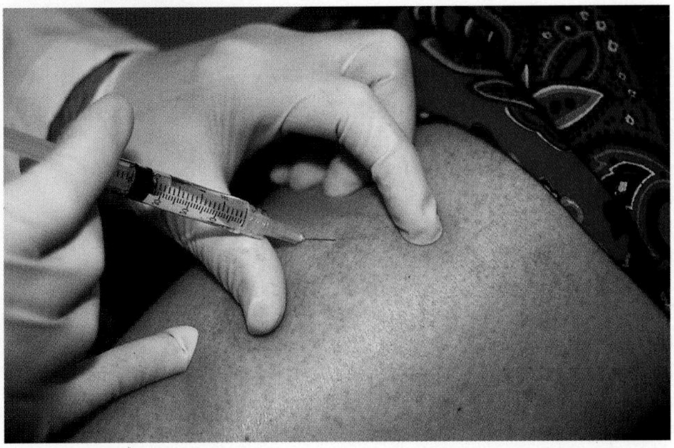

Figure 8-8
For the beginning sclerotherapist treating reticular veins or in any case where the question of the intravenous status of the needle and the sclerosant is in question, aspiration of a small amount of blood into the hub of the syringe will verify that the needle is within the vein.

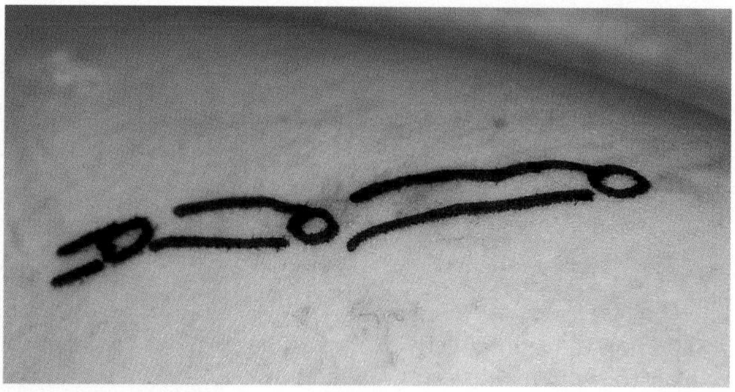

Figure 8-9

Marking of points of reflux at 5- to 7-cm intervals prior to the treatment of a reticular vein is helpful in finding injection sites for larger-diameter reticular veins.

side of the table, or the patient may be standing if the vein is not visible in a supine position.

4. A 25-gauge butterfly needle (Becton Dickinson, Franklin Lakes, NJ, U.S.A.) attached to a 3-mL syringe is used to rapidly cannulate the cutaneous surface and subsequently the endothelium in a rapid biphasic motion, as described in the classic supine technique.
5. Upon vessel puncture, the intravascular position of the needle is confirmed by aspirating blood into the butterfly tubing and then reinjecting in order to prevent the tube from clogging.
6. The needle is then taped into position with paper tape (Fig. 8-10A).
7. The procedure is then repeated along the entire course of the treated reticular vein at 5- to 7-cm intervals.

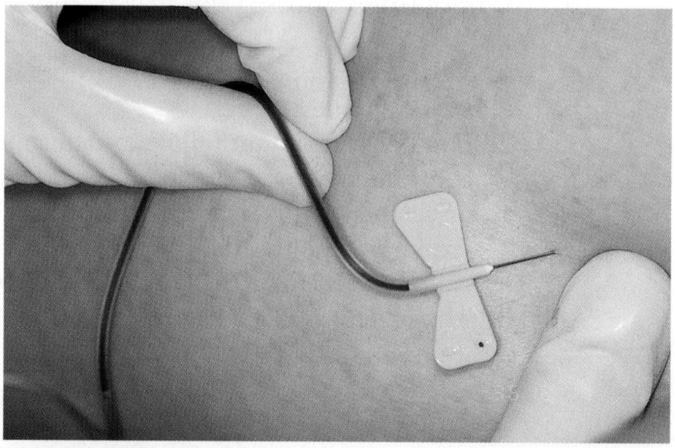

A

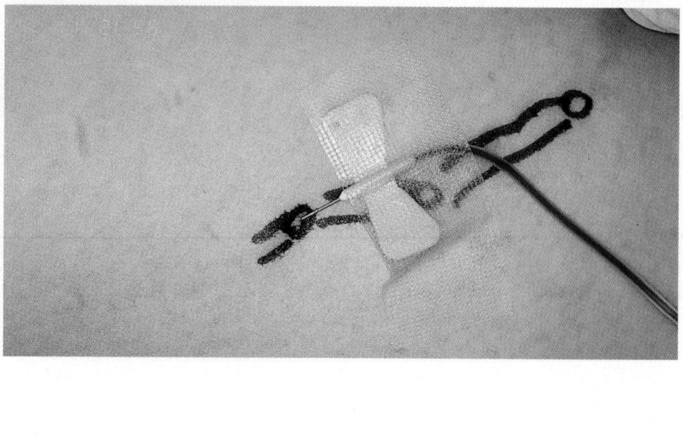

B

Figure 8-10

The butterfly cannulation technique for the treatment of large reticular veins. A 25-gauge butterfly is inserted into the reticular vein with the leg dependent, and intravascular position is confirmed by blood aspiration into the hub of the syringe. The needle is taped in place **(A)** and the leg is elevated to empty the vein before injecting 0.5 mL of sclerosant at each injection site (5- to 7-cm intervals) **(B)**.

8. The patient is then placed supine with the leg elevated 30 degrees to ensure emptying of blood from the vein. This allows improved contact of the sclerosant with the vein wall and prevents dilution of the sclerosant.
9. The position of the needle in the vein lumen is again confirmed by aspirating blood into the tubing.
10. Then 0.5 mL of sclerosant is injected at each site (Fig. 8-10B).
11. The sclerosant is then gently kneaded into the surrounding vein segment to ensure uniform distribution.

This injection technique for large reticular veins is similar to that utilized in treating large varicosities (Chapter 9).

Regardless of technique, reticular veins undergo spasm immediately after treatment. Inflammation may be noted. If associated telangiectasia blanch or become erythematous during treatment of reticular veins, this points to passage of sclerosant into these vessels and indicates that no further treatment is indicated at this time. If these vessels do not disappear in the expected time, they can be reinjected at a later date. If injection is carried out and these veins are already inflamed secondary to filling via treatment of associated reticular veins, this will lead to an increased incidence of postsclerotherapy pigment dyschromia and ulceration.

Posttreatment Compression of Reticular Veins

Local compression is immediately applied to treatment sites, utilizing cotton balls or gauze pads and hypoallergenic elastic tape (Fig. 8-11). Large, protuberant reticular veins or those that are located in the posterior aspect of the thigh or popliteal fossa may also benefit from $\frac{1}{2}$-inch gauze pads (STD-E pads) (Hereford, England). These are cut to the length of the treated vein and beveled, so that the center has the highest diameter.

Several sclerotherapists apply Dermafit, a cotton stockinette available in several diameters, over the entire treated extremity.

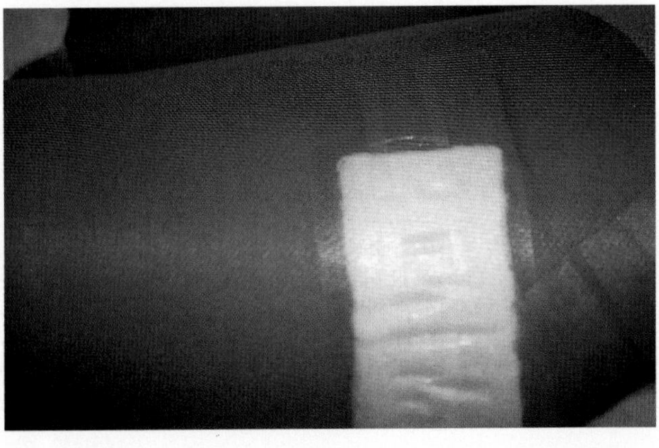

Figure 8-11

Local spot compression, utilizing gauze pads, of the treated bulging reticular varicosity is commonly employed.

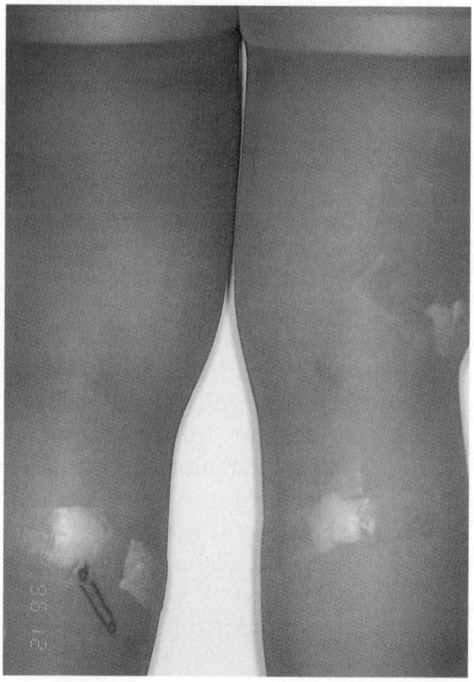

Figure 8-12

A class II graduated compression stocking is placed while the patient is on the treatment table following treatment of a reticular varicosity. This is recommended to ensure effective endosclerosis.

In the treatment of intermediate and larger veins, compression is a mainstay of therapy. Class II (30 to 40 mm Hg) graduated compression stockings are strongly encouraged in the setting of treatment of reticular and large-diameter veins (Fig. 8-12).

All compression devices should be applied while the patient is still on the treatment table, prior to leaving the sclerotherapist's office. Again, because of the fragility factor in treating reticular veins, this is of paramount importance in order to minimize the postsclerotherapy increase in bruising, pigmentation, and potential reticular vein fragility-related ulceration. Adequate compression is also helpful in minimizing postinjection pain.

The major question, again, is how long the optimal compression period should be. Based upon the author's recently published studies, a period of 3 weeks of compression is recommended (*Dermatology Surgery*, 1999).

The author has his patients adhere to the following postsclerotherapy guidelines (Table 8-3).

TABLE 8-3. COMPRESSION CONSIDERATIONS IN THE TREATMENT OF RETICULAR VARICOSE VEINS

1. Removal of local spot-compression pads the morning after the sclerotherapy procedure.
2. Class II (30–40 mm Hg) compression stockings worn continuously for a period of 21 days.
3. If patient is intolerant of this regimen, compression stockings may be removed nightly starting with the second night; however, they are worn during the day for a period of 21 days.

Repeat Treatment Sessions

Treatment sessions as for telangiectasia should be spaced at 4- to 6-week intervals for a given vessel to ensure that maximum endosclerosis has occurred and in order to properly assess the results of the preceding treatment session. If expected results do not occur after 1 or 2 treatments, hidden sources of reflux, such as occult perforators feeding involved reticular veins, should be sought.

If no source of hidden reflux can be found by continuous-wave Doppler evaluation, one may try a slightly increased concentration of the previously employed sclerosant or, alternatively, a different sclerosant agent may be tried.

If no obvious source of treatment failure can be isolated by these maneuvers, then duplex ultrasound examination should be carried out in order to assure that an atypical anatomic source of reflux not confirmed by the above, simpler measures has not been missed.

Pitfalls in the Treatment of Reticular Veins

Vein Depth

This may be the most difficult aspect of the treatment of reticular veins. It is often difficult to determine the depth of these vessels, and misjudgments may lead to inadvertent vessel transection. Utilization of the blood-aspiration technique, as previously described, and the proper utilization of venoscopy may help to bypass this difficulty.

Vein Fragility

As stated previously, reticular veins have fragile walls; this often leads to sclerosant diapedesis, with an increased propensity for postsclerotherapy hyperpigmentation, bruising, and extravasation necrosis.

This consideration may be alleviated somewhat by employing minimal sclerosant concentrations and low injection pressures.

Determining the Appropriate Treatment Sequence of Reticular Veins

Reticular veins feeding clusters of telangiectasia, as stated previously, should be treated first in order to assess the results of treating these feeder vessels. This often decreases the number of treatment sessions and the number of injections necessary to treat a given reticular vein-telangiectatic complex.

In addition, by using a minimal number of injections to treat small-diameter telangiectasias, the sclerotherapist can diminish his or her complication profile in terms of pigmentary dyschromia and ulceration, which are seen more commonly with microsclerotherapy.

Reflux Considerations

Finally, any reticular vein 2 to 5 mm or more in diameter in the vicinity of telangiectatic flares should be considered incompetent. This phenomenon may be substantiated by continuous-wave Doppler examination.

Conclusion

The treatment of reticular veins may be challenging because of previously stated considerations. However, if therapy is approached in an appropriate, systematic fashion, excellent results in terms of functional and symptomatic improvement may be accomplished. In addition, cosmetic satisfaction may be achieved in the appropriate setting. Finally, improved results in the treatment of telangiectasia associated with underlying reticular veins may be noted, with decreased numbers of treatment sessions producing improved long-term results and a low complication profile.

BIBLIOGRAPHY

De Groot WP. Practical phlebology-sclerotherapy of large veins. *J Dermatol Surg Oncol* 1991;17:589–595.

Gallagher PG. Varicose veins—primary treatment with sclerotherapy. *J Dermatol Surg Oncol* 1992;18:39–42.

Goldman MP. Advances in sclerotherapy treatment of varicose and telangiectatic leg veins. *Am J Cosmet Surg* 1992;9:235–240.

Goldman MP. Regional sclerotherapy techniques for leg telangiectasia. *J Dermatol Surg Oncol* 1993;22:933.

Tournay R. How should resistant varicose veins be sclerosed? *Phlebology* 1990;5:151–155.

Weiss RA, Goldman MP. Advances in sclerotherapy. *Dermatol Clin* 1995;13:431–445.

Weiss RA, Sadick NS, Goldman MP, Weiss MA. Post-sclerotherapy compression: controlled comparative study of duration and its effect on clinical outcome. *Dermatol Surg* 1999;25:106–108.

CHAPTER 9

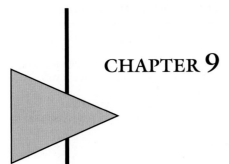

TREATMENT OF VARICOSE VEINS

In North America, the traditional approach to treating large varicose veins and complicated venous pathology has been surgical. However, in the last decade, the concept of compression sclerotherapy has gained increased popularity in the treatment of larger-diameter vessels. Varicose veins are superficial dilated veins that may be troublesome for cosmetic reasons or because they are symptomatic; however, in all settings, they are always the result of increased venous pressure. The sources of the high-pressure reflux that leads to the development of varicosities (either through surgical or sclerotherapy techniques) must be addressed before treatment of associated feeding varicosities can begin. It is with these thoughts in mind that this chapter on the treatment of larger-diameter vessels, including perforating veins and truncal varicosities, has been written. The treatment of axial varicosities (i.e., the greater and lesser saphenous veins and associated saphenofemoral and saphenopopliteal junction incompetence) is addressed in Chapter 10 (Table 9-1).

Diagnostic Approaches

In order to understand the approach to the treatment of large-diameter varicosities, one must go back to the anatomic variations that may present as large-diameter (usually 2- to 10-mm) veins (Table 9-2).

Lower extremity varicosities may be divided into four types.
The first type is the most common.

Type I

The patient presents with varicose veins that are only in the lower leg and receive their reflux from an incompetent saphenofemoral junction in the groin, which may be demonstrated by Doppler examination (Fig. 9-1). The long saphenous

TABLE 9-1. BASIC CONCEPTS IN THE TREATMENT OF LARGE-DIAMETER VARICOSE VEINS

1. The highest point of reflux should be treated first and the entire treatment should proceed from above down.
2. The highest point of reflux is very often the saphenofemoral or saphenopopliteal junction for varicose veins of the long saphenous and short saphenous system respectively.
3. Incompetent perforators are subsequently treated.
4. Sclerotherapy of large-diameter truncal varicosities is subsequently instituted.
5. Sclerotherapy of reticular veins (often associated with arborizing foci of telangiectasis) is carried out.
6. Finally, residual telangiectasia and venulectasia are addressed.

TABLE 9-2. CLASSIFICATION OF LARGE-DIAMETER VARICOSE VEINS

Greater and lesser saphenous veins and associated axial junctions
Truncal/branch varicosities
Perforators

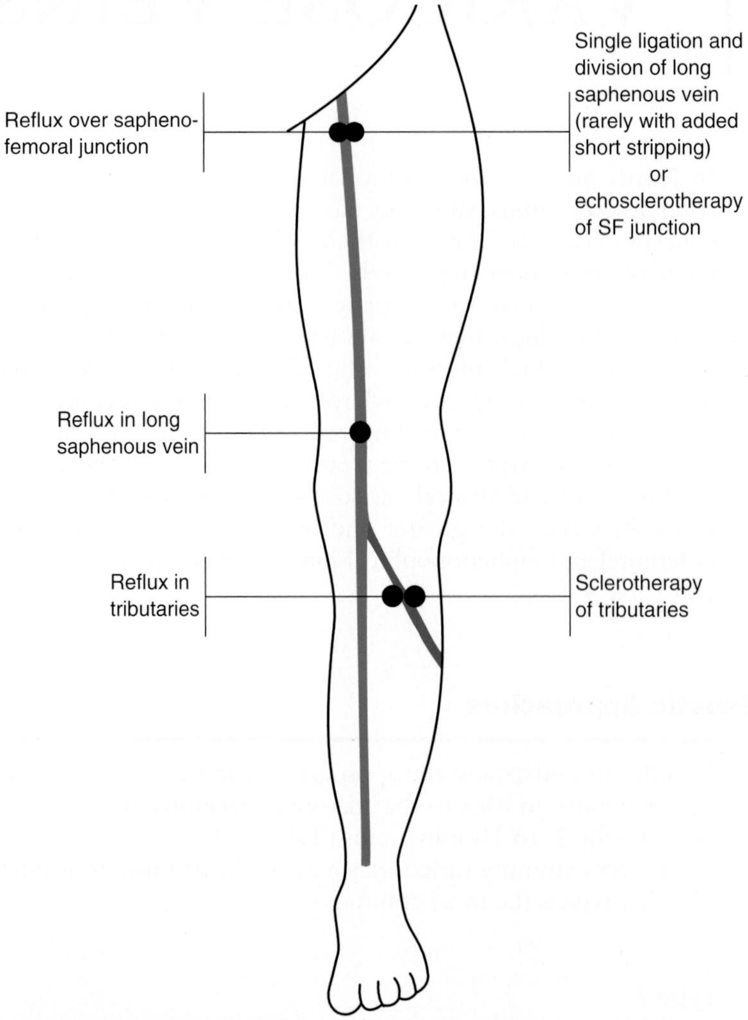

Figure 9-1

Type I varicose veins. Lower leg varicosities associated with reflux from an incompetent saphenofemoral junction in the groin. The saphenous vein may be diseased and subsequently dilated in the thigh.

trunk itself may also be visibly varicose; often, however, the long saphenous vein appears normal and serves as a passive conduit for the reflux originating from the saphenofemoral junction.

The first step in the treatment of this pattern is the abolishment of the reflux by surgical ligation and division of the long saphenous vein (the long saphenous vein is disconnected from the femoral vein at the saphenofemoral junction) with, a short stripping from the groin to the knee of the long saphenous trunk itself if it is degenerated. An alternative approach is continuous-wave Doppler-guided injection of the incompetent saphenofemoral junction. The approach to this type of varicose vein formation is surgical flush ligation of the saphenopopliteal junction or duplex-guided obliteration by sclerotherapy of this reflux site (Chapter 10).

After the surgery or junctional sclerosant obliteration, many varicose veins may partially or completely disappear. Remaining varicosities are treated with sclerotherapy, as described in the present chapter.

Type II

The patient presents with varicose veins localized to the lower leg. They arise from an incompetent short saphenous vein (saphenopopliteal incompetence) and its associated tributaries (Fig. 9-2) (Chapter 10).

Type III

Truncal varicose veins present in the thigh or entire lower limb. This varicose tributary also receives its reflux from an incompetent saphenofemoral junction (Fig. 9-3). However, the varicose tributary, which is usually the anterior saphenous vein or another major tributary, takes off immediately at the junction without a segment of the long saphenous vein transmitting the reflux. Upon clinical and Doppler examination, the long saphenous vein is completely normal and there are minimal distal varicose tributaries (Fig. 9-3).

The treatment approach here is ligation and division of the long saphenous vein or duplex-guided sclerotherapy to obliterate the incompetent junction. Residual varicose veins are subsequently treated by sclerotherapy.

Type IV

This type represents all cases of varicose veins that, on Doppler examination, have no relationship with an incompetent saphenofemoral or saphenopopliteal junction. These varicosities may present at any place on the lower limb. This means that they receive their reflux from incompetent perforators (Fig. 9-4). Treatment consists of sclerotherapy only. One attempts to isolate these perforators by physical examination (fascial gaps), Doppler, and/or duplex ultrasound evaluation and to treat these sources first whenever possible. In most cases, from a selective point of view, sclerotherapy of the varicose vein as it presents itself will often adequately treat associated incompetent perforators.

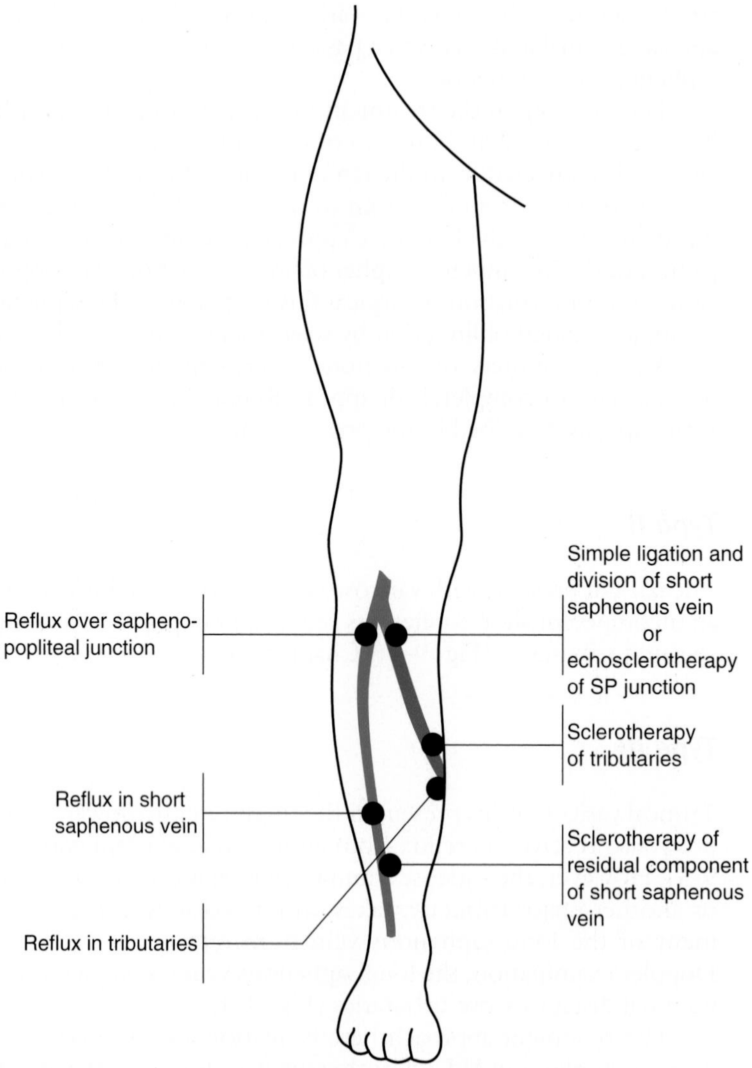

Figure 9-2

Type II varicose veins. Lower leg varicosities associated with incompetence at the saphenopopliteal junction.

Pretreatment Evaluation

With the utilization of proper technique and careful pretreatment evaluation, sclerotherapy is an effective treatment modality for eradicating large-diameter varicose veins. However, treatment of these larger-diameter vessels requires greater and more precise attention to detail concerning anatomic and reflux considerations. These factors will minimize the risk of posttreatment recurrences and complications, which are of greater concern in dealing with larger-diameter vessels. Factors of importance in the treatment of large-diameter varicose veins are as follows:

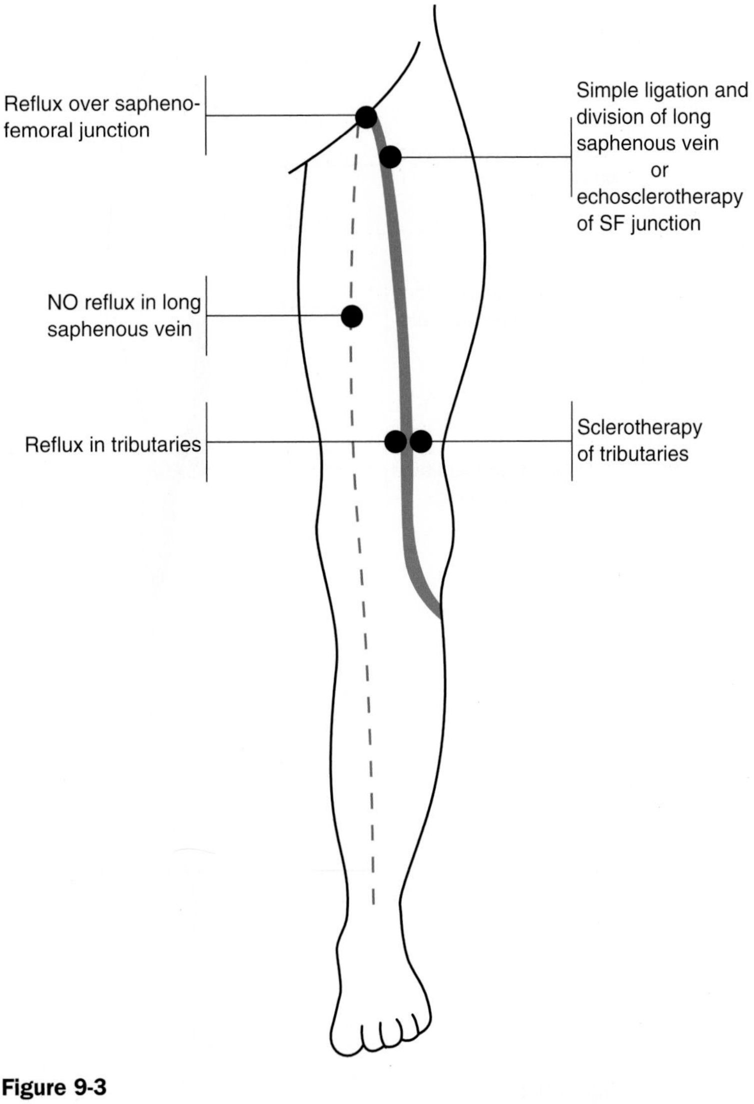

Figure 9-3

Type III varicose veins. Anterior saphenous vein tributary in the thigh associated with an incompetent saphenofemoral junction but normal greater saphenous vein.

1. *An understanding of the precise anatomy of the varicosity under treatment consideration.* Even when performed by an experienced sclerotherapist, clinical examination cannot always elucidate intricate relationships among anatomic vessels and degrees of incompetence. Anatomic variations are particularly important when treating vessels in relation to the axial junctions (saphenofemoral, saphenopopliteal) or feeding perforating veins. Bidirectional Doppler ultrasound and plethysmography are also limited in making these precise determinations. In this setting duplex ultrasonography is an important tool for visualizing vessel morphology and anatomic irregularities, particularly the origin of complex varicose veins, and clari-

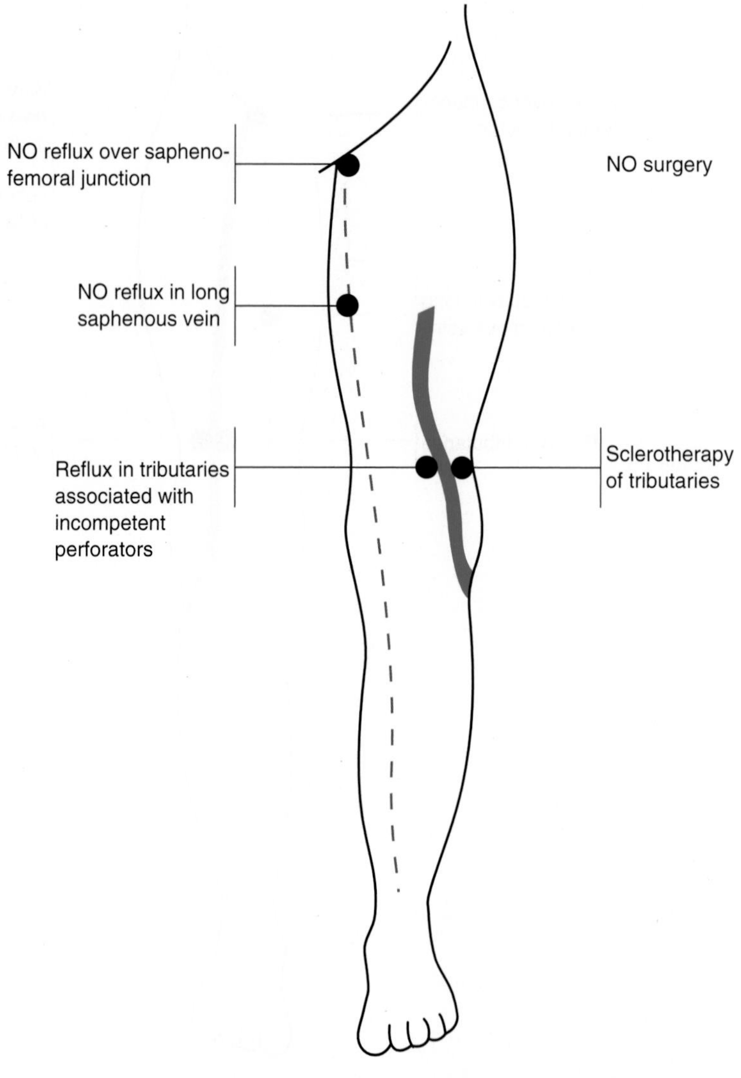

Figure 9-4

Type IV varicose veins. Varicose veins that present as sources of secondary reflux in association with incompetent perforators.

fying the relationship between the target treatment veins and nearby structures.

2. *Adherence to a rational treatment plan of beginning injections at the highest point of reflux and progressing to the next highest point in a proximal-to-distal direction.* Only by assuring that proximal points of reflux have been addressed can the sclerotherapist hope to achieve satisfactory results in obliterating large-diameter veins. After precisely locating the highest point of incompetence, the physician should verify the target vein's relationship to surrounding structures, particularly arteries, as accidental injection of these vessels can lead to serious complications. Finally, in

large-vein sclerotherapy, injection should be as close as possible to the point of incompetence.

3. *Determination of the point of reflux in the deep venous system.* In 91% of cases, the greater saphenous vein (GSV) terminates in the common femoral vein (CFV). In 9% of cases, the GSV and its upper tributaries share a common termination in the CFV.

   The short saphenous vein (SSV) shows even more anatomic variation. It may terminate in the popliteal fossa in approximately 65% of cases. Alternatively, it may empty into the gastrocnemius vein (12%), the superficial femoral vein (7%), the deep femoral vein (3%), or other variations of venous termination (10%). It may also terminate in multiple veins (4%). These reflux patterns may be determined by duplex ultrasound evaluation.
4. *Diameter of the treatment vein determined by duplex ultrasonography.* In general it is easier to sclerose a large thin-walled vein than a minimally dilated thick-walled vein.
5. *Venous compressibility.* The more compressible the vein, the easier it will be to sclerose. Veins with extensive wall damage and minimal reflux are easiest to sclerose.
6. *Valvular leaflet competency.* By means of duplex ultrasound, valve leaflets may be assessed with respect to mobility and coaptation capabilities. Frozen or immobile valves are commonly the result of posttraumatic or postphlebitic syndromes.
7. *Degree of reflux.* Both the extent and degree of reflux in a large vein may be adequately visualized by duplex scanning. Distal compression or Valsalva maneuvers may be employed. Vessels with greater degrees of reflux are more difficult to eradicate and are associated with an increased recurrence rate.

As can be seen from the preceding discussion, Duplex ultrasound graphic guidance is of help in treating larger-diameter vessels, particularly those cases where the anatomy is so intricate that the points of reflux would otherwise by inaccessible.

However, in most cases that are not complex, Doppler evaluation and careful physical examination are sufficient to deal with the majority of large-vein problems encountered in a sclerotherapy practice.

There are also several problems that are of greater importance in performing large-vein sclerotherapy with either the compression or duplex-guided techniques. These are listed in Table 9-3 and are discussed in greater detail in this chapter.

TABLE 9-3. PROBLEMS INHERENT IN LARGE-VEIN SCLEROTHERAPY

1. Frequent recurrences
2. Lack of successful results
3. High incidence of thrombophlebitis
4. Increased incidence of hematoma
5. Pulmonary embolus

Techniques of Large-vein Sclerotherapy

Patient Position

Marking of veins to be treated is normally carried out with the patient in a standing position. Subsequently, injection is usually carried out in a supine position. Standing injection leads to instillation of sclerosant against the hydrostatic forces associated with gravitational blood flow. Theoretically, this could lead to uneven distribution of sclerosant, increased vessel inflammation and subsequently increased risk of thrombophlebitis. Secondly, standing instillation of sclerosant may lead to retrograde flow of sclerosant through perforators, causing inadvertent damage to the deep venous system. Finally, the risk of vasovagal reaction and subsequent injury is increased when injections are carried out with the patient standing. For these reasons, large-vein sclerotherapy is normally carried out with the patient supine.

Four basic techniques are employed for the treatment of large varicose veins:

1. *Fegan technique—dependent cannulation.* This is the major technique with minor variations; it is employed by most sclerotherapists today (Fig. 9-5). With the patient standing or sitting at the end of the examination table, the varicose vein is cannulated with a needle or butterfly angiocath. Tape may be applied to keep the needle in a steady position. The leg is then elevated for 1 to 2 minutes by either the physician or an assistant in order to ensure maximal vessel emptying. Before injection, a small amount of blood is aspirated in order to make sure that the needle remains correctly positioned. Injection is subsequently carried out utilizing 0.5 to 1.0 mL of sclerosant, followed by finger kneading 2 to 3 cm above and below the site of injection for 30 to 60 seconds in order to localize sclerosant action and ensure maximal endothelial-sclerosant contact. This is followed by immediate application of a beveled compression foam pad secured by elastic tape or an inelastic wraparound bandage such as Medi-Rip (Conco, Rockhill, SC, U.S.A.).

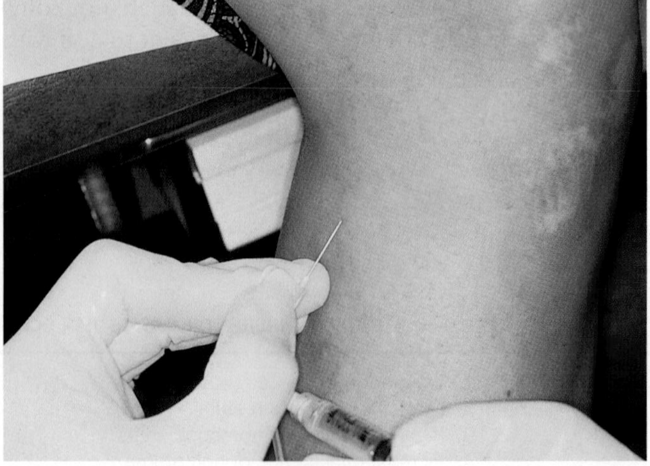

Figure 9-5

Fegan technique. Injection is carried out in a supine position following dependent cannulation.

A

B

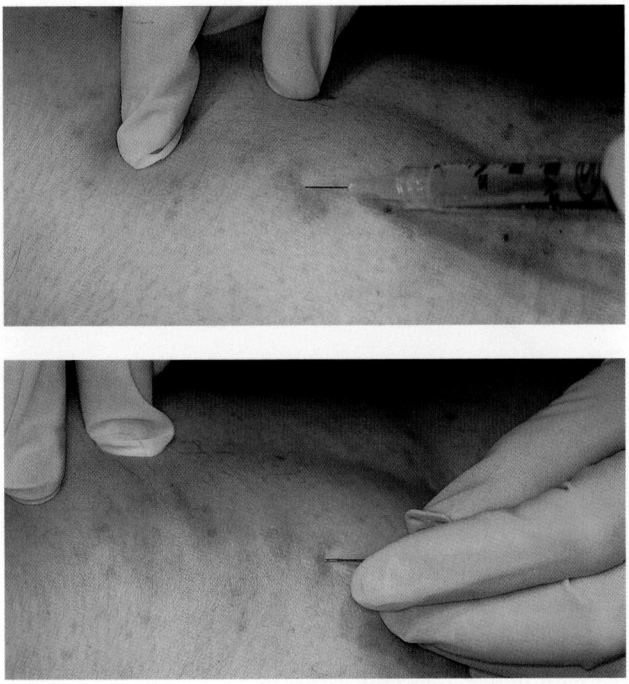

Figure 9-6

Fegan variant. Needle insertion is carried out in the recumbent or reverse Trendelenburg position utilizing a 30-gauge needle (A) or 25-gauge angiocath (B).

2. *Fegan variant—needle insertion with the patient in the recumbent or reverse Trendelenburg position (Fig. 9-6).* This is also a commonly employed technique. As in the traditional technique, the varicosity is marked with the patient in the standing position. However, needle insertion occurs with the patient lying supine or in a slight reverse Trendelenburg position. This variant in technique is more rapid and efficient to perform and minimizes movement of the leg while the needle is being inserted. After injection, the leg can be elevated and direct compression applied. However, the author feels that presclerotherapy elevation of the limb to be treated is of great importance in order to empty it of blood and thus improve the physical aspects of sclerosant-endothelial interaction. For this reason the more conventional Fegan technique is preferred by the author.
3. *Hobbs technique—multiple punctures (Fig. 9-7).* Multiple puncture sites are placed at 4- to 6-cm intervals along the entire treated varicosity. Intravascular spasm, a negative aspect of this technique, may be minimized by multiple cannulations before injection is actually carried out.

   The author has found this technique to be associated with frequent vascular spasm and lower rates of treatment success.
4. Sigg technique—open needle cannulation with the needle attached to the syringe (Fig. 9-8).

   A needle is inserted into the treated vessel and positioned until blood return occurs.

   Optionally, blood may be withdrawn until the vessel is emptied.

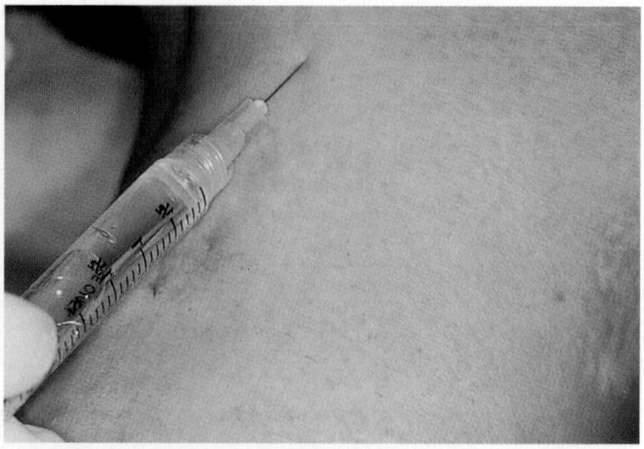

Figure 9-7

Hobb technique. Multiple punctures are performed at 4- to 6-cm intervals, doing the entire treated varicosity.

The author has found the latter step to be associated with an increased incidence of vascular spasm and less satisfactory results as well.

Regardless of technique employed, the important factors to be kept in mind in treating large varicose veins include:

- Marking of the treated vein in a dependent position
- Emptying blood from the vessel prior to treatment
- Ensuring intravascular location of the needle prior to injection
- Kneading of sclerosant around the injection site immediately postcannulation to ensure even distribution of sclerosant and maximal endothelial-sclerosant contact
- Proximal-to-distal treatment approach
- Treatment of an entire varicosity at a given treatment session
- Immediate and adequate postsclerotherapy compression

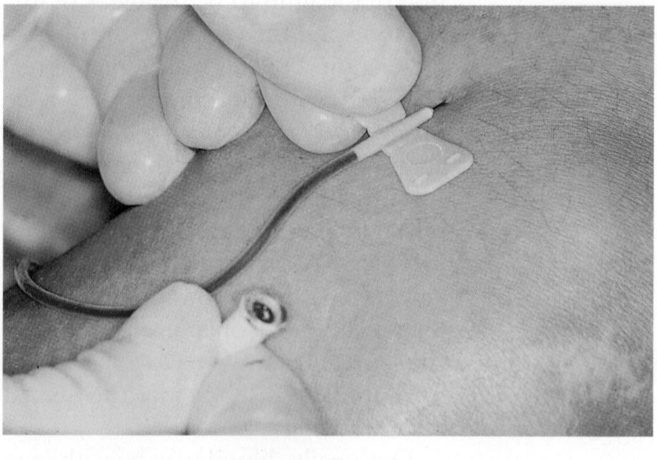

Figure 9-8

Open-needle Sigg technique. Cannulation is carried out with the needle attached to a syringe. It is positioned in the treated vessel until the sclerotherapist notes blood return and the subsequent instillation of sclerosant is carried out.

Treatment Protocols—Compression Sclerotherapy

For the treatment of truncal (long and short saphenous) or nontruncal (non-saphenous) varicose veins, the following technique is used:

1. The patient stands for a few minutes in order to allow the veins to fill.
2. All visible and palpable vein segments in areas to be injected are marked by an indelible marker such as the Sharpee fine point (Fig. 9-9A).
3. The patient is then placed on the treatment table in a comfortable sitting position with the legs flat and the back elevated 30 degrees.
   a. Anterior veins are injected in the aforementioned position.
   b. Lateral veins are injected in a slightly rotated position.
   c. Posterior veins are injected in a prone position.
4. The patient's leg is then elevated to empty it of residual blood for 1 to 2 minutes (Fig. 9-9B).
5. Sclerosant is injected. This is done with the patient in a supine position, employing the multiple puncture technique.

   A 3-mL syringe (Becton Dickinson, Franklin Lakes, NJ, U.S.A.) (Fig. 9-9C) ⅝ inch long with attached 30-gauge needle or 23-gauge angiocath (Figure 9-9D) (Becton Dickinson, Franklin Lakes, NJ, U.S.A.) is used for injection.

   Sotradecol (STS) is the primary sclerosant employed by the author for the treatment of large varicose veins. The dose of STS depends on the site of the veins. Initial recommended dosages for treatment of vessels of various sizes are presented in Table 9-4. A maximal volume of 10 mL of sclerosant is employed for a given treatment session.

   Cannulation sites for leg injection are spaced 5 to 7 cm apart along the course of the treated vessel in order to permit adequate perfusion of sclerosant along the length of the treated vein.

   Blood is always withdrawn before an injection is made in order to ascertain that the tip of the needle is inside the vein. *If no blood can be withdrawn, no injection is made.*

   The injection pressure is gentle in order to prevent extravasation or potential neoangiogenic matting.

6. The sclerosant is immediately massaged distally into the surrounding treatment area for a distance of 5 to 10 cm (Fig. 9-9E).
7. Large cotton ball or beveled foam rubber compression pads such as STD pads (STD Pharmaceutical, Hereford, England) are applied immediately at each injection site. Bulging areas of varicose dilatation are then wrapped with either Elastoplast (Beiersdorf, Norwalk, CT, U.S.A.) or Medi-Rip (Conco, Rockhill, SC, U.S.A.).

A midthigh graduated compression stocking class II (30- to 40-mm Hg compression) is applied and worn for a period of 48 to 72 hours day and night and then for 3 weeks hence during waking hours.

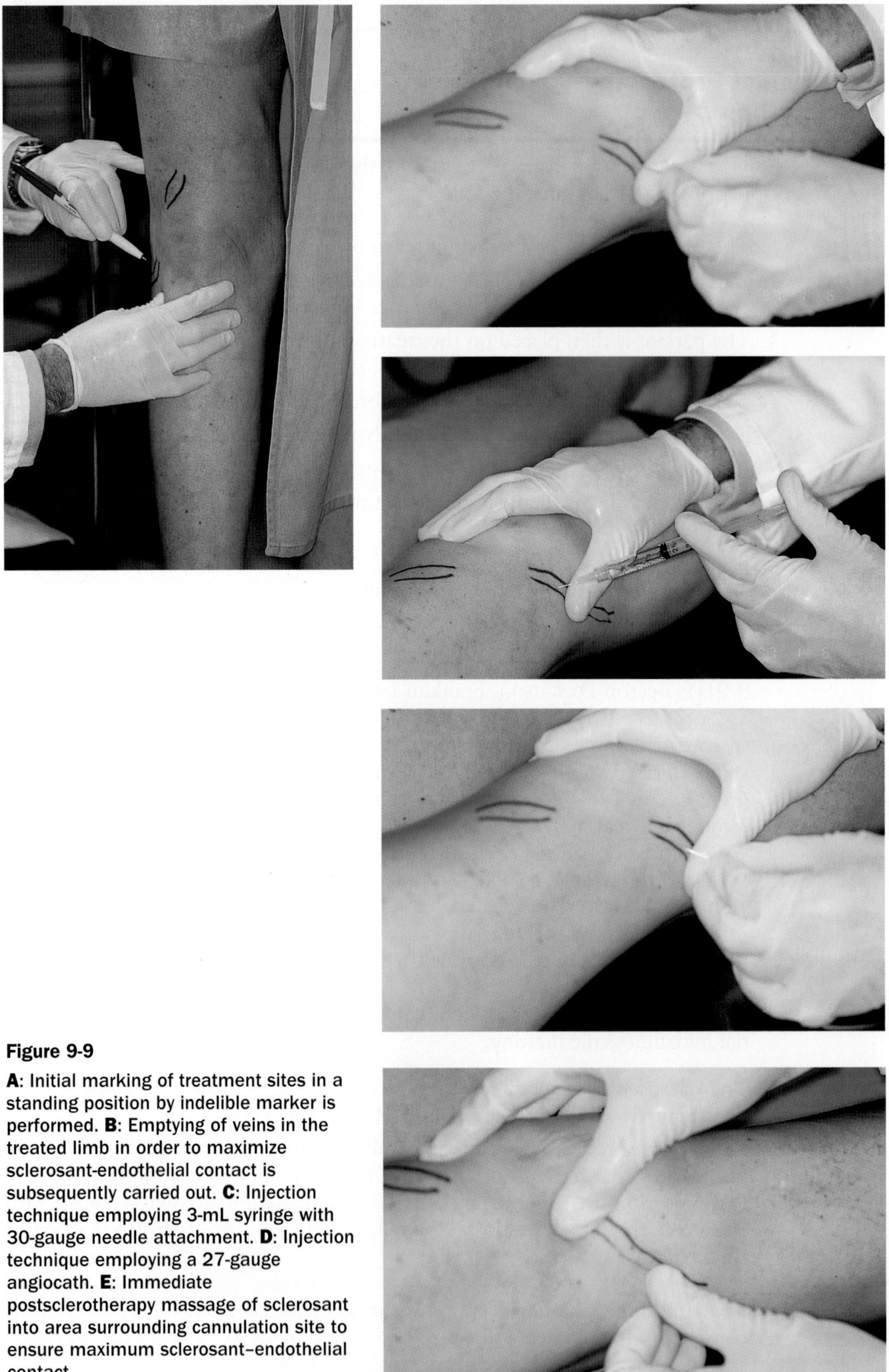

A B C D E

Figure 9-9

A: Initial marking of treatment sites in a standing position by indelible marker is performed. **B**: Emptying of veins in the treated limb in order to maximize sclerosant-endothelial contact is subsequently carried out. **C**: Injection technique employing 3-mL syringe with 30-gauge needle attachment. **D**: Injection technique employing a 27-gauge angiocath. **E**: Immediate postsclerotherapy massage of sclerosant into area surrounding cannulation site to ensure maximum sclerosant–endothelial contact.

TABLE 9-4. INITIAL CONCENTRATION AND VOLUME OF SOTRADECHOL EMPLOYED FOR TRUNCAL (LONG AND SHORT SAPHENOUS) OR NONTRUNCAL (NONSAPHENOUS) VARICOSE VEINS

Vein Size	Saphenous	Nonsaphenous
10 mm	1.0 mL 3%	0.5 mL 3%
8 mm	1.0 mL 2%	0.5 mL 2%
6 mm	1.0 mL 1%	0.5 mL 1%
5 mm	0.8 mL 0.5%	0.4 mL 0.5%
4 mm	0.8 mL 0.3%	0.4 mL 0.3%
3 mm	0.3 mL 0.2%	0.25 mL 0.2%
2 mm	0.3 mL 0.1%	0.25 mL 0.1%

8. Patients are encouraged to ambulate actively immediately after treatment (high-impact exercise is discouraged for a period of 3 days after each treatment session).
9. Patient follow-up. Patients are usually seen for follow-up in 1 to 2 weeks

   One of the following five outcomes may be noted by the sclerotherapist:

   a. The vein disappears completely. A scarring action was effected by successful endosclerosis.
   b. The vein disappears partially. The injection worked, but further injections are needed with the same concentration or a slightly stronger one.
   c. The vein remains exactly as it was before the injection. This means that the patient's vein requires a stronger concentration of sclerosant. If there has been no response to the initial injection session, the concentration of sclerosant is increased by 25% to 50% (i.e., STS 0.05% to 0.1% increments). The patient is then seen at 2- to 4-week intervals. The concentration of sclerosant is increased by 25% to 50% at each injection session until the threshold concentration is achieved to close the treatment vein under consideration.

      Once the minimal sclerosant concentration (MSC) has achieved a successful sclerotherapeutic response, the concentration usually remains constant for the treatment of similar sized vessels.
   d. A cordlike firm structure is palpated. This indicates that the vein has scarred down as desired but the scar has not yet dissolved, as it will within a few weeks.
   e. The vein swells; it is tender, lumpy, and hyperpigmented. The vein looks worse than before treatment. This is usually due to an intravascular hematoma, which may be evacuated employing an 11-inch Bard Parker blade (Becton Dickinson, Franklin Lakes, NJ, U.S.A.).

Most truncal and branch varicosities can be treated with STS concentrations between 0.25% and 1.0%, provided that preexisting junctional and perforator insufficiency has been addressed.

Utilizing this protocol and employing MSCs for treating truncal and branch varicosities will produce optimal results that minimize postsclerotherapy complications.

How much can maximally be injected safely during one treatment session? French sources state that 3 mL of 5% STS is the maximum dose per session. However, there are no adequate scientific studies to substantiate these claims.

However, as 3% STS is the highest concentration available in the United States, this translates into 5 mL of 3% solution. Therefore, the concentrations, dosage, and number of injections recommended above by the author are well within this safety zone.

Treatment of Perforator Veins

Perforating veins are marked with the patient in the standing position.

1. They are identified by palpation as fascial gaps that manifest as soft, compressible foci or by Doppler examination and are marked as such with an indelible pen (Fig. 9-10).
2. These perforators and their associated anatomic connections may be further substantiated by Doppler and/or duplex ultrasound.

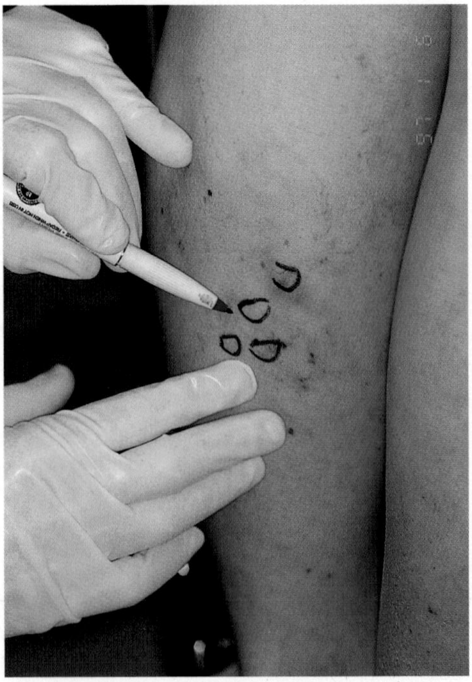

Figure 9-10

Marking of perforator vein and feeding surface varicosity with indelible marker is carried out in a vertical position. The perforator has been assessed as a localized fascial defect by physical examination and subsequently confirmed by Doppler evaluation.

3. Techniques for injection are similar to those presented in the previous section. Suggested initial concentrations of STS for the treatment of perforator veins of the lower extremity are as follows:

Vein Size	Concentration of STS
4–6 mm	0.5%
6–8 mm	0.75%
7–8 mm	1.0%

4. If varicosities are present on the skin surface in anatomic proximity to feeding perforator veins, these are treated at the same treatment session.
5. Postsclerotherapy compression and activity considerations are similar to those presented in the previous section on truncal and branch varicosities.

Duplex Ultrasound–guided Injection Technique

Duplex ultrasound is a helpful tool in the treatment of large nonjunctional varicose veins in selected circumstances.

1. Obese patients in whom varicose veins are not easily palpable on physical examination.
2. Perforator veins with a deep location not obvious on physical examination.
3. Complex anatomic structures in which the point of proximal reflux is not obvious by physical examination and/or Doppler evaluation.
4. Cases of treatment failure where a hidden source of reflux may not be obvious by physical examination, photoplesythmography, or Doppler maneuvers.
5. Patients with previous varicose vein surgery in whom administration of a sclerosant might otherwise be difficult.

Duplex ultrasound–guided needles, 18 or 20 gauge, are commercially available (Smart Needle, Advanced Cardiovascular Systems Inc., Temecula, CA, U.S.A.).

Duplex-guided injection is also helpful in:

1. Ascertaining intravenous localization (avoiding intraarterial injection). This is particularly helpful in obese patients and in those whose veins, obvious in a standing position, become inconspicuous in the recumbent state.
2. Assessing treatment responses. Incomplete endosclerosis presents as a partial intravascular thrombosis (multiple echoes) with the vein lumen remaining partially patent. When sclerotherapy has been successful, the vein wall is thickened and noncompressible (nonechogenic).

Technique

Once the extent of venous disease and source of reflux has been isolated, duplex ultrasound (echography) is carried out to guide the physician to the target vein and monitor the injection. It is also used to confirm correct needle placement (Fig. 9-11).

The vein is punctured briskly with the patient in the supine position. Echography confirms needle placement, which is double checked by blood aspiration into the hub of the syringe.

If pulsating, bright-red blood appears or if echography does not confirm proper needle positioning, the needle is withdrawn.

If the needle is in correct position, a small amount of sclerosant is slowly injected.

Echography confirms that sclerosant is entering the target vein. If the display shows an arterial flow disturbance or extravasation of fluid into tissues, the needle is immediately withdrawn.

If the patient complains of pain, indicating extravascular or intraarterial injection, the needle is removed. STS does not cause pain upon intraarterial injection and thus is often mixed with a pain-producing sclerosant in performing echosclerotherapy. At this point, blood is reaspirated to reconfirm correct needle positioning and the rest of the dosage is administered in rapid fashion.

Adjuvants to Echographic Guidance

1. Echo-enhanced contrast agents. These agents produce enhanced, clutter-free echographic signals and thus improve therapeutic results. One of the most common products in SHU508, a galactose/palmitic acid–based microbubble preparation.

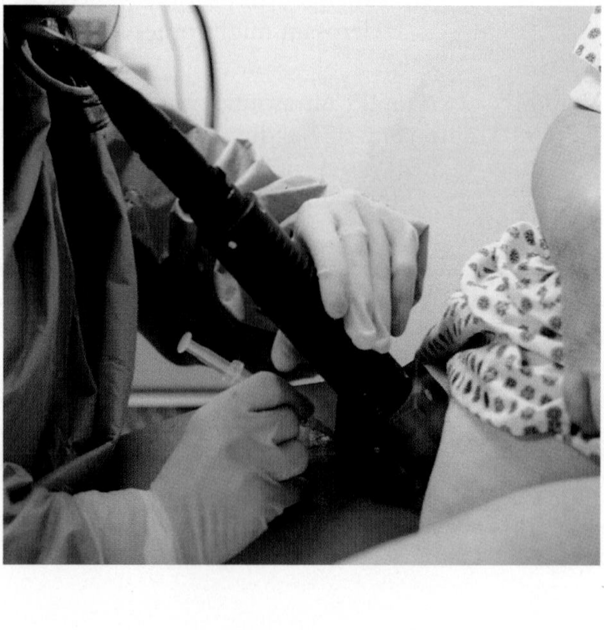

Figure 9-11

Duplex ultrasound-guided injection technique employing an 18-gauge ultrasound-guided needle. (Courtesy of Pauline Raymond-Martimbeau, M.D.)

2. Improved needle visualization techniques. Two new techniques have improved needle visualization:
   - Smart Needle. Visualization is enhanced by a Doppler probe incorporated in the needle's tip, which is used to guide the needle toward the target vein and confirm proper intravascular position.
   - Color Mark System. Needle location is indicated by a colored line generated by piezoelectrically induced flexural waves.

Doppler-guided Sclerotherapy

A hand-held Doppler is an effective tool in large-vein sclerotherapy, particularly when access to duplex ultrasound is not readily available.

Doppler may pick up points of occult reflux and perforator veins not obvious on physical examination. Change in position of varicose veins from a standing to a supine position, which may occur in up to 25% of cases, may also be assessed by this technique. Finally, it may also provide a guide to accurate instillation points for sclerosing solutions.

Utilizing the 8-MHz probe, the point of maximal reflux is assessed and the probe is placed approximately 1 cm distal or proximal to that point (Fig. 9-12).

With an assistant holding the Doppler probe in place, injection may be carried out utilizing the aforementioned techniques.

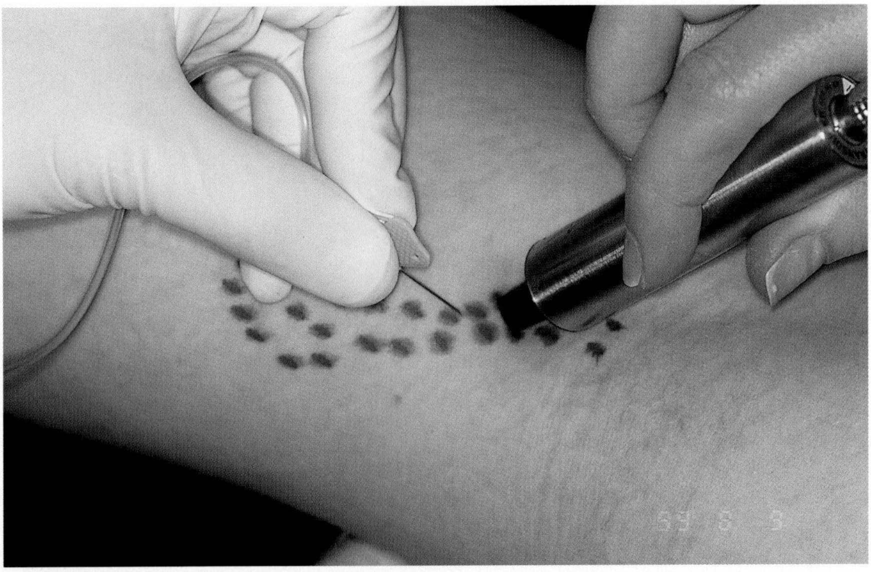

Figure 9-12

Doppler guided sclerotherapy. Doppler-guided injection is carried out 1 cm distal to point of reflux as ascertained by Doppler examination.

Conclusion

Sclerotherapy of large truncal, branch, and perforating varicose veins, although associated with increased risk and morbidity in comparison with treatment of reticular and telangiectatic veins, may produce a gratifying results when careful consideration of anatomic variation, reflux principles, fastidious technique, and adequate compression are adhered to.

Compression sclerotherapy with Doppler- and duplex-guided assistance is well accepted by patients and may provide effective and permanent results.

BIBLIOGRAPHY

Cornu-Thenard A, De Cottreau H, Weiss RA. Sclerotherapy—continuous-wave Doppler-guided injections. *Dermatol Surg* 1995;21:867–870.

DeGroot WP. Practical phlebology—sclerotherapy of large veins. *J Dermatol Surg Oncol* 1991;17:589–595.

Gallagher PG. Varicose veins—primary treatment with sclerotherapy. *J Dermatol Surg Oncol* 1992;18:39–42.

Goldman MP. Advances in sclerotherapy treatment of varicose and telangiectatic leg veins. *Am J Cosmet Surg* 1992;9:235–281.

Goldman MP, Weiss RA, Bergan JJ. Diagnosis and treatment of varicose veins: a review. *J Am Acad Dermatol* 1994;31:393–413.

Marley WM, Marley NF. Sclerotherapy treatment of varicose veins. *Semin Dermatol* 1993;12:98–101.

Raymond-Martimbeau P. Advanced sclerotherapy treatment of varicose veins with duplex ultrasonographic guidance. *Semin Dermatol* 1993;12:123–128.

Thibault PK, Lewis WA. Recurrent varicose veins: Part 2. Injection of incompetent perforating veins using ultrasound guidance. *J Dermatol Surg Oncol* 1992;18:895–900.

CHAPTER 10

TREATMENT OF REFLUX OF THE SAPHENOFEMORAL AND SAPHENOPOPLITEAL JUNCTIONS

All physicians involved in the treatment of varicose vein disease agree that obliteration of axial reflux (i.e., reflux of the saphenofemoral or saphenopopliteal junctions), when present, is the first step in the treatment of lower extremity venous dysfunction; however, the most appropriate approach to this end has remained somewhat controversial. The important issue is whether surgery of saphenofemoral and saphenopopliteal incompetence is superior to injection therapy. Many previous studies have cited recurrence rates of greater than 50% when injection sclerotherapy is employed as a therapeutic intervention in junctional incompetence, compared with 10% to 20% recurrence rates when surgical ligation with or without short ligation procedures are performed. However, experienced phlebologists have claimed successful obliteration of the saphenofemoral and saphenopopliteal junction in 50% to 90% of patients. Both surgeons and phlebologists agree that saphenous varicose veins with diameters of equal to or greater than 10 mm as determined by color-flow duplex ultrasound tend to have inferior cure rates by injection techniques. With injection sclerotherapy, symptoms are commonly improved after treatment; however, long-term follow-up is necessary before adequate judgment concerning results of treatment can be exercised.

Major concerns for treatment of an incompetent saphenofemoral junction (SFJ) and saphenopopliteal junction (SPJ) are listed in Table 10-1. With more re-

TABLE 10-1. MAJOR COMPLICATION CONCERNS IN THE TREATMENT OF INCOMPETENT SAPHENOFEMORAL AND SAPHENOPOPLITEAL JUNCTIONS

1. Deep venous thrombosis
2. Pulmonary embolism
3. Intraarterial injection
4. Damage to the deep venous system (femoral vein, popliteal vein)
5. Treatment failures

cent experience with appropriate sclerosing agents and utilization of proper dosages and minimal sclerosant concentrations (MSCs)—protocols for treating the SFJ and SPJ have become more standardized.

Principles of Injection of the Saphenofemoral and Saphenopopliteal Junctions

Several basic principles are important to adhere to in treating axial vein incompetence with associated junctional reflux:

1. Duplex ultrasound examination should be performed prior to treatment. The exact nature of the anatomy in considered treatment areas should be elucidated. Major points to be considered are the following:
   a. Dilation of the greater saphenous vein equal to or greater than 10 mm may be better approached with surgical intervention.
   b. Is an accessory greater saphenous vein present?
   c. The lesser saphenous vein has a variable anatomy at the SPJ, showing a variable termination in up to 50% of cases.
2. It has become apparent over the last decade that in order to avoid accidental injection into the deep venous or arterial systems, it is preferable to administer a single injection of a major sclerosing agent (iodine solution, sodium tetradecyl sulfate, sodium salicylate) a few centimeters (4 to 5 cm) below rather than at the SFJ (Fig. 10-1).
3. Other areas of advancement in the treatment of saphenofemoral and saphenopopliteal incompetence include utilization of the "sequestration technique." Compression both at the SFJ and below the injection site localizes the effectiveness of the sclerosant at the injection site while also preventing retrograde movement of sclerosant into the femoral vein or other branches of the deep venous system.
4. Injection of the SFJ and SPJ should always be performed under duplex guidance or by means of endoscopic (angioscopic) visualization.

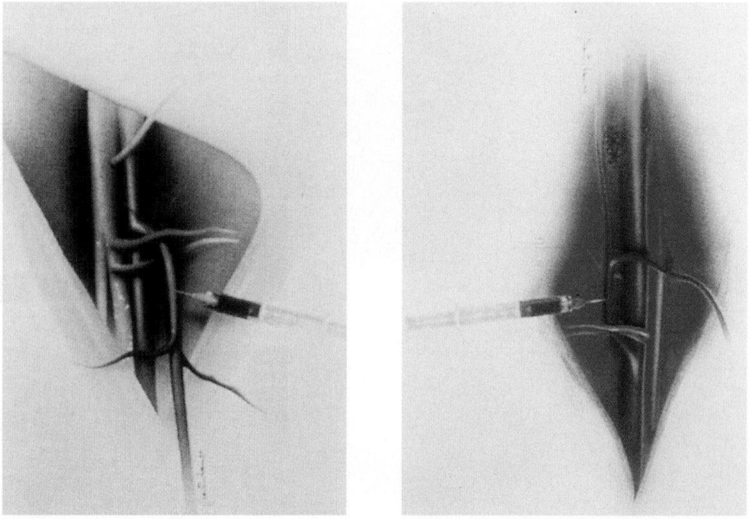

Figure 10-1
Injection of the greater saphenous vein 4 to 5 cm below the saphenofemoral junction.

Treatment Protocols

Most sclerotherapists prefer to inject patients in the supine or sitting position (Fig. 10-2A), although others utilize the standing position (Fig. 10-2B and C). The author prefers the former, utilizing the empty vein technique outlined below.

Technique of Injecting the Incompetent Saphenofemoral Junction

1. With the patient in a standing position on a sclerotherapy stool as previously described in Chapter 9, injection sites are marked off under duplex ultrasound guidance with an indelible marker.
2. The greater saphenous vein is then emptied by elevation of the treated extremity for a period of 5 minutes.
3. The patient is placed in a supine position and the leg abducted and rotated externally, with the knee flexed at a 90-degree angle.
4. Injection is administered under duplex guidance approximately 4 to 5 cm below the SFJ, utilizing either a standard 25-gauge, $\frac{5}{8}$-inch needle or a 25-gauge, $\frac{3}{4}$-inch butterfly needle with 3 inches of tubing.
5. Intravascular localization is confirmed by duplex evaluation.
6. Utilizing the sequestration technique, digital pressure is applied at the junction and below the injection site (Fig. 10-3).
7. Pressure at the junction is maintained throughout the injection and held for a few minutes afterwards, whereas distal pressure is released as soon as injection is complete.

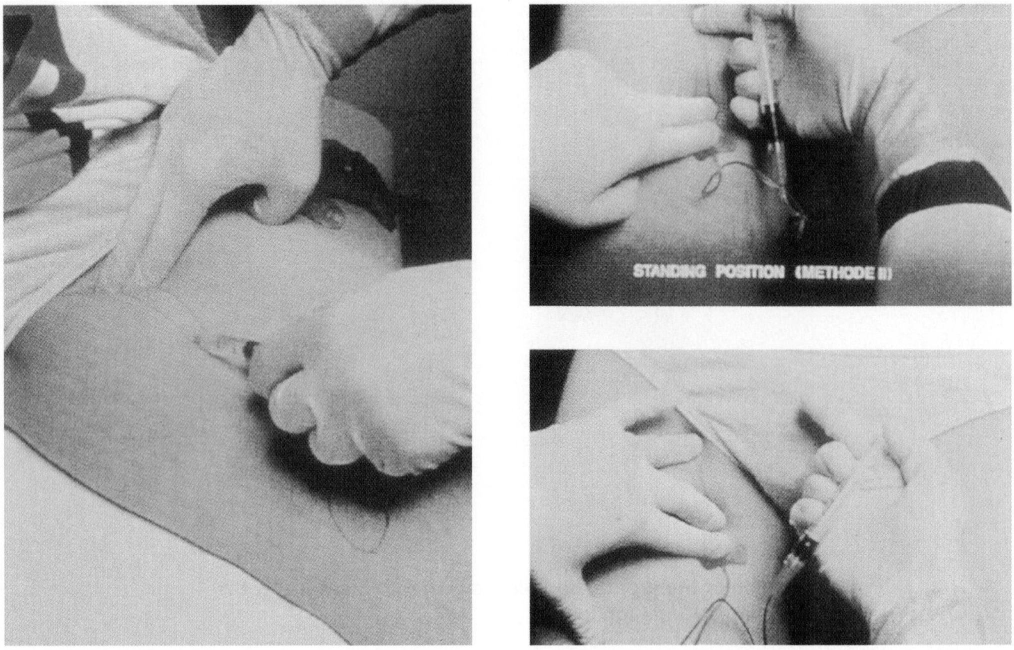

A B C

Figure 10-2

A. Injection of the incompetent saphenofemoral junction with the patient in sitting position. **B** and **C.** Injection of the incompetent saphenofemoral junction with the patient in a standing position.

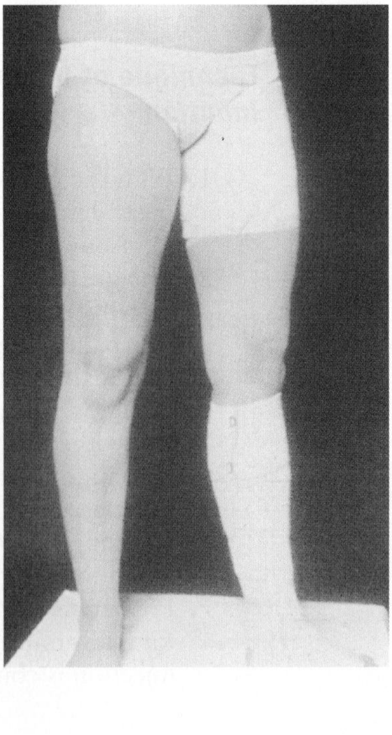

Figure 10-3

Postsclerotherapeutic compression dressing and elastic bandage.

8. The limb is elevated while pressure at the junction is maintained.
9. A beveled compression pad, elastic bandage, and class II 30-mm Hg support hose are immediately applied to the injection site (Fig. 10-3).

Compression bandages are removed after a period of 24 hours, while support hose are worn for 2 weeks following each treatment session.

Choice of Sclerosant

Sodium tetradecyl sulfate (STS) in 3% concentration or iodine sodium iodide 2% to 6% are the major sclerosants employed in the treatment of saphenofemoral incompetence. Suggested treatment protocols are presented in Tables 10-2 and 10-3.

Several points are noteworthy:

1. STS is approved by the U.S. Food and Drug Administration (FDA) versus iodine sodium iodide (NaI); however, it is slightly weaker in a 3% STS concentration versus 5% to 6% NaI concentration and thus may be associated with a lower rate of success in junctional obliteration.
2. If occlusion does not occur after injection, patients are re-treated according to the previously described treatment protocols at 3- to 6-week intervals.
3. Following sclerosant instillation, the treated vein will feel indurated at the treatment site. This is not to be confused with the development of thrombophlebitis.
4. Patients should be followed up at 3, 6, and 12 months and then at yearly intervals in order to look for evidence of recurrences.

Technique of Injecting of the Incompetent Saphenopopliteal Junction

Injection of the lesser saphenous vein at the SPJ is similar to that of the SFJ. Injection techniques are often more successful in this location and are more uni-

TABLE 10-2. SCHEDULE AND DOSAGE OF SODIUM TETRADECYL SULFATE (SOTRADECOL) INJECTIONS FOR TREATING GREATER SAPHENOUS VEIN INCOMPETENCE SECONDARY TO SAPHENOFEMORAL JUNCTIONAL MALFUNCTION

Visit	Dosage	Site
1	2 mL at 3% concentration	Below SFJ[a]
2	2 mL at 3% concentration	Below SFJ
3	2 mL at 3% concentration	Below SFJ
4	2 mL at 3% concentration	Below SFJ
	1 mL at 3% concentration	Midthigh level
5	2 mL at 3% concentration	Below SFJ
	1 mL at 3% concentration	Midthigh level
	1 mL at 2% concentration	Knee level

[a] Saphenofemoral junction.

TABLE 10-3. SCHEDULE AND DOSAGE OF IODINE SODIUM IODIDE (SCLERODINE, VARIGLOBAN) INJECTION IN TREATING GREATER SAPHENOUS VEIN INCOMPETENCE SECONDARY TO SAPHENOFEMORAL JUNCTION MALFUNCTION

Visit	Dosage	Site
1	2 mL of 2% concentration	Below SFJ
2	2 mL at 3% concentration	Below SFJ
3	2 mL at 4% concentration	Below SFJ
	or	
	2 mL at 3% concentration	Midthigh level
	1 mL at 3% concentration	Below SFJ
4	2 mL at 5% concentration	Below SFJ
	or	
	2 mL at 3% concentration	Below SFJ
	1 mL at 3% concentration	Midthigh level
	1 mL at 2% concentration	Knee level
5	2 mL at 6% concentration	Below SFJ
	1 mL at 3% concentration	Midthigh level
	1 mL at 2% concentration	Knee level

[a] Saphenofemoral junction.

formly accepted as an initial modality of therapy because of the fact that the variable termination of the lesser saphenous vein makes this a difficult area to approach surgically. With surgery, there are failure rates of 90% to 95% with 1-year follow-up after attempted ligation of the SPJ.

Sclerotherapy has the advantage of destroying abnormal feeding veins into this region as well.

Injection technique is duplex-guided with the patient in a supine position or standing (the author prefers the former) after marking of the intended injection site while the patient is standing (Fig. 10-4).

Emptying of the vein to be treated is again of importance, as in treatment of all large varicose veins.

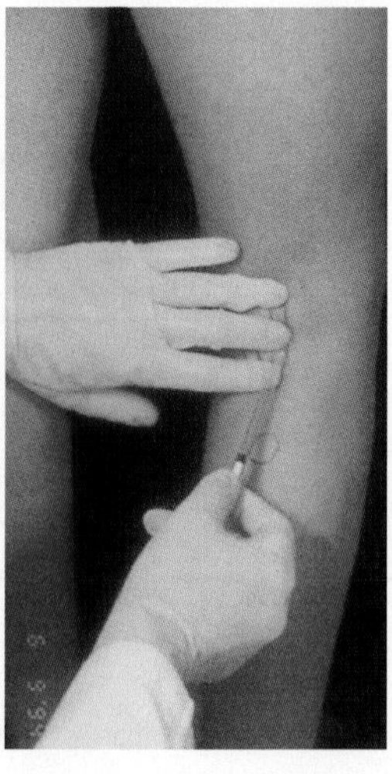

Figure 10-4

Injection of the saphenopopliteal junction using the "sequestration technique."

TABLE 10-4. SCHEDULE AND DOSAGE OF SODIUM TETRADECYL SULFATE (SOTRADECOL) INJECTIONS FOR TREATING LESSER SAPHENOUS VEIN INCOMPETENCE SECONDARY TO SAPHENOPOPLITEAL JUNCTION MALFUNCTION

Visit	Dosage	Site
1	2 mL of 2% concentration	Below SPJ[a]
2	2 mL at 2% concentration	Below SPJ
3	2 mL at 3% concentration	Below SPJ
4	2 mL at 3% concentration	Below SPJ
5	2 mL at 3% concentration	Below SPJ

[a] Saphenopopliteal junction.

Choice of Sclerosant

The sclerosants of choice for the treatment of the short saphenous vein and associated junctional incompetence are STS at 1% to 3% concentrations and NaI at 3% to 6% concentrations (Tables 10-4 and 10-5).

Repeat treatment sessions, as stated for SFJ incompetence, are performed at 4- to 6-week intervals.

The protocol for compression is identical to that utilized for treatment of the greater saphenous vein.

Complication Profiles

As stated previously, the major complications of concern in treating the saphenofemoral and saphenopopliteal junctions are arterial injection and thrombophlebitis with its associated risk of pulmonary embolus. Injection technique 4 to 5 cm below the SFJ, as stated, will minimize inadvertent arterial injection, as the femoral artery is less likely to be cannulated in this anatomic location. Duplex guidance by the experienced phlebologist will also help to minimize this adverse sequela. Immediate and adequate ambulation may help to lessen the risk of inadvertent thromboembolic phenomena.

TABLE 10-5. SCHEDULE AND DOSAGE OF IODINE SODIUM IODIDE (SCLERODINE, VARIGLOBAN) INJECTION FOR TREATING LESSER SAPHENOUS VEIN INCOMPETENCE SECONDARY TO SAPHENOPOPLITEAL JUNCTION MALFUNCTION

Visit	Dosage	Site
1	2 mL of 3% concentration	Below SPJ[a]
2	2 mL of 4% concentration	Below SPJ
3	2 mL of 5% concentration	Below SPJ
4	2 mL of 6% concentration	Below SPJ
5	2 mL of 6% concentration	Below SPJ

[a] Saphenopopliteal junction.

Of note, a toxic iodide hypersensitivity-type reaction—characterized by fever, flulike symptoms, and shortness of breath—has been described as well. Utilization of the sequestration technique and appropriate duplex guidance will help to minimize retrograde damage to the deep venous system.

Other complications, including ulceration and pigmentary dyschromia, are comparable to those of treating other large-diameter varicosities.

Conclusions

The role of sclerotherapy in the treatment of saphenofemoral vein incompetence is controversial, with a variable success rates of 50% to 90% and a high recurrence rate of up to 50%. Duplex guidance, angioscopic visualization, and utilization of the "sequestration" and "empty vein" techniques in association with adequate compression have helped to improve results and decrease morbidity associated with this technique. Long-term follow-up results and standardization of injection treatment protocols will help to determine the place of duplex-guided sclerotherapy in the treatment of saphenofemoral vein incompetence versus the surgical approach, which continues to remain the "gold standard" of care at this time.

Treatment of SPJ incompetence, with its relatively poor surgical outcome, is another issue. Here, sclerotherapy is much more effective and remains the cornerstone of therapy.

BIBLIOGRAPHY

Biegeleisen K, Nielsen RP. Failure of angioscopically guided sclerotherapy to permanently obliterate greater saphenous varicosities. *Phlebology* 1994;9:21–24.

Cornu-Thenard A, DeCottreau H, Weiss DA. Sclerotherapy—continuous wave doppler–guided injections. *Dermatol Surg* 1995;21:867–870.

Kanter A, Thibault P. Saphenofemoral incompetence treated by ultrasound guided sclerotherapy. *Dermatol Surg* 1996;22:648–652.

Raymond-Martimbeau PR. Two different techniques in sclerosing the incompetent saphenofemoral junction—a comparative study. *J Dermatol Surg Oncol* 1990;16:626–631.

Raymond-Martimbeau P. Advanced sclerotherapy treatment of varicose veins with duplex ultrasonographic guidance. *Semin Dermatol* 1993;12:123–128.

CHAPTER 11

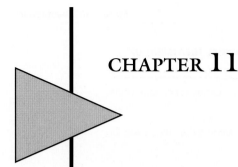

WHEN TO ASK FOR SURGICAL CONSULTATION

Although a detailed discussion of surgical approaches to the treatment of varicose veins of the superficial and deep venous system is beyond the scope of this text, it is important for the sclerotherapist to understand indications for surgical intervention so that appropriate referrals may be instituted. He or she should also have a rudimentary understanding of the many options and have a basic idea of the various operative techniques employed to treat both superficial and deep venous insufficiency.

The physician involved in the treatment of venous pathology needs this knowledge in order to have a broad based understanding of all available treatment options, regardless of his or her capability or desire to perform these procedures. Only in this way can he or she offer patients the most optimal treatment program for their particular venous problem.

Surgical Treatment of Chronic Venous Insufficiency

The surgical approach to the treatment of venous pathology may be divided into four basic categories as related to the anatomic localization of the specific venous pathology.

- Saphenous incompetence (greater or lesser saphenous veins)
- Perforator incompetence
- Deep venous vascular incompetence
- Truncal incompetence

TABLE 11-1. ANATOMIC INDICATIONS FOR THE SURGICAL TREATMENT OF VARICOSE VEINS

1. Determination of axial reflux in the greater or lesser saphenous veins
2. Large diameter of varicosities
3. Varicosities in the medial or anterior thigh
4. Dilated vein in a site vulnerable to trauma, such as the shin, ankle, or dorsum of the foot
5. A combination of these factors

The essential principle in the treatment of each of these venous pathologies is elimination of the source of venous incompetence as completely as possible. It is with these basic principles in mind that this chapter is presented.

Surgical Indications

Indications for surgical treatment of varicose veins may be divided into anatomic, functional (pathophysiologic), and cosmetic indications. The major focus of the present discussion is on the treatment of superficial venous insufficiency. The major anatomic indications for surgical treatment of varicose veins are listed in Table 11-1. When these problems have been identified by appropriate noninvasive laboratory testing—i.e., physical examination, Doppler, photoplesythmography (PPG), and/or duplex ultrasound evaluation, consideration of a surgical consultation is indicated. There are also various functional (pathophysiologic) signs and symptoms that may indicate that surgery should be considered as a therapeutic option. These are listed in Table 11-2.

Finally, many patients who are asymptomatic may seek treatment of large varicosities for cosmetic reasons only. This occurrence is less common, as most individuals seek treatment of smaller-caliber "spider telangiectasias" in this setting.

Contraindications to Surgery

As important as understanding indications for varicose vein surgery is an understanding of the relative contraindications to surgery in varicose veins. This will circumvent unnecessary referrals in the managed care era and also will avoid any pos-

TABLE 11-2. FUNCTIONAL PATHOPHYSIOLOGIC INDICATIONS FOR SURGICAL TREATMENT OF VARICOSE VEINS

1. Chronic and persistent pain unresponsive to compression therapy
2. Stasis changes
   - Skin pigment dyschromia
   - Dermatitis
   - Ulceration
3. History of sudden hemorrhage from a dilated varicosity
4. Dilated veins in athletes who fear the risk of traumatic hematoma or superficial thrombophlebitis

TABLE 11-3. CONTRAINDICATIONS TO VARICOSE VEINS SURGERY

Pregnancy
Peripheral arterial disease
Any contraindication to general anesthesia
Bleeding diathesis (coagulopathy)
Infection of the lower extremity
Lymphedema
Venous claudication
Congenital malformation
Oral contraceptives
These should be stopped 4 weeks before surgery and restarted at the next convenient period 2 weeks afterwards

sible morbidity associated with potential surgical interventions in such settings. Contraindications to varicose vein surgery are presented in Table 11-3.

Basic Surgical Principles in the Treatment of Superficial Venous System Incompetence

Several basic principles are adhered to regardless of the surgical technique employed in the treatment of incompetent superficial varicose veins. The four basic components that must be addressed are as follows:

1. Elimination of the source of incompetence. This usually involves ligation of the incompetent vein flush with the deep vein from which it arises. This is usually the source of retrograde flow, such as the termination of the long saphenous vein with the femoral vein or the short saphenous vein with the popliteal vein.
2. Remove the entire pathway of the incompetent vein. This is usually a single channel, such as the long or short saphenous vein, which is usually removed by either a stripping procedure (passing of a stripper with eversion and exteriorization of the involved vein) or stab avulsion (phlebectomy) techniques.
3. Remove as many as possible of the associated feeding varicosities (tributaries in the pathway of incompetence).

   Many varicose veins that are smaller in diameter are not amenable to removal by stripping procedures. In this setting, stab avulsion (phlebectomy) techniques, as discussed in Chapter 14, employing hook dissection through small incisions, may be employed to remove as many of the feeding tributaries as is possible.
4. Elimination of incompetent perforating veins. In most cases of superficial vein incompetence, perforator veins are acting as passive conduits communicating between the deep and superficial venous systems. However, perforators may occasionally become extremely dilated and may in themselves become sources of distal incompetence of communicating larger veins lower down in the affected extremity.

   This is particularly common in the midthigh perforating veins connecting with the long saphenous vein and the short saphenous vein in the midcalf. This may be accomplished by open ligation or microincision stab avulsion phlebectomy procedures. Duplex- or echo-guided injections (echosclerotherapy) with appropriate compression considerations are nonsurgical alternatives.

Surgical Options/Superficial Venous System

With these principles in mind, the following surgical techniques employed in the treatment of superficial varicose veins are presented.

"Classic" Saphenous Vein Ligation and Stripping

- This has been the "gold standard" of treatment of the greater saphenous vein in the past.
- The technique involves making incisions in the groin over the saphenofemoral junction with ligation of all branches in association with flush saphenofemoral junction ligation.
- Greater saphenous vein ligation is carried out at the level of the medial malleolus and the vein is subsequently stripped.
- Ligation of perforating veins and excision of large truncal branches and tributaries are performed concomitantly.
- The long-term reproducible result is a recurrence rate of less than 10% per year.
- Morbidity—including scarring, persistent neuritis, and removal of normal vein segments—are major adverse sequelae.

Limited Saphenous Vein Stripping

This procedure (Fig. 11-1) has gradually replaced the classic saphenous vein ligation and stripping procedure for the treatment of saphenofemoral vein incompetence.

- This is similar to the classic saphenous vein procedure.
- Flush saphenofemoral ligation is carried out.
- However, the greater saphenous vein distally is ligated and stripped more proximally at the level of the knee.
- This removes thigh tributaries as well.
- Smaller truncal and tributary branches are excised or treated by the stab avulsion phlebectomy technique.
- Alternatively, associated branches may be treated by compression sclerotherapy at a later date.
- Results are comparable to those of the classic operative procedure.
- There is less morbidity associated with this technique, including persistent neuritis, scarring, and removal of normal venous segments.

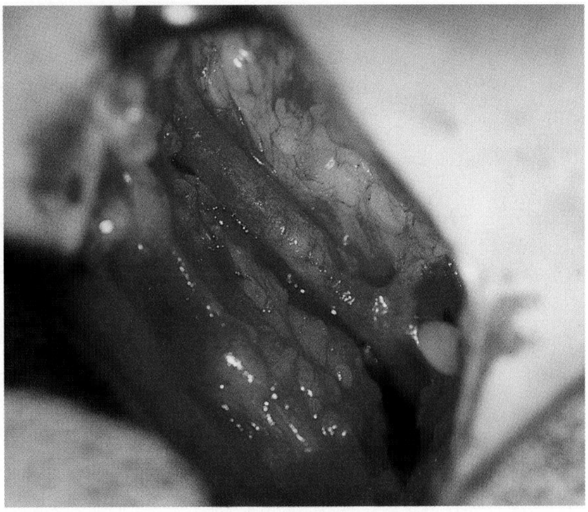

Figure 11-1

Greater saphenous vein. Limited saphenous vein stripping procedure with flush saphenofemoral ligation and proximal stripping at the level of the knee. A lateral circumflex iliac vein is noted. The junction will be closed and the vein stripped by the inversion technique. (Courtesy of Lawrence Tretbar, FACS.)

Saphenopopliteal Vein Ligation and Stripping

- In this technique (Fig. 11-2) ligation of the lesser saphenous vein at the saphenopopliteal junction is carried out
- Division of the vein is performed at the posterior border of the medial malleolus in conjunction with full length stripping
- Venous tributaries and truncal branches are simultaneously excised or treated at a later date with injection sclerotherapy

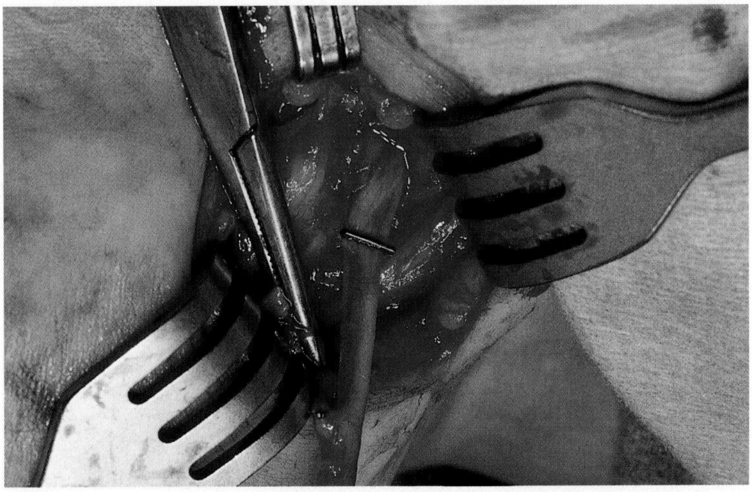

Figure 11-2

Saphenopopliteal vein ligation and stripping with flush ligation at the saphenopopliteal junction and excision of venous truncal tributaries. (Courtesy of Lawrence Tretbar, FACS.)

- Variable anatomy in the saphenopopliteal junction and the deep location of vessels in this anatomic location with limited access makes this procedure less effective and associated with a higher recurrence rate (30–40%) than the same procedure performed at the saphenofemoral junction

Isolated Saphenofemoral/Saphenopopliteal Vein Ligation

- Utilized to stop reflux at the saphenofemoral or saphenopopliteal junction
- Provides long-term results by itself
- Efficacious when performed in combination with injection compression sclerotherapy or ambulatory phlebectomy procedures

Saphenofemoral/Saphenopopliteal Vein Ligation and Stab Phlebectomy (Ambulatory Phlebectomy)

- This technique has become the "gold standard" of surgical treatment of saphenofemoral and saphenopopliteal vein incompetence.
- It consists of ligation of the saphenofemoral or saphenopopliteal junctions.
- This is combined with stab avulsion microincision phlebectomy of associated dilated varicosities.
- Residual varicose veins may be removed by injection compression sclerotherapy at a later date.
- This technique eliminates reflux with removal of all associated dilated veins (truncal and perforators) by a technique that produces minimal trauma and excellent cosmesis.

Ligation of Truncal/Perforating Veins

- Ambulatory phlebectomy is rapidly becoming the treatment of choice in this setting because of its low morbidity, excellent cure rate, and superb cosmesis.
- Alternate techniques in this setting include open and percutaneous ligation procedures.

Venous Banding

- This is a relatively new technique, where surgical cuffs are implanted circumferentially at the sites of incompetent valves.
- It may be utilized to abolish saphenofemoral reflux.
- Long-term results of this procedure are not known.

Combination of Surgery with Sclerotherapy

Surgical or sclerotherapy techniques are not mutually exclusive. As in the above discussion, sclerotherapy is commonly employed after varicose vein surgery when dilated varicosities have not been eradicated with the previously described surgical techniques. In addition, veins may sometimes be too fragile for surgical removal, in which case sclerotherapy becomes the treatment of choice for removal of such residual veins. Finally, in the debilitated patient, the surgeon may opt for a restricted surgical procedure, in which case sclerotherapy becomes part of the armentarium for the treatment of pathologic venous reflux.

In all of the situations outlined above, one must keep in mind that surgical techniques as well as sclerotherapy may be employed concomitantly in selected clinical situations to produce therapeutic results that are superior to those of either modality alone.

Conclusion

As stated above, the practicing sclerotherapist should have a good understanding of when to refer a patient for surgical consultation. Most physicians agree that saphenofemoral incompetence with large dilated saphenous veins greater than 10 mm in diameter and poor hemodynamic function as proven by PPG and duplex ultrasound techniques is a definitive indication for surgical consultation.

Other cases of lesser saphenofemoral incompetence, as stated in Chapter 10, may be treated by either surgery, as described in the present chapter, or duplex-guided compression sclerotherapy.

For the practicing clinician not well trained in the technique of axial vein sclerotherapy or not wishing to deal with the potential complication profile associated with these techniques, the surgical consultation is of the essence.

Truncal and perforating venous disease is more commonly treated by ambulatory (microstab avulsion) phlebectomy at the time of this writing, although compression and echosclerotherapy techniques are perfectly suitable treatment options.

Finally, an integrated understanding of all treatment options for specific venous problems will allow the practicing physician dealing with venous disease to provide his or her patients with optimal management and subsequently produce the best available clinical results.

BIBLIOGRAPHY

Campanello M, Hammarsten J, Forsberg C, Berland P, Henrikson O, Jensen J. Surgery for primary varicose veins. *Phlebology* 1996;11:45–49.

Fratila A, Rabe E. The differentiated surgical treatment of primary varicosities. *Semin Dermatol* 1993;12:102–116.

Georgiev M. The femoropopliteal vein—ultrasound anatomy, diagnosis and office surgery. *Dermatol Surg* 1996;22:57–62.

Goren G, Yellen AE. Invaginated axial saphenectomy by a semisurgical stripper perforate-invaginate stripping. *J Vasc Surg* 1994;20:970–977.

Hubner K. The out-patient therapy of trunk varicosities of the greater saphenous vein by means of ligation and sclerotherapy. *J Dermatol Surg Oncol* 1991;17:818–823.

Ricci S, Georgiev M. Office varicose vein surgery under local anesthesia. *J Dermatol Surg Oncol* 1992;18:55–58.

Trempe J. Long-term results of sclerotherapy and surgical treatment of the varicose short saphenous vein. *J Dermatol Surg Oncol* 1991;17:597–600.

CHAPTER 12

Compression Considerations in Sclerotherapy

Compression following sclerotherapy of varicose veins is essential to optimize both short- and long-term treatment results. The role of compression in the treatment of cosmetic telangiectasia and venulectasia remains somewhat more controversial. There are several benefits on both a theoretic as well as clinical basis in employing postsclerotherapy compression. These include the following:

1. Direct contact of the sclerosant with the inner walls of the veins, which results in more effective fibrosis; this, aided by external compression, may allow for utilization of lower concentrations of sclerosing agents (Fig. 12-1).
2. The reduced extent of thrombosis formation should decrease the risk of recanalization.
3. Decreased vascular mass should, theoretically, lead to diminished inflammation.
4. More direct contact of sclerosing agents with endothelium should lead to diminished retrograde flow of blood, which can lead to damage of the deep venous system.
5. A decrease in the extent of thrombus formation and postsclerotherapy inflammation should also diminish the incidence of postsclerotherapy pigmentation.
6. Lowered risk of telangiectatic matting (formation of neoangiogenic vessels <0.2 mm in diameter) in the treatment sites.
7. Improved efficiency of the calf-muscle pump, which provides both the physiologic benefit of improved venous circulation and increased patient comfort.
8. More rapid diffusion of the sclerosant from the deep venous system reducing the risk of deep-venous thrombosis.

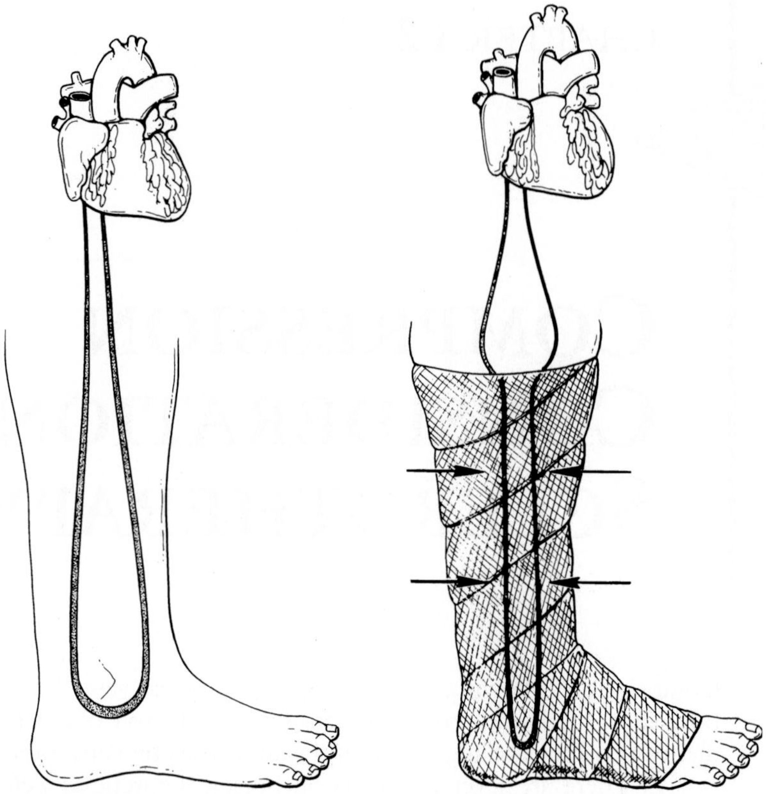

Figure 12-1

Direct contact of sclerosant with the vein walls due to adequate compression produces more effective endofibrosis and subsequent vein resolution.

Indications

Most phlebologists agree that compression is an essential part of the treatment program of enlarging varicose veins for the reasons stated above. Several studies that have sought to ascertain the optimal duration of compression following sclerotherapy of varicose veins have shown no difference in results between 3 weeks, 3 days, or 8 hours versus 6 weeks of compression. French phlebologists in general use more limited compression after sclerotherapy than do the Irish and British. Further studies are needed to define such duration parameters more precisely. The fact remains that by decreasing vein diameter, increasing venous return, and suppressing superficial inflammation and thrombus formation, local and graduated compression remains an essential part of the treatment protocol of varicose veins. However, the role of compression in the treatment of reticular veins and telangiectatic vessels remains somewhat more controversial. Patients being treated for cosmetic spider veins will often be less tolerant of unfashionable compression protocols. However, there are several theoretical as well as clinical reasons why postsclerotherapy compression of telangiectasia makes sense.

1. Telangiectasias have been demonstrated both radiographically as well as with duplex ultrasound evaluation to arise from larger subcutaneous and subfascial veins. Thus, graduated compression of these vessels should theoretically minimize venous flow retrograde into the treated telangiectasias.
2. Previous studies have shown that, after sclerotherapy of distal (calf or ankle) leg telangiectasias less than 1 mm in diameter, there is greater resolution after utilization of 30 to 40 mm Hg of graduated compression for 72 hours.
3. A decrease in hyperpigmentation from 40.5% to 28.5% has been described in studies where compression (30 to 40 mm Hg) stockings were worn continuously for 72 hours following sclerotherapy of telangiectasia.
4. Ankle and calf edema has been shown to be diminished when graduated compression stockings were worn immediately following sclerotherapy of telangiectasias.

In summary, compression makes sense from a theoretical as well as a clinical point of view. The author's recommendation is that if a patient will wear support hose following sclerotherapy of vessels of any diameter, it is wise to have him or her do so. The exact role of compression in the treatment of telangiectasia remains controversial. Many phlebologists feel that it is impossible to compress telangiectasias adequately. The author has concluded a multicenter clinical trial looking at the optimal duration of compression and its role in decreasing such postsclerotherapy sequelae as pigment dyschromia, neoangiogenesis, and thrombophlebitis. The results of this trial (Weiss et al., 1999) showed that clinical improvement was significantly improved and hyperpigmentation markedly decreased in patients wearing compression hose 3 for weeks after sclerotherapy as compared with controls. Even compression for as little as 3 days showed some benefit. The author strongly recommends compression in the treatment of small-vessel disease. This measure takes on increased importance in the following types of patients:

1. Patients who manifest a mixture of telangiectasias and large-diameter vessels
2. Patients who are on their feet a good part of the day
3. Patients with a history of edema, aching or fatigue of the legs
4. Patients who are menstruating

Finally, it is important to educate patients that compression will not only improve the results of their sclerotherapy treatments but may also prevent the emergence of newer large varicosities and help stabilize the appearance of smaller ones.

Types and Amounts of Compression

Compression materials for use after sclerotherapy may be divided into those intended for general compression and those suitable for localized or spot compression (Table 12-1). The theory of utilizing a dual or bilayered approach to postscle-

TABLE 12-1. COMPRESSION CONSIDERATIONS AFTER SCLEROTHERAPY

General
- Support stockings
- Elastic wraps

Spot
- Strapping over padding
  - Shaped gauze sponges
  - Foam compression pads
    - Small (4 × 13 × 1.75 cm)
    - Large (5 × 13 × 2.5 cm)

rotherapy compression is that the leg is not a uniform cylinder. Areas of disproportionate irregularity are based upon subcutaneous bone and muscular variations. Adipose tissue acts as a shock absorber and will diminish compression pressure, while areas of bony prominence tend to increase compression pressures. The amount of compression that is theoretically critical to diminish retrograde blood flow is 30 mm Hg. Because of these considerations, localized specific point compression is an important part of the postsclerotherapy compression approach and may be of greater importance in treating localized, small-diameter, nonbulging telangiectasias and reticular veins.

Therefore, the initial step in the biphasic approach is localized or spot compression, which may be accomplished by several modalities:

1. Cotton balls (Fig. 12-2A) or gauze pads (Fig. 12-2B) plus tape occlusion provide minimal compression, depending upon the number of cotton balls or gauze pads applied as well as the degree of stretch on the skin exerted by the tape. Micropore Tape (5 mm, ½ inch) or Microfoam Surgical Tape (3M Medical–Surgical Division, St. Paul, MN, U.S.A.) is preferred by the author. Exact degrees of compression have not been studied clinically.
2. Beveled foam rubber pads (STD Pharmaceuticals, Hereford, England; Delasco, Council Bluffs, IA, U.S.A.) (Fig. 12-3) have also been applied under graduated compression bandages and stockings. These have been shown to increase cutaneous and subcutaneous pressures up to 50%. They also have the advantage of improving patient comfort by decreasing abrasion from pressure stockings and tape. Their major drawback is their expense. The author utilizes these foam pads in treating bulging varicosities where more precise spot compression is indicated. One can also create such pads by dissecting large foam rubber pads and then shaving them down to achieve the beveled configuration, which leads to more uniform compression. How much extra compression these foam pads give is a matter of debate.
3. Elastic wraps such as Medi-Rip (Conco, Bridgeport, CT, U.S.A.) (Fig. 12-4) or Duoderm (Bristol Meyers Squibb, Princeton, NJ, U.S.A.) may achieve a still greater degree of local compression and are particularly effective in treating solitary varicosities or postcompression sclerosis of the axial junctions (saphenofemoral, saphenopopliteal). They may be applied

A

B

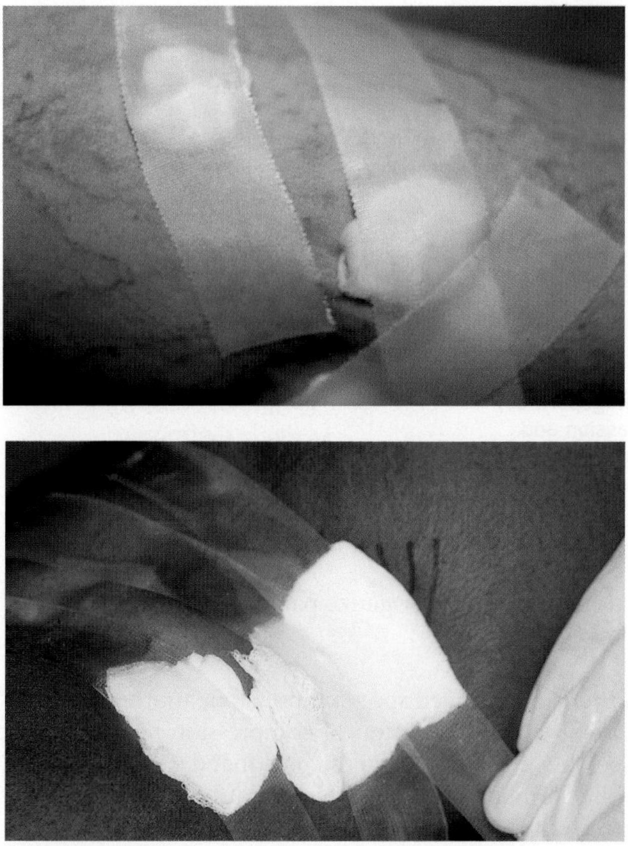

Figure 12-2

Cotton balls (**A**) or gauze pads (**B**) applied under occlusion deliver localized spot compression, which, when tightly secured by stretch tape (i.e., Micropore-3M), provides some degree of localized compression.

Figure 12-3

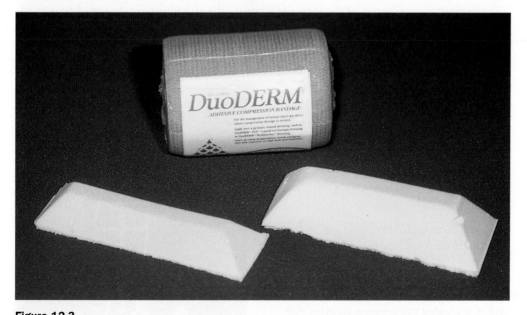

Beveled foam pads (STD Pharmaceuticals, Hereford, England; Delasco, Council Bluffs, IA, U.S.A.) may be applied under tape occlusion, theoretically increasing spot compression pressure over that achieved with cotton balls or gauze pads yet they have less abrasive potential than other modalities.

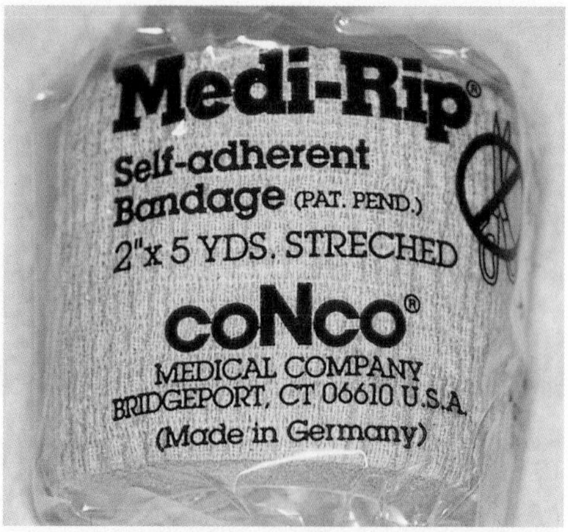

Figure 12-4
Elastic wraps such as Medi-Rip (Conco, Bridgeport, CT, U.S.A.) improve the effects of spot compression and are particularly useful for the treatment of bulging, solitary varicosities of the saphenofemoral or saphenopopliteal junctions.

alone or in conjunction with cotton or gauze pads, which may provide some degree of additive effect.

In addition to these methods of localized spot compression, another aspect of the compression approach involves the utilization of compression hosiery. Apart from its limitations, discussed above, it can still exert a prolonged resting pressure, which varies depending on the garment's class of compression. Modern compression hosiery has two-way stretch capability (the garments are elastic in both length and width) in order to prevent a tourniquet-type effect. To reproduce the normal hydrostatic pressures of the lower extremity, the stockings are designed to provide graduated pressures that decrease from the ankle upward (Fig. 12-5), ensuring unidirectional flow to the heart.

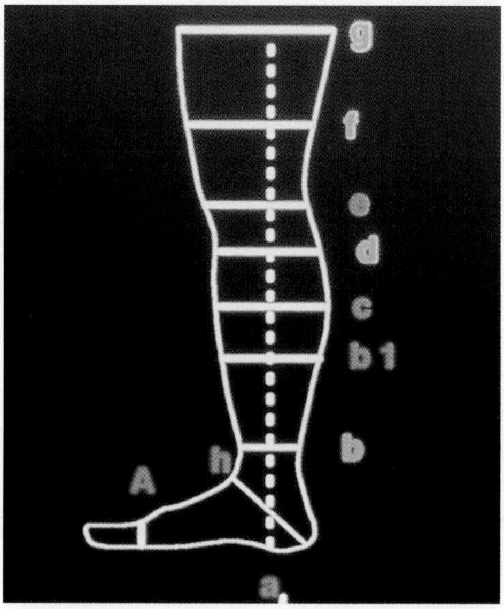

Figure 12-5
Schemata of graduated compression garment that provides for maximal compression at the ankle and a diminishing pressure gradient superiorly, reproducing the physiologic hydrostatic force gradient present in the venous circulation of the lower extremity.

TABLE 12-2. COMPRESSION CLASSES AND INDICATIONS

Class	Pressure in Ankle Area	Indications
Nonprescription fashion	15–20 mm Hg	Postsclerotherapy Telangiectasia/venulectasia where patients will not comply with class I support hose
Class I—mild compression	20–30 mm Hg	Postsclerotherapy Telangiectasia/venulectasia Small reticular veins Menstrual edema Pregnancy
Class II—moderate compression	30–40 mm Hg	Varicose veins Postsclerotherapy large reticular veins Postambulatory phlebectomy ulcerations
Class III—strong compression	40–50 mm Hg	Postambulatory phlebectomy > 4 mm diameter vessels Postsclerotherapy of saphenofemoral or saphenopopliteal junctions or postsurgical ligation of saphenofemoral/saphenopopliteal junction Postthrombotic venous insufficiency Dermatosclerosis Atrophie blanche
Class IV—extra strong compression	50–60 mm Hg	Lymphedema Elephantiasis

An accepted outline of compression classes and their associated indications is presented in Table 12-2. (The hosiery represented by these classes is presented in Fig. 12-6). As stated, most telangiectasia/venulectasia and small-diameter reticular veins may be compressed with class I hose (20 to 30 mm Hg). If the patient cannot tolerate such hose, then nonprescription 15 to 20-mm Hg support hose, available in numerous fashions and colors, may be worn (Fig. 12-7). Class II 30- to 40-mm Hg compression is recommended for treatment of larger-diameter reticular veins, truncal varicosities, and postambulatory phlebectomy of vessels 2 to 6 mm in diameter. Class III 40 to 50-mm Hg compression may be employed in attempting to achieve interruption of the saphenofemoral/saphenopopliteal junction or following ambulatory phlebectomy of vessels greater than 6 mm in diameter.

As stated previously, the usefulness of compression in the treatment of class I to II telangiectasia/venulectasia has been shown in the author's multicenter study, as it improves clinical results and decreases postsclerotherapy dyschromia.

A listing of support hosiery manufacturers is provided in Table 12-3. Associated styles and compression pressures are listed in the compression hosiery prescription shown in Table 12-4.

Custom-designed compression hose available by prescription are commonly employed and may save the physician time in his or her management of the sclerotherapy patient.

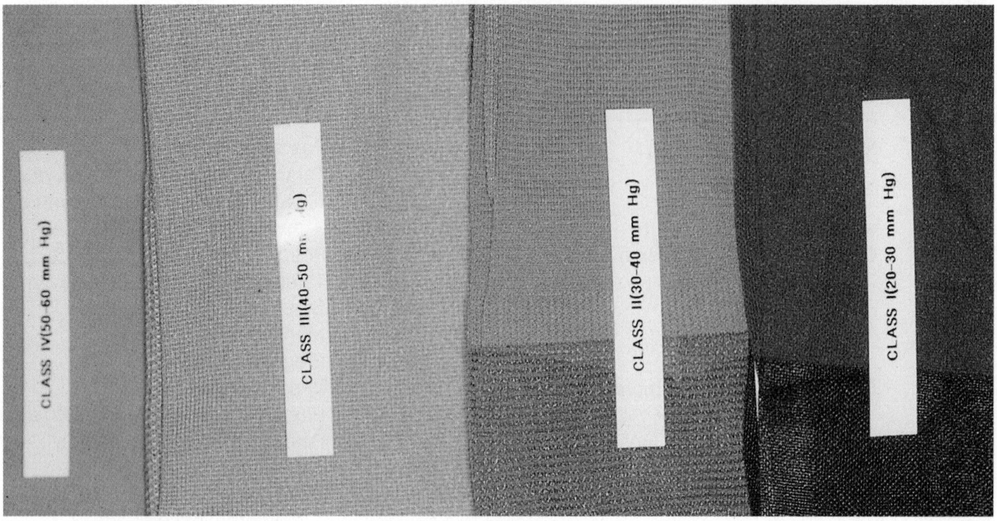

Figure 12-6
A clinical sampling of classes I to IV compression hosiery.

In addition, the following details must be given when one is prescribing compression hosiery:

1. The number of hosiery garments
2. Style of hosiery required
3. Compression class
4. If necessary, "made to measure"
5. If necessary, the prescribing of hosiery accessories

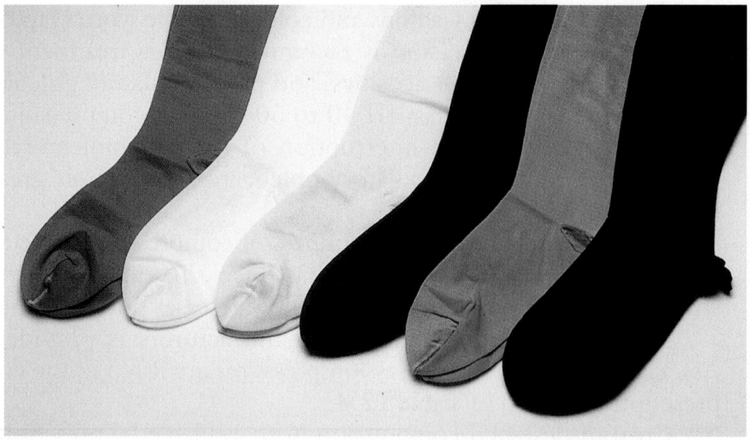

Figure 12-7
Class I (20 to 30 mm Hg) support hose are now available in a number of sheer and colorful varieties that are cosmetically acceptable to patients.

TABLE 12-3. ADDRESS LISTINGS OF COMPRESSION STOCKING COMPANIES

Medi USA
76 W. Seegers Road
Arlington Heights, IL 60005
(847) 640–8400

International Medi-Surgical
P.O. Box 300187
Houston, TX 77230
(800) 745–8346, or (713) 794–0115

Jobst
5825 Carnegie Boulevard
Charlotte, NC 28209
(704) 551–7163, or (704) 554–9933

Juzzo
P.O. Box 1088
Cuyahoga Falls, OH 44223
(216) 923–4999

Sigvaris, Inc.
1119 Highway 74
Peachtree City, GA 30269

Venosan
1617 N. Fayetteville Street
P.O. Box 4068
Asheboro, NC 27203–4068

TABLE 12-4. SAMPLE COMPRESSION HOSIERY PRESCRIPTION

For ______________________________	Date ____________
Fashion Hose (15–20 mm Hg)	
Medi—Comfort	Below knee (calf)
International Medi Surgical—IMS16/IMS22S	Above knee (midthigh)
Juzzo—Lite Line	Thigh length
Jobst—Ultrasheer/Sheer/Future Sheer/Relief/Fastlift	Panty hose
Venosan—Legline	Maternity
Sigvaris—Delilah, Samson	
Class I (Mild) (20–30 mm Hg)	
Medi—Mediven, Medi 75, Medi Plus	Open toe
International Medi Surgical—IMS2J, IMS30	Closed toe
Juzzo—Hostess 2501, Hostess 2581, Varin Super 3531	
Jobst—Maternity, Medi, Future Firm	
Venosan—2030	
Sigvaris—801, 901	
Class II (Moderate) (30–40 mm Hg)	
Medi—Mediman, Medi 32, Medilastex	
International Medi Surgical—IMS40	
Juzzo—Hostess #2502, Varin Soft #3512, Varin Custom, Varin-Soft-In, Varin Soft-n-Silk, Varin Super 3532	
Jobst—Medi 75, Med, Ultimate, Varisox	
Venosan—3040	
Sigvaris—202, 503, 702, 802, 902	
Class III (Strong) (40–50 mm Hg)	
Medi—Medi 33	Stays
Juzzo—Varin Super 3533, Varin Soft S3513	Hose Caddy
Sigvaris—504	Garter Belt
Class IV (Extra Strength) (50–60 mm Hg)	Cast Saver
Juzzo—Helastic 3024	
Sigvaris—505	

6. Diagnosis
7. Any additional remarks—e.g., brand name, etc.

A sample compression hosiery prescription is illustrated.

Duration of Compression

At present the author employs guidelines for compression based on his personal experience and published clinical studies. Local spot compression may be removed within 24 to 72 hours after a given treatment session. Such spot compression may not be necessary in following treatment of telangiectasia.

Telangiectasia/Venulectasia

Class I support hose (20 to 30 mm Hg) or nonprescription fashionable (15 to 20 mm Hg) hose, if the former are not tolerated, are worn for 72 hours after treatment, including at night, and then worn for 3 weeks during waking hours.

This is especially important for vessels larger than 0.5 mm in diameter, vessels located at the distal calf and ankle, the vessels of women on hormone-replacement therapy, treatment of resistant cases, or when previous treatment has produced adverse sequelae such as pigment dyschromia or neo-angiogenesis.

Reticular Veins

Patients are asked to maintain day- and nighttime compression (class I, 20 to 30 mm Hg, for small-diameter reticular veins below 2 mm in diameter; Class II, 30 to 40 mm Hg, for large-diameter reticular veins above 2 mm in diameter) day and night for 3 days after a given treatment session and then continue daytime wear for 3 weeks or until all signs of inflammation dissipate.

Truncal Varicosities/Perforator Veins, Axial Veins of the Saphenofemoral or Saphenopopliteal Junctions

Patients are asked to wear class III (40 to 50 mm Hg) support hose for 4 to 6 weeks during waking hours after each treatment session.

In addition, the following measures are often carried out:

1. In cases where hyperpigmentation or telangiectatic matting has occurred, patients may be encouraged to wear support hose at night or for prolonged periods of time or to wear an increased compression class.
2. Patients with widespread or recurrent telangiectasias are advised to wear class I (20 to 30 mm Hg) stockings over the long term in an attempt to minimize recurrences.

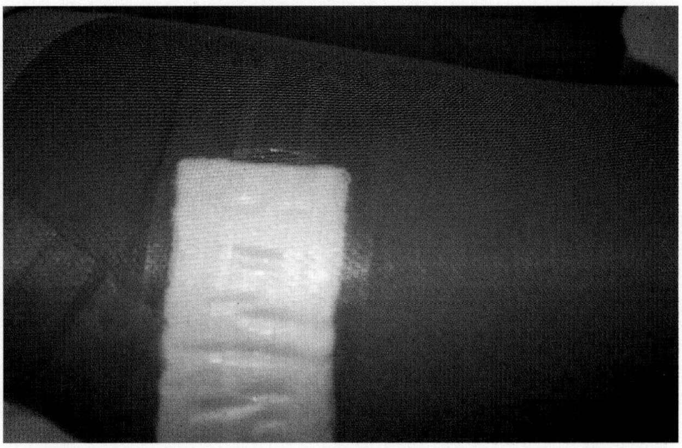

Figure 12-8
Localized spot compression may be applied using simple gauze pads and elastic adhesive tape prior to putting on graduated compression hose.

How to Apply Compression

The exact methods for applying compression may vary among phlebologists. Comparable results may be achieved in different hands by different compression methods.

Local and Segmental Compression

As stated previously, local or segmental compression (Fig. 12-8) may be achieved by using cotton balls, gauze pads, or—in the case of larger-diameter vessels—beveled foam rubber pads fixed in place with elastic adhesive tape such as Micropore (3M Medical Surgical Division, St. Paul, MN, U.S.A.).

In flexural areas such as the popliteal fossa or at the lateral or medial malleoli, the utilization of Microfoam (3M Health Care, St. Paul, MN, U.S.A.) under the Micropore tape may minimize the incidence of irritant and occlusive dermatitis.

Such localized compression devices should be applied by the sclerotherapist's assistant immediately after a given injection has been carried out.

These localized compression modalities may be removed within 24 to 72 hours after a given treatment session.

General Compression Measures

In patients with larger telangiectasia or venulectasia, wrapping the legs with compression or Ace-type adhesive bandages may be employed (Medi-Rip, Conco, Bridgeport, CT, U.S.A.).

In other circumstances, as stated, a full-length compression garment is preferable. These support hose are applied while the patient is still on the sclerotherapy table immediately after a given treatment (Fig. 12-9).

For these reasons, a decision as to type and length of compression garment must be made at the initial consultation session.

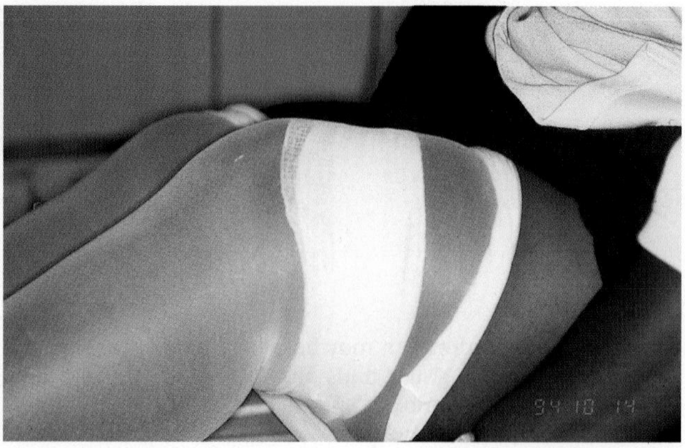

Figure 12-9
Graduated compression hose should be put in place while the patient is still on the sclerotherapy table, immediately following a treatment session.

The compression stocking is normally worn during the day and taken off in the evening after 48 to 72 hours of round-the-clock usage. Practice and education are needed to properly apply and remove compression hosiery (particularly class III). Attachment devices and application caddy frames are available from most manufacturers (Fig. 12-10).

The sclerotherapist's office staff should be available to educate patients on the use of these compression devices at the time of the sclerotherapy treatment session. A second pair of light sheer hose may be worn under the prescribed compression garment, which will make it easier to put on the prescribed garment.

The author has found the pantyhose length of compression hose to be most practical in the large majority of cases.

Conclusion

Compression considerations are an important part of the sclerotherapy treatment approach, gaining greater importance with treatment of larger-diameter vessels. The concepts of local segmental as well as graduated compression maneuvers

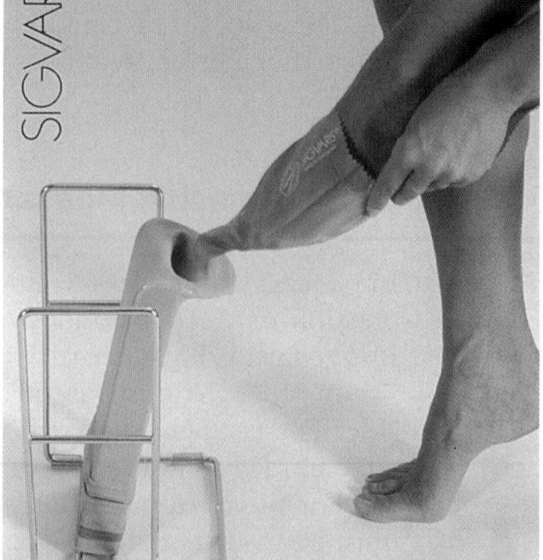

Figure 12-10
Application devices such as stocking caddies are helpful in putting on compression hosiery, particularly the heavier hose such as those of classes III to IV. (Courtesy of Sigvaris Corp., Peachtree, GA, U.S.A.)

should be mastered by all physicians involved in the treatment of varicose vein disease. The theoretic advantages of compression practices cannot be challenged, as substantiated by recent clinical studies, and should be incorporated into the setting of telangiectatic and varicose vein treatment in order to minimize complications and optimize treatment results.

Addendum 1

Washing Compression Hosiery

1. Water should be lukewarm, not more than 105°F.
2. Use a mild soap for delicate fabrics (not Woolite).
3. Rinse well in lukewarm water.
4. Roll in towel.
5. Dry in an airy, shady place.
6. Do not dry the stocking in dryer.

Addendum 2

Commonly Asked Questions Concerning Compression Hosiery

Q: I wore the hose regularly and I developed blisters on my feet. What should I do?

A: Discontinue the use of the hose until you can have them adapted to your feet.

Q: I began developing cramps in the middle of my foot after wearing the hose. What should I do?

A: Since patients cannot tolerate the pressure exerted on the lateral aspect of the feet, which simply pushes the bones together, you may need custom hosiery. Consider wearing the lighter hose.

Q: Can I wear two pairs of hosiery?

A: This is a good method for patients who have difficulty putting on the hose. Usually the inner part of the hosiery has a closed toe and the outer an open toe.

Q: Will my insurance pay for hosiery?

A: This depends on your insurance policy. If the hosiery is considered a medical device, some plans will pay for it.

Q: I find it almost impossible to put on compression hosiery. What should I do?

A: Consider the purchase of a hose caddy, which makes it simpler to put on the hosiery.

BIBLIOGRAPHY

Christopoulos D, Nicolaides AN, Belcaro G. The long term effect of elastic compression in the venous haemodynamics of the leg. *Phlebology* 1991;685–693.

Goldman MP. Utilization of localized compression to optimize sclerotherapy. *J Am Acad Dermatol* 1994;31:101–103.

Goldman MP, Beaudoing D, Marley W, Lopez L, Butie H. Compression in the treatment of telangiectasia—a preliminary report. *J Dermatol Surg Oncol* 1990;16:322–325.

Partsch H. Compression therapy of the legs—a review. *J Dermatol Surg Oncol* 1991;17:799–805.

Stanley PRW, Bickerton DR, Campbell WB. Injection sclerotherapy for varicose veins—a comparison of materials for applying local compression. *Phlebology* 1990;6:37–39.

Veraart JCJM, Neumann HAM. Interface pressure measurements underneath elastic and non-elastic bandages. *Phlebology* 1996;1:52–53.

Veraart JCJM, Koster D, Neumann HAM. Compression therapy and the pressure in the deep venous system. *Phlebology* 1996;1(suppl):56–59.

Weiss RA, Sadick NS, Goldman MP, Weiss MA. Post-sclerotherapy compression: controlled comparative study of duration and its effect on clinical outcome. *Dermatol Surg* 1999;25:106–108.

CHAPTER 13

Minimizing Complication Profiles in Sclerotherapy

Sclerotherapy of telangiectatic and varicose veins remains one of the safest of all cosmetic procedures. Adverse sequelae are not uncommon but usually are relatively minor and self-limiting. The esthetic imperfections that may result are usually nominal compared with the esthetic improvement achieved by eradication of the treated veins. Minor complications include hyperpigmentation, telangiectatic matting (TM) localized urticaria over injection sites, contact dermatitis related to local compression techniques, and hirsutism (Table 13-1). More severe adverse sequelae associated with greater morbidity are fortunately rare. These major complications include ulcerations; systemic allergic reactions; thrombophlebitis of the injected vessel; deep venous thrombosis (DVT), which may result in chronic deep venous insufficiency or the development of pulmonary emboli; and arterial injection, resulting in ischemic necrosis (Table 13-2).

There are three major considerations in understanding and managing complications noted in sclerotherapy practice. The first is that fastidious technique will minimize the incidence of side effects, as discussed below. Second, an appropriate understanding of maneuvers that may be instituted if something is felt to have gone wrong (i.e., inadvertent extravascular injection of sclerosant is paramount). Immediate remedial measures will help to minimize the possible progression of adverse sequelae from eventuating in more deleterious consequences. Finally, an understanding of the management options of adverse sequelae and their order of institution is of major importance in minimizing and ameliorating the spectrum of complications occurring in the management of sclerotherapy patients.

The following discussion summarizes the pathophysiology, prevention, and therapeutic options relevant to the management of sclerotherapy complications.

TABLE 13-1. MINOR COMMON SCLEROTHERAPY COMPLICATIONS

Hyperpigmentation
Telangiectatic matting (neoangiogenesis)
Syncope
Localized urticaria
Bruising
Edema
Compression-related problems (folliculitis, contact dermatitis)
Hirsutism
Needle phobia
Scotomata

Common (Minor) Side Effects

Postsclerotherapy Pigmentation

The incidence of postsclerotherapy hyperpigmentation varies from 10% to 30% in various studies. More controlled scientific trials are indicated in order to define a more exact incidence. Hyperpigmentation usually presents 3–4 weeks after a given treatment session. There are two distinct patterns of postsclerotherapy hyperpigmentation. The first is a diffuse purple–brown pigmentation that runs along the entire treated vessel (Fig. 13-1). The second pattern is that of a punctate pigmentation, which usually appears at sites of discrete venous needle transections (Fig. 13-2). It is exceptional to find persistent postsclerotherapy pigmentation. Studies have found a 70% resolution within 6 months and a 98% to 99% resolution within 1 year (Fig. 13-3A to C). In some cases, hyperpigmentation may occasionally be present over superficial varicosities, telangiectasias, and foci of chronic venous insufficiency prior to treatment. Therefore preoperative photographic documentation is of significant importance.

Studies utilizing iron (Perls) and melanin (Fontanna-Masson) stains have defined the pigment as consisting of iron metabolite products (hemosiderin) (Fig. 13-4). This ignores the fact that extravascular diapedesis of erythrocytes is the major pathophysiologic factor responsible for postsclerotherapy pigmentation.

The role of melanin in postsclerotherapy hyperpigmentation is solely theoretical, with free radical formation causing melanocyte stimulation resulting from local iron accumulation being hypothesized; but this has not been proven. Predisposing factors to postsclerotherapy hyperpigmentation are listed in Table 13-3.

TABLE 13-2. MAJOR UNCOMMON SCLEROTHERAPY COMPLICATIONS

Ulceration
Systemic allergic reactions
Thrombophlebitis
Deep venous thrombosis/Pulmonary embolus
Arterial injection
Nerve damage

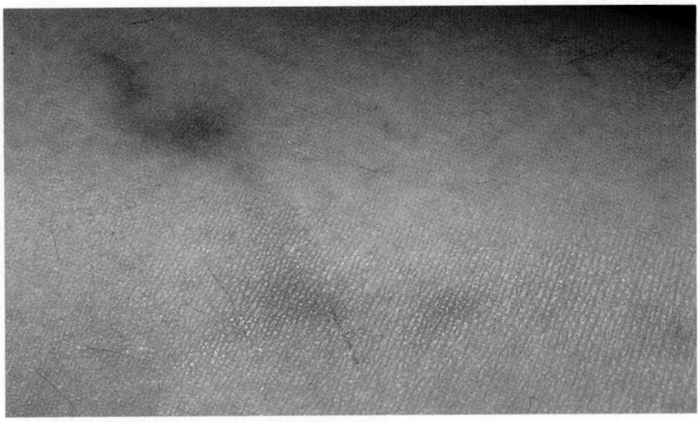

Figure 13-1
Diffuse pattern of brown–purple postsclerotherapy hyperpigmentation, which is usually due to vessel perforation, vessel inflammation, and erythrocyte diapedesis.

Several factors have been shown to influence or predispose patients to postsclerotherapy hyperpigmentation. These include:

1. A genetic predisposition to postinflammatory hyperpigmentation.
   a. Skin types IV to V.
   b. Increased total body iron stores—elevated ferritin levels as well as defective iron-transport mechanisms.
2. Vascular fragility syndromes (i.e., antithrombin III, protein C or S deficiency; antiphospholipid antibody syndrome; elevated histamine states; hormones; salicylates; nonsteroidal antiinflammatory drugs; elderly population.
3. Sclerotherapy techniques involving selection of inappropriate solution and concentration.
4. Gravitational and elevated intravascular pressures following sclerotherapy treatments. These factors are theoretically ameliorated by postsclerotherapy compression.
5. Vessel location and diameter. The inner thigh and medial malleolus appear to be associated with an increased incidence of postsclerotherapy

Figure 13-2
Punctate pattern of postsclerotherapy hyperpigmentation, which is usually due to erythrocyte leakage secondary to local vein puncture.

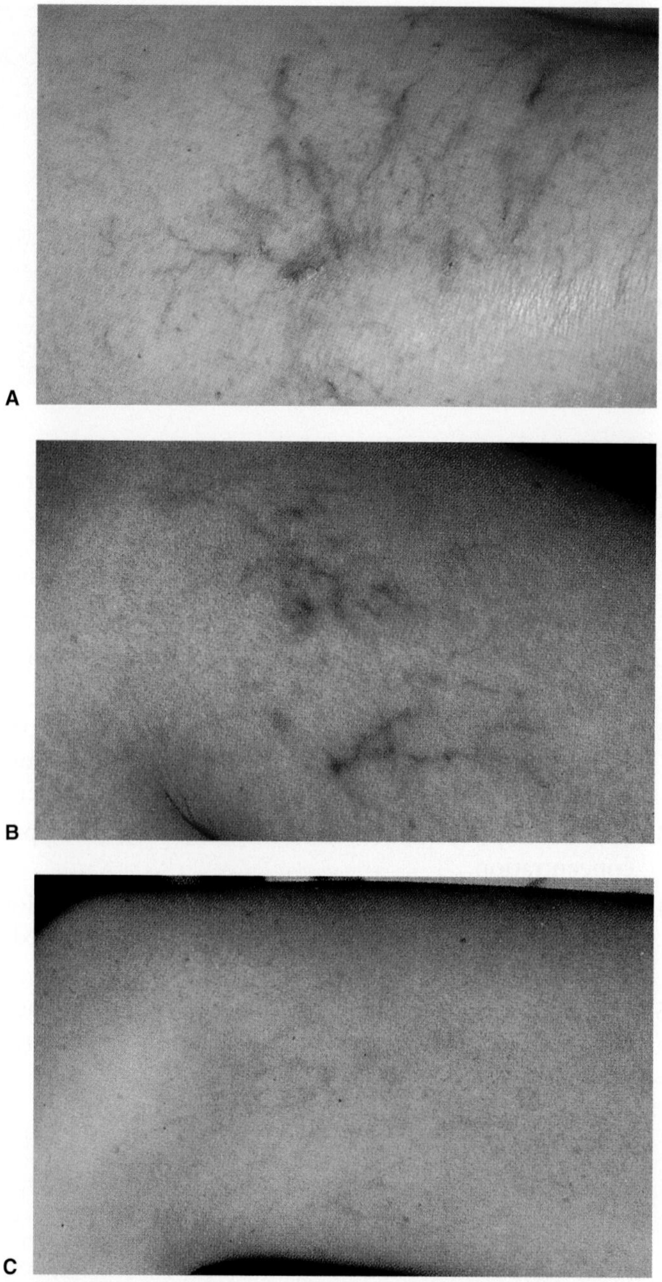

Figure 13-3

A: Sclerotherapy-induced hyperpigmentation, which is diffusely distributed along the entire treated vessel. **B:** Fading of pigmentation at 1 month. **C:** Total resolution of postsclerotherapy hyperpigmentation at 12 months, which usually occurs in 98% to 99% of cases.

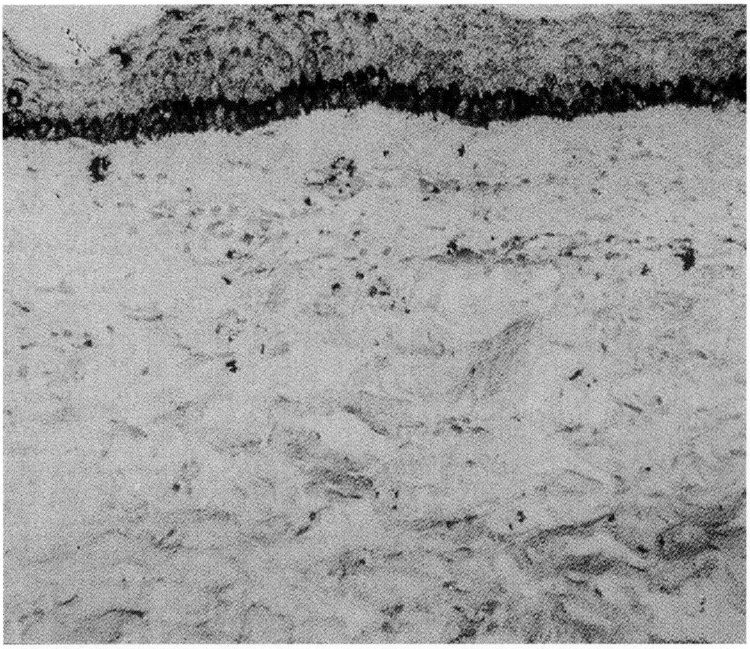

Figure 13-4
Perls stain (original magnification, ×40) of postsclerotherapy pigmentation reveals hemosiderin as the major pigment involved in this setting.

TABLE 13-3. PREDISPOSING FACTORS TO POSTSCLEROTHERAPY HYPERPIGMENTATION

Genetic predisposition to postinflammatory hyperpigmentation
Skin types IV–V
Increased body iron stores
Vascular fragility syndromes
Antithrombin III deficiency
Protein C or S deficiency
Antiphospholipid antibody syndrome
Medications—hormones, salicylates, NSAIDs, estrogens
Elevated histamine states
Old age
Sclerotherapy techniques
Choice of sclerosant
Sclerosant concentrations
Gravitational factors
Vessel location and diameter
Esp: inner thigh and medial malleolus

hyperpigmentation. Finally, injecting linear microtelangiectasias as well as reticular veins may be associated with an increased risk of postsclerotherapy dyschromia.

Measures that Help to Minimize Postsclerotherapy Hyperpigmentation

The major measure of importance in minimizing postsclerotherapy hyperpigmentation (Table 13-4) is the restriction of vascular endothelial rupture, which leads to diapedesis of erythrocytes. This is accomplished by fastidious technique. Sclerosing agents such as polidocanol have been associated in the literature with a slightly diminished incidence of hyperpigmentation, while agents such as sodium tetradecyl sulfate (STS; Sotradecol) have been associated with a greater tendency for pigment dyschromia. However, in the author's opinion, other factors such as choosing the appropriate minimal sclerosing concentrations (MSCs) for a given vessel diameter, avoiding excessive syringe pressures, decreasing the amount of sclerosant injected at a given cannulation site (0.5 to 1 mL), and minimizing intravascular pressures by elevating the treated extremity during treatment (especially important for treatment of larger diameter vessels) are of paramount importance in decreasing postsclerotherapy pigmentation.

Other mechanisms—such as identification and elimination of sources of proximal reflux as well as the utilization of proper graduated compression—also help to minimize venous pressures and subsequent stasis of erythrocytes.

Finally, recognition and incision and drainage of postsclerotherapy thrombi, utilizing a number 11 blade, within 48 hours evolution may decrease the incidence of pigmentation. Persistent thrombi may induce chronic venular inflammation; thus all coagula, when identified, should be drained for up to 2 months postsclerotherapy.

Treatment

There is no known effective treatment for postsclerotherapy hyperpigmentation (Table 13-5). As stated, the majority of patients improve within 12 to 18 months.

TABLE 13-4. TIPS TO MINIMIZE POSTSCLEROTHERAPY HYPERPIGMENTATION

Fastidious technique—minimize vessel rupture
Choice of a sclerosant with minimal inflammatory potential
Use of minimal sclerosant concentration for a given vessel diameter
Prior elimination of sources of reflux into treatment site
Utilization of graduated compression immediately posttreatment
Prompt removal of postsclerotherapy coagula
Identification of patients with vascular fragility syndromes (protein C, protein S, antithrombin III deficiency, antiphospholipid antibody syndrome)
Avoid medications associated with pigmentation predilection or vascular fragility i.e., minocycline, aspirin, NSAIDs, conjugated estrogens)
Treatment of central focus of arborizing clustered vessels in order to minimize number of injections
Avoidance of treating patients with defects in iron transport mechanisms

TABLE 13-5. TREATMENT MODALITIES FOR POSTSCLEROTHERAPY HYPERPIGMENTATION

Exfoliants (20%–40%) trichloracetic acid
Chelating agents
  Disodium ethylenediaminetetraacetic acid
  150 g/mL ointment (Star Pharmaceuticals, Pampano Beach, FL, U.S.A.)
Tretinoin (Retin A) (Ortho, Raritan, NJ, U.S.A.)
  Retin A Micro 0.1% (preparation recommended)
  Differen Gel 0.1% (Galderma, Fort Worth, TX, U.S.A.)
Alpha hydroxy acids
  Glycolic acid (Glyderm, ICN, Costa Mesa, CA, U.S.A.)
  Lactic acid (Lachydrin, Westwood Squibb, New York, NY, U.S.A.)
  Pyruvic acid
Stanazolol (Sanofi, Winthrop Pharmaceuticals, New York, NY, U.S.A.)
Lasers/flash-lamp sources
  Ruby laser (694 nm) (Palomar, Inc., Lexington, MA, U.S.A.)
  Alexandrite laser (755 nm) (Cynasure, Chelmsford, MA, U.S.A.; E.S.C./Sharplan, Needham, MA, U.S.A.)
  Photoderm VL (500–1,200 nm) (E.S.C./Sharplan, Needham, MA, U.S.A.)
  Flashlamp Excited Pulsed Dye Laser (510 nm) (Candela, Wayland, MA, U.S.A.)
Cryotherapy
  Liquid nitrogen
  Solid CO_2

Photographic documentation of this improvement will allay the anxiety of most patients. The utilization of antimelanin agents such as hydroquinone, kojic acid, and azelaic acid have not been shown to be effective in minimizing postsclerotherapy hyperpigmentation, as expected in a clinical setting where melanin is not the major pigment responsible for the dyschromia.

The utilization of exfoliants such as trichloroacetic acid is associated with its own intrinsic risks of scarring and hyperpigmentation. Tretinoin and alpha-hydroxy acid preparations may have a similar although milder mechanism of exfoliating activity; in the author's experience, these are associated with a lower incidence of morbidity.

Lasers—ruby (694 nm) and alexandrite (755 nm)—and noncoherent flashlamp light sources (500–1,200 nm) have produced variable degrees of success, with reports of 45% to 69% efficiency. Although these lasers have shown predictable (positive) interaction with hemosiderin (maximum 410 to 415 nm absorption peak followed by a gradually sloping curve throughout the visible spectrum), melanin, which has a higher absorption coefficient at these wavelengths, causes nonspecific interaction. Lasers are hypothesized to fragment pigment granules, which are subsequently reabsorbed by phagocytosis.

In summary, there are modalities that are effective in the treatment of selective cases of postsclerotherapy hyperpigmentation, which has been defined as a hemosiderin deposition phenomenon. All of these modalities induce reabsorption of ferritin particles by means of macrophage digestion over time. Appropriate measures—i.e., fastidious injection technique and appropriate graduated compression—remain the cornerstones of prevention.

Telangiectatic Matting (Neoangiogenesis)

TM is defined as a network of very fine blushes of red telangiectasis less than 0.2 mm in diameter that occur surrounding sites of previously sclerosed telangiectases or surgical ligation of varicose veins. Up to 90% of patients have spontaneous resolution of TM within 12 months (Fig. 13-5A and B). However, because up to 10% of TM may be permanent, it should be included in the presclerotherapy informed consent. Presclerotherapy photography is helpful in documenting the degree of TM resulting from treatments rather than residual microtelangiectasias remaining after treatment of larger-diameter vessels. Sites of predilection include the thighs, medial malleolus, and medial and lateral calves (with the inner thighs being the most common sites).

The incidence of TM has been estimated from 5% to 24% in various series. TM has been hypothesized to occur from either inflammatory or neoangiogenic

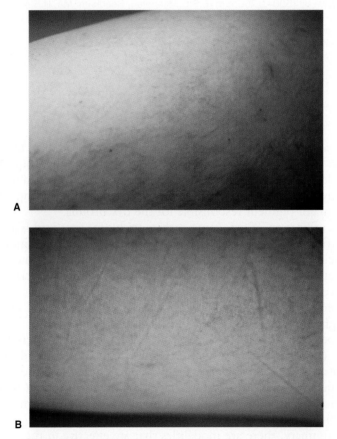

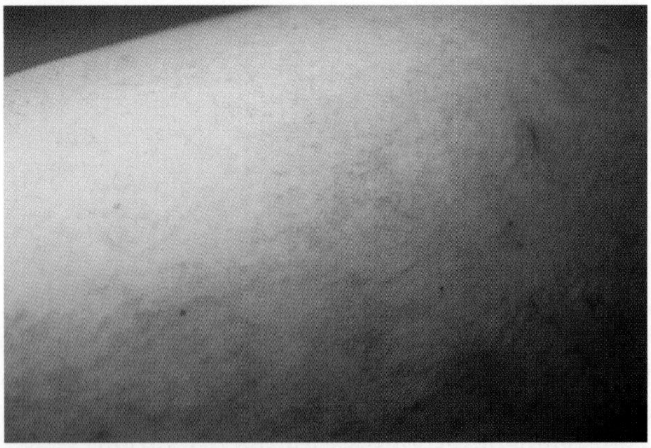

A

B

Figure 13-5

A: Telangiectatic matting consists of vessels less than 2 mm in diameter that appear at sites of previously treated vessels or foci of surgical vein ligation. **B:** The majority of neoangiogenesic vessels, as shown in this case, resolve within a period of 6 to 12 months.

TABLE 13-6. PREDISPOSING FACTORS OF TELANGIECTATIC MATTING

Exogenous/endogenous estrogen
Obesity (>20% normal body weight)
Family history of telangiectasia/telangiectatic matting
Increased duration of vascular ectasia

mechanisms. Induction of an inflammatory state by sclerosant-induced endothelial irritation with subsequent mast-cell heparin generation may lead to microvascular proliferation.

In the angiogenic theory endothelial damage leads to increased mast cell proliferation and the release of various cytokines and growth factors, stimulating new vessel formation. Endothelial cell growth factor (ECGF), fibroblast growth factor (FGF), and transforming growth factor beta (TGF-β) are three active angiogenic peptides felt to play a major role in this regard; they are presently being studied in the author's laboratory.

Predisposing Factors for Telangiectatic Matting

Risk factors for the development of TM (Table 13-6) is a controversial topic. Estrogens are known to be angiogenic in nature; the author has studied their presence in TM and has been unable to isolate them in this setting by monoclonal antibody techniques. However, these agents may produce these changes by secondary indirect vasodilatory mechanisms. Other less studied factors that have been described in the literature include obesity, a family history of TM, and a prolonged duration of pretreatment vessels. Further studies by the author are presently in progress, looking at angiogenic cytokines that are likely responsible for the development of TM as stated in the previous discussion on pathogenesis.

Measures to Help Minimize Telangiectatic Matting

The measures helpful in minimizing TM are listed in Table 13-7. Technique modifications including utilization of MSCs; low-volume, low-pressure injection techniques; and early treatment of foci of proximal reflux are probably the most helpful factors in minimizing these difficult-to-treat complications. Physiologic modifications, including discontinuance of estrogen therapy, 1 month prior and 2

TABLE 13-7. MEASURES TO HELP MINIMIZE TELANGIECTATIC MATTING

Utilize minimal sclerosant concentrations
Use low injection pressures, particularly in high-risk anatomic locations
Use no more than 1 mL of sclerosant per injection site
Limit injection blanch to 1–2 cm
Encourage patients to discontinue oral contraceptive therapy for 1 month prior and 2 months following sclerotherapy treatment
Encourage normalization of body weight
Eliminate points of reflux prior to treatment of associated telangiectasias

months following planned treatments as well as normalization of body weight in obese individuals are probably also helpful maneuvers.

Treatment of Telangiectatic Matting

Of greatest importance is that approximately 90% of TM will resolve spontaneously in 3 to 12 months. Because of the limited scope of treatment modalities, preventive measures listed in Table 13-8 assume greater importance. The author has had good success in treating these neoangiogenic vessels with both the extended-duration pulse dye laser (Candela Corp., Wayland, MA, U.S.A.) using a 600-nm wavelength and employing a new dynamic cooling device with a 5- or 7-mm round spot handpiece and a fluence of 18 to 20 J/cm^2. Good results have also been obtained with flash-lamp therapy (a noncoherent light source such as Photoderm (E.S.C./Sharplan, Needham, MA, U.S.A.) 550-nm (light skin types I to II) or 570-nm (dark skin types III to IV) cutoff filters with a pulse duration of 6 ms and fluences of 30 to 40 J/cm^2). Alternately a double-pulse modality may be employed, utilizing a pulse duration of 2.5/6.0 ms with a 20-ms delay and energy fluences of 45 to 50 J/cm^2. Approximately 60% to 70% of patients may have resolution of their TM after an average of two treatment sessions spaced 4 weeks apart in cases that do not resolve spontaneously. Laser and flash-lamp options are the treatments of choice when blushes of neoangiogenic vessels appear.

Alternately, microinjections of these small-diameter vessels utilizing small-gauge needles (31- to 33-gauge disposable or autoclavable), employing low injection pressures, have also been helpful in selected settings. Disposable insulin syringes (0.5 mL; Becton Dickinson and Company, Rutherford, NJ, U.S.A) utilizing microgauge needles (33-gauge) have been successful in selected patients with refractory TM. These disposable needles are stiffer and sharper than autoclavable needles of similar gauge.

More recently, microangiocath devices (previously described), including the 33-gauge small vein infusion system (Kawasumi Labs America Inc., Tampa, FL, U.S.A.) and the 30-gauge STD microsclerotherapy infusion system (STD, Hereford, England) have been found to be extremely helpful in treating isolated foci of neoangiogenic microtelangiectases (Fig. 13-6).

Injection of reticular veins feeding areas of TM has also been found to be helpful. These veins may lie below the epidermal surface; improved identification may be accomplished by transepidermal illumination (venoscopy).

TABLE 13-8. TREATMENT OF TELANGIECTATIC MATTING

Probably effective
Laser/flash-lamp therapy
Pulsed dye/extended-duration pulsed dye laser (595–600 nm) (Candela Corporation, Wayland, MA, U.S.A.)
Photoderm (E.S.C./Sharplan, Needham, MA, U.S.A.)
Microneedle/microcannula injections
Injection of reticular veins feeding areas of telangiectatic matting
Possibly effective
Antiangiogenins
Protamine
β-xylosides
β-cyclodextrin tetradeasulfate

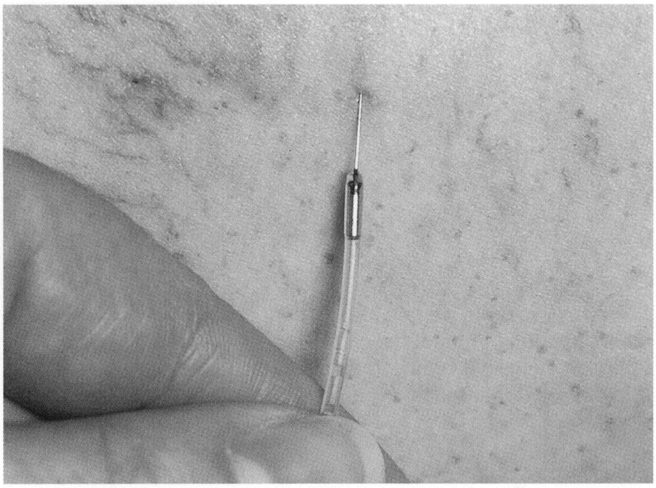

Figure 13-6
Treatment of telangiectatic matting may be accomplished with microinfusion systems, such as the one illustrated, which incorporates small-diameter tubing and a 33-gauge needle (Kawasumi Labs America Inc., Tampa, FL, U.S.A.).

Finally; investigative trials presently in progress are employing antiangiogenins such as protamine, beta xylosides, and cyclo-dextrin tetradeosulfate, which, when added to sclerosing solutions, may help to minimize the incidence of TM.

Syncope

Syncope is an infrequent but important to recognize complication occurring in the sclerotherapy setting. Recognition of this syndrome is the most important facet of this stress-related finding. It must be differentiated from type I anaphylactic hypersensitivity reactions.

Light-headedness, nausea, sweating, and disorientation are the classic clinical findings.

Prevention

Several measures (Table 13-9) may be instituted in order to prevent sclerotherapy-related syncope. Perhaps the most important is documentation of vasovagal tendencies. In such individuals, presclerotherapy monitoring of blood pressure and heart rate may be instituted.

Other helpful measures include instructing the patient to eat a light meal prior to each treatment session; adequate ventilation, and consideration of treatment of predisposed patients in a totally supine position. In addition, careful physician and patient communication takes on greater importance in the treatment of such predisposed individuals.

TABLE 13-9. PREVENTION/TREATMENT OF SYNCOPE

A light meal eaten by the patient prior to treatment sessions
Documentation of vasovagal tendencies
Presclerotherapy monitoring of blood pressure and heart rate
Adequate ventilation
Careful physician–patient communication
Consideration of treatment with patient in a totally supine position

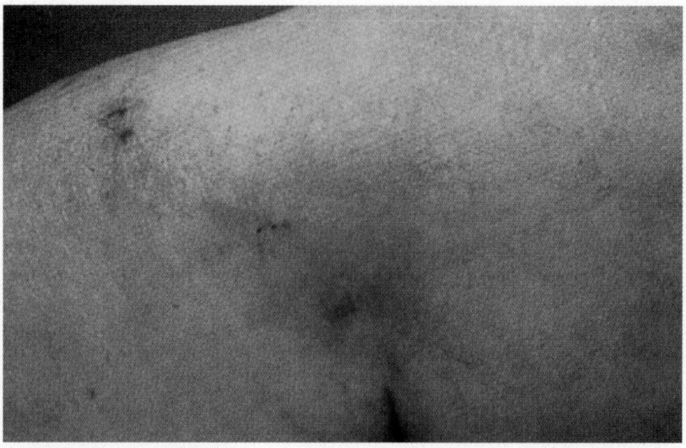

Figure 13-7
Localized urticarial wheals at injection sites appearing immediately after injection of class II venulectasia with 23.4% hypertonic saline.

Treatment

If a syncopal episode is documented, the patient should be placed in a supine Trendelenburg position. Assurance and/or moist compresses and ammonia inhalants (James Alexander Corp., Blairstown, NJ, U.S.A.) may be helpful.

Utilization of sclerosants associated with decreased pain, such as STS and polidocanol, is preferred in this setting.

Localized Urticaria

Localized urticaria present as erythematous wheals that may occur after instillation of any sclerosing agent in a susceptible individual (Fig. 13-7). The fact that it usually occurs at all treatment sites and with the instillation of unadulterated 23.4% hypertonic saline (HS) mitigates against systemic or localized antigen-mediated allergy. More likely it is the result of sclerosant-mediated endothelial inflammation with subsequent release of histamine and other inflammatory cytokine mediators. It usually resolves in 30 to 60 minutes. Several patterns are recognized. First of all, in susceptible individuals, it is usually recurrent with subsequent treatment sessions. This is a generalization but not an absolute rule. In susceptible individuals, the urticaria tends to be more intense with increased sclerosant concentrations. Of importance is differentiation of this phenomenon from a true immunologic hypersensitivity reaction.

Treatment

Factors shown to be helpful in the treatment of localized urticaria (Table 13-10) include pretreatment with H_1 antihistamines and topical twice-daily application of a medium-potency topical steroid cream such as fluocinolone acetonide (Dermik, Collegeville, PA, U.S.A.).

Finally, utilization of minimal sclerosant concentrations (MSC) and limiting injection quantities per injection site may ameliorate the urticaria, when recognized, in subsequent treatment sessions.

TABLE 13-10. TREATMENT OF LOCAL URTICARIA

Pretreatment with H_1 antihistamines
Medium-potency topical corticosteroids
Utilization of minimal sclerosant concentrations
Limitation of injection quantities per injection site

Bruising

Bruising is a common phenomenon after all forms of sclerotherapy treatment. It is related to vascular inflammation and subsequent direct extravasation of erythrocytes. It is temporary and should not be alarming to either the patient or the sclerotherapist. It presents as a purple ecchymotic mat surrounding treated vessels (Fig. 13-8).

Predisposing factors of bruising include vascular fragility states, as stated in the previous section on hyperpigmentation.

Prevention

Prevention (Table 13-11) is best accomplished by practicing fastidious technique and minimizing the number of puncture sites utilized during a given treatment session, as endothelial transection is a major factor related to the development of bruising. Low sclerosant injection pressures and utilization of MSCs are other adjuvant factors that may be helpful in minimizing these sequelae.

Finally, discontinuation of medications such as nonsteroidal antiinflammatory drugs (NSAIDs) prior to performing sclerotherapy is indicated.

Treatment

Treatment (Table 13-12) may include the application of vitamin K cream (Merck and Company, Inc., West Point, PA, U.S.A.; LaRoche Labs, Inc., Nutley, NJ, U.S.A.) (Fig. 13-9). It is applied twice daily for 5 days prior to sclerosant sessions and continued for 3 days after each session in order to minimize the amount of bruising that occurs in susceptible individuals. Adequate postsclerotherapy compression may also be helpful.

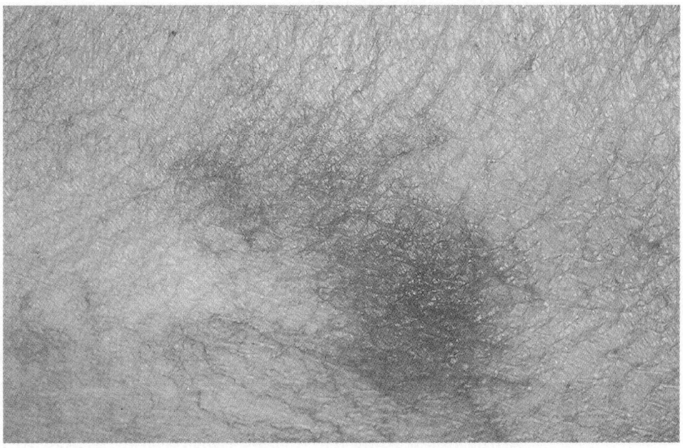

Figure 13-8

Postsclerotherapy bruising presenting as ecchymotic purple patches along sites of treated vessels.

TABLE 13-11. PREVENTION OF POSTSCLEROTHERAPY BRUISING

Fastidious technique
Application of minimal sclerosant concentration
Use of low injection pressures
Recognition of vascular fragility states
Discontinuance of medications such as salicylates, warfarin, and NSAIDs prior to treatment

Edema

Lower extremity edema is related to hydrostatic considerations and endothelial permeability as well as perivascular inflammatory factors. It is most common when veins below the ankle are treated by sclerotherapy. It may also be a consequence of the utilization of nongraduated compression.

Prevention

Prevention (Table 13-13) of lower extremity edema may be accomplished by limiting the quantity of sclerosing solution to 1 mL per ankle. In addition, the use of postsclerotherapy graduated compression hosiery with a gradient of 30 to 40 mm Hg (class II) may minimize edema, particularly when treating veins in the feet.

Treatment

Edema is self-limited and requires no specific therapy, although elevation of the affected extremity may ameliorate it. The edema usually resolves within 18 to 72 hours.

Compression-Related Problems

The most common problems related to bandaging include:

Ulcers
Pressure bullae
Contact dermatitis
Folliculitis

Pressure ulcers and bullae are most commonly related to tight occlusive dressings or pressure pads over areas of friction-related mobility such as the ankle, posterior calf, medial thigh, and popliteal fossa. Atrophic skin is most susceptible to such changes.

TABLE 13-12. TREATMENT OF POSTSCLEROTHERAPY BRUISING

Vitamin K cream
Apply twice daily for 5 days before and 3 days after treatment
Adequate postsclerotherapy compression

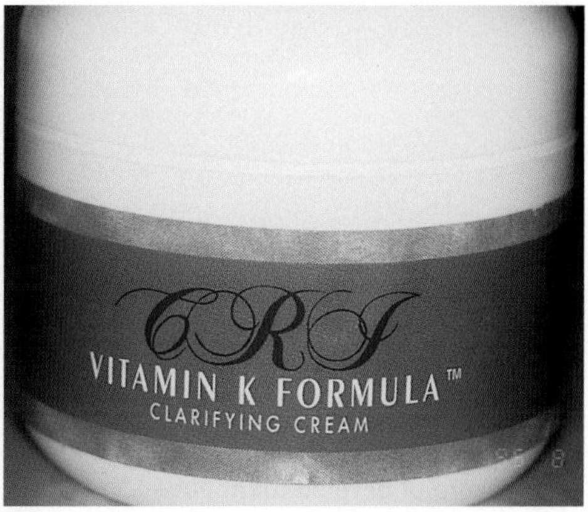

Figure 13-9
Vitamin K cream may be applied twice daily. 5 days before and 3 days after sclerotherapy sessions in order to minimize postsclerotherapy bruising by improving vascular integrity.

Ulcers are usually superficial (middermal) (Fig. 13-10) and must be distinguished from extravasation necrosis reactions, where the ulcerations are deeper (reticular dermis → subcutaneous fat → fascia) and associated with more significant necrotizing changes.

Blisters are usually flaccid and superficial and may be noted with any adhesive preparation. Like ulcers, they occur more commonly in fragile atrophic cutaneous sites.

Contact dermatitis (Fig. 13-11) may present as patchy erythema or a papulovesicular dermatitis. Adhesives are the major irritant source.

Folliculitis, when present, occurs as a pustular or papulopustular eruption, usually sterile in nature, although occasionally *Staphylococcus aureus, Pseudomonas aeruginosa,* or *Candida albicans* may be isolated. It is usually due to occlusive phenomena and is more common during the warm summer months.

Prevention

Blisters and ulcers may be minimized (Table 13-14) by checking the tightness of bandages, particularly if the patient complains of increasing pain.

Hypoallergenic paper tape (Dermilite II, Johnson & Johnson, New Brunswick, NJ, U.S.A) may be utilized as an alternative over foam pads or cotton balls.

The utilization of beveled rubber foam pads (STD, Hereford, England) may decrease pressure over treatment sites of large veins.

Tubigrip tubular support bandages (Seton Products, Inc., Montgomeryville, PA, U.S.A.) may be utilized over compression pads in place of standard graduated support hose in order to decrease pressure phenomena.

Finally, folliculitis may be minimized by changing dressings every 24 to 48 hours, particularly during the summer months.

TABLE 13-13. PREVENTION/TREATMENT OF LOWER EXTREMITY EDEMA

Limit the quantity of sclerosing solution to 1 mL per ankle
Use of postsclerotherapy (class II) 30–40 mm Hg graduated compression

Figure 13-10

Superficial erosions secondary to pressure of beveled foam pads after sclerotherapy treatment.

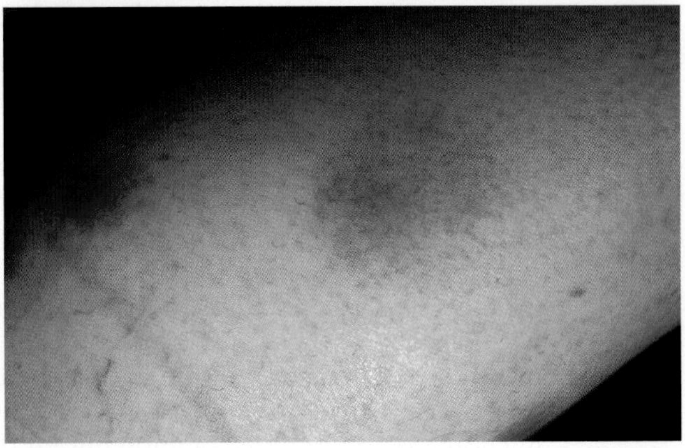

Figure 13-11

Contact dermatitis presenting as erythema and purple hyperpigmentation secondary to use of 3M Microfoam tape (3M Medical Surgical Division, St. Paul, MN, U.S.A.).

TABLE 13-14. PREVENTION OF COMPRESSION-RELATED ULCERS, BLISTERS, CONTACT DERMATITIS, AND FOLLICULITIS

Check tightness of bandages if patient complains of increasing pain
Use of beveled rubber foam pads
Use Tubigrip tubular support bandages (Seton Products Inc., Montgomeryville, PA, U.S.A.)
Change occlusive dressings at 24–48 hours, particularly during summer months
Utilize hypoallergenic paper tape

TABLE 13-15. TREATMENT OF COMPRESSION-RELATED ULCERS, BLISTERS, CONTACT DERMATITIS, AND FOLLICULITIS

Aluminum acetate 1%–5% Domeboro Solution (Bayer Corporation, West Haven, CT, U.S.A.)
Medium-potency corticosteroid lotions and creams
Hydrocolloid dressings (i.e., Duoderm, Convatec, Princeton, NJ, U.S.A.)
Mupirocin ointment (Bactroban, SmithKline Beecham Pharmaceuticals, Philadelphia, PA, U.S.A.)

Treatment

Ulcers and blisters may be treated (Table 13-15) by routine reepithelializing therapies such as desiccating wet to dry dressings [Domeboro Solution (5% aluminum acetate), Bayer Corporation, West Haven, CT, U.S.A.] and antibacterial ointments such as Bactroban (SmithKline-Beecham Pharmaceuticals, Philadelphia, PA, U.S.A.).

In more severe areas of ulceration, hydrocolloid dressings such as Duoderm (Convatec, Princeton, NJ, U.S.A.) may be utilized.

Contact Dermatitis

Contact dermatitis reactions may be treated by a minimally sensitizing medium-potency steroid such as hydrocortisone butyrate (Loccoid Cream 0.1%, Ferndale Labs, Ferndale, MI, U.S.A.).

Inclusive inflammatory folliculitis may be treated with 1% to 2% hydrocortisone lotion (Hytone, Dermik Labs, Collegeville, PA, U.S.A.). Secondary infectious folliculitis may be treated with application of Mupirocin (Bactroban, SmithKline Beecham Pharmaceuticals, Philadelphia, PA, U.S.A.) ointment twice daily.

Hirsutism

Hirsutism is a rare occurrence (Fig. 13-12) and is probably related to changes in hemodynamics that occur at vessel treatment sites. It is usually temporary and the hair usually falls out 3 to 4 months after presentation with no special therapy. Usually it presents with local hypertrichosis of terminal hairs at treatment sites.

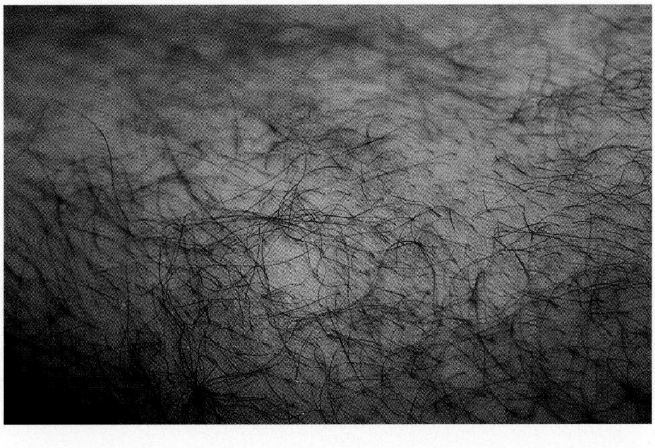

Figure 13-12

Localized hirsutism. Localized hypertrichosis of terminal hairs is usually temporary, with fallout occurring within 3 to 4 months.

Needle Phobia

Needle phobia is a phenomenon that must be recognized by the physician at the time of the initial consultation and dealt with either by utilizing visual blindfolds or another modality of therapy such as flash-lamp or laser intervention when deemed applicable.

Scotomata

Many physicians including the author have described temporary blindness or unusual visual disturbances after sclerotherapy. Ischemia of the calcarine cortex, either through vasospasm or embolism of the ophthalmic arteries, has been hypothesized. These findings are usually associated with a benign outcome and the condition resolves spontaneously in 30 to 60 minutes. It is recommended, however, that such patients be examined by an ophthalmologist to rule out other more significant conditions.

Uncommon (Major) Sclerotherapy Complications

Ulceration

Cutaneous ulcerative necrosis may occur with the injection of any sclerosing agent, although several agents pose a greater risk in this respect. Although the majority of cases are probably related to technique, this is not always the case. The major hypothesized etiologic factors of postsclerotherapy cutaneous necrosis are:

- Extravasation of sclerosing solution into perivascular tissue
- Intradermal arteriolar injection or injection into an arteriovenous malformation
- Vascular spasm
- Extravasation secondary to vascular fragility syndromes
- Compression- or bandage-related necrosis

Technique-related cutaneous necrosis is related to extravasation of sclerosing solution into perivascular soft tissue. It is related to vessel wall disruption and is probably the most important factor related to extravasation necrosis. Of commonly utilized sclerosing agents, the relative incidence of necrosis is felt to be as follows:

Hypertonic saline → STS → Polyiodide iodine → Polidocanol → Chromated glycerine

Injection of telangiectasias associated with dermal arterioles may also be a cause of extravasation necrosis. The incidence of this pathophysiologic factor is unknown.

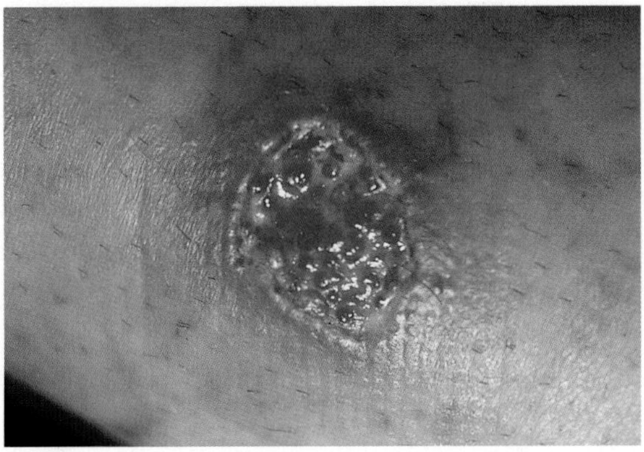

Figure 13-13

Postsclerotherapy necrotic ulceration following extravasation of hypertonic saline.

The role of vascular spasm in producing ulceration is also unknown, although it is felt that arterial spasm may be a predisposing factor to this untoward sequela.

Vascular fragility states such as protein C and S deficiency as well as antiphospholipid antibody states may predispose individuals to vascular leakage of sclerosant and subsequent cutaneous ulceration.

Finally, overzealous compression of the skin overlying treated veins may lead to anoxia, with the subsequent development of ischemia-induced ulceration.

Ulceration usually manifests as blanching in perivascular tissue, often presenting with a porcelain white appearance. Pain may be an associated finding, particularly when dealing with sclerosants such as hypertonic saline and polidocanol. A hemorrhagic bulla usually forms over this area within 2 to 48 hours and then usually progresses to form a necrotic ulcer (Fig. 13-13). In vascular fragility states, multiple ulcerations may occur at individual treatment sites (Fig. 13-14). During the healing phase, a dry eschar with surrounding erythema usually appears. Ulcerations usually take 6 to 12 weeks to reepithelialize, depending on the depth of cutaneous involvement.

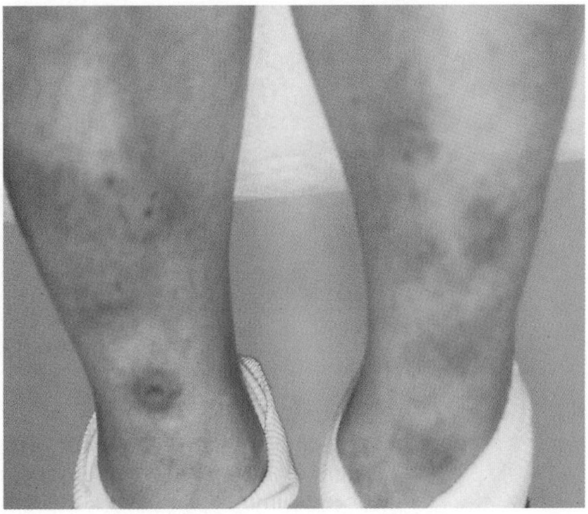

Figure 13-14

Multiple ulceration sites after sodium tetradecylsulfate sclerotherapy in a patient with protein C deficiency not previously diagnosed.

TABLE 13-16. MEASURES HELPFUL IN PREVENTING ULCERATIVE NECROSIS

Fastidious technique
  Nitroglycerin ointment 2%
Dilution of hypertonic sclerosants with normal saline
Hyaluronidase (Wydase, Wyeth–Ayerst Laboratories, Philadelphia, PA, U.S.A.)
    75–150 U USP
Utilization of double compression hose (each 15–20 mm Hg) in order to keep
    supine compression below 30 mm Hg
Recognition of vascular fragility states
  Protein C deficiency
  Protein S deficiency
  Antiphospholipid antibody syndrome

Prevention

If extravasation is suspected or perivascular whitening occurs which suggests vasospasm, several clinicians have advocated rubbing in a small amount of 2% nitroglycerin ointment (generic) into the involved area (Table 13-16; Fig. 13-15).

In addition, one should immediately attempt to dilute the sclerosant at the site of extravasation. If hypertonic solutions have been employed, these should be diluted by immediate instillation of normal saline. In addition, if detergent sclerosing agents such as STS are utilized, dilution with lyophilized hyaluronidase 150 USP U/mL (Wydase, Wyeth–Ayerst Laboratories, Philadelphia, PA, U.S.A.) has been shown—via a mechanism that promotes diffusion of solution through tissues and subsequent absorption—to decrease the incidence of subsequent ulcerative necrosis (Fig. 13-16). Doses of 75 to 150 USP units diluted in 5 mL of 0.9% sodium chloride are recommended to be instilled immediately at sites of suspected extravasation.

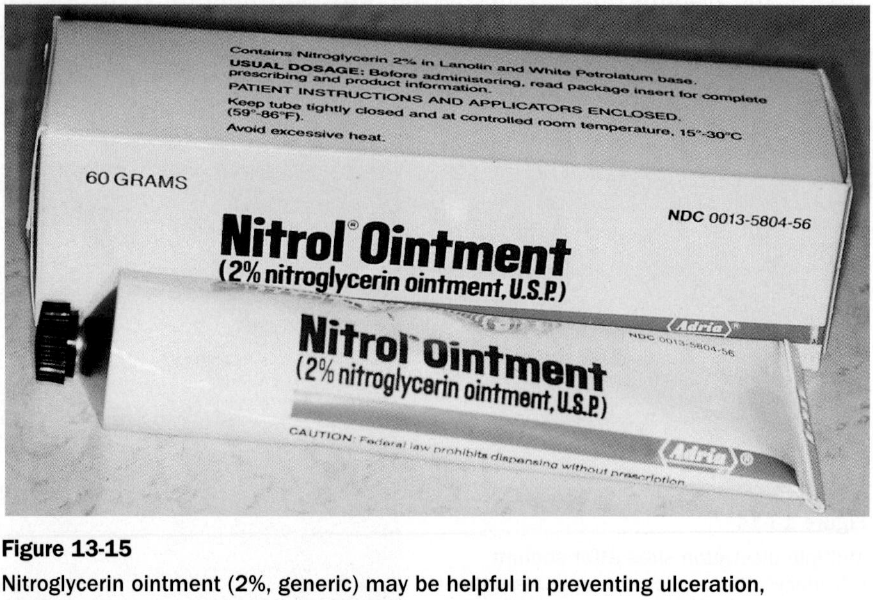

Figure 13-15

Nitroglycerin ointment (2%, generic) may be helpful in preventing ulceration, particularly when vasospasm or arteriolar communications are suspected as evidenced by immediate postsclerotherapy blanching.

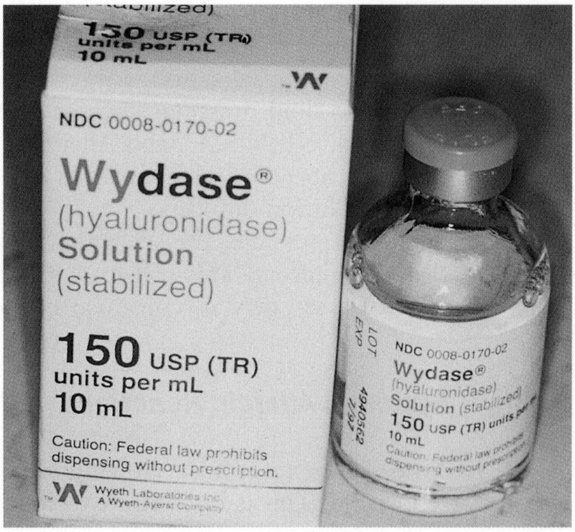

Figure 13-16
Hyaluronidase (Wydase, Wyeth–Ayerst Laboratories, Philadelphia PA, U.S.A.) in dosages of 75 to 150 U USP diluted in 5 mL of 0.9% sodium chloride may be instilled immediately after suspected extravasation of detergent sclerosants in order to minimize extravasation necrosis by changing tissue diffusion coefficients, thus increasing absorption of extravasated sclerosant.

Urticarial reactions have been described following hyaluronidase instillation. Finally, because of its limited stability, hyaluronidase should be reconstituted with 0.9% sodium chloride.

Recognition of vascular fragility states is helpful in identifying patients at increased risk for developing postsclerotherapy ulcerations.

Finally double-layer graduated compression hose (two stockings with 15 to 20 mm Hg compression) may prevent excess compression over treated vessels, as it is felt that external pressure greater than 30 to 40 mm Hg in a prolonged supine position may cause muscle ischemia.

Removal of the second set of compression stocking while the patient is recumbent would subsequently decrease cutaneous pressures to 20 to 30 mm Hg at the ankle, which would theoretically prevent cutaneous ischemia.

Treatment

Treatment options for ulcerations due to extravasation are geared toward maximizing healing parameters (Table 13-17).

If ulcerations are small, less than 4 mm in diameter, they may be allowed to heal by secondary intention.

Wet to dry compresses utilizing an antibacterial astringent such as Domeboro Solution (1% to 5%) (Bayer Corporation, West Haven, CT, U.S.A.), with subse-

TABLE 13-17. TREATMENT OF NECROTIZING ULCERATIONS

Ulcerations of less than 4 mm heal well by primary intention
Burow's (Domeboro, Bayer Corporation, West Haven, CT U.S.A.) solution 1%–5%
Mupirocin (Bactroban, SmithKline Beecham Pharmaceuticals, Philadelphia, PA, U.S.A.) ointment
Ulcerations greater than 4 mm should be excised with primary closure, when possible, at the earliest possible time
Hydrocolloid dressings
Duoderm (Convatec, Bristol Meyers Squibb, Princeton, NJ, U.S.A.)
Allervyne (Smith and Nephew, Largo, FL, U.S.A.)

quent application of an antibacterial ointment such as Mupirocin (Bactroban, SmithKline Beecham Pharmaceuticals, Philadelphia, PA, U.S.A.) may aid in promoting reepithelialization. Larger ulceration may also benefit from the application of hydrocolloid dressings such as Duoderm (Convatec, Bristol Meyers Squibb, Princeton, NJ, U.S.A.) and Allervyne (Smith and Nephew, Largo, FL, U.S.A.). These agents may decrease pain as well as increase wound healing, leading to more rapid resolution of ulcers.

When possible, the sclerotherapist may also consider excision with primary closure of ulcers. This will lead to rapid resolution of the complication and, in selected cases, may also produce a superior cosmetic result.

Systemic Allergic Reactions

True allergic reactions following sclerotherapy treatments are extremely rare and reportable. This is in contrast to localized urticarial reactions, which occur with greater frequency and are not a sign of systemic hypersensitivity. In addition, these reactions must be distinguished from vasovagal reactions, which are more frequent. Diaphoresis, bradycardia, and changing mentation, as previously described in the discussion of syncopal episodes, characterize this untoward event.

True allergic reactions may be characterized as mild, moderate, or severe. Mild cutaneous manifestations usually occur on a delayed basis some 8 to 16 hours after a single sclerotherapy treatment session. These reactions may be urticarial in nature or may present as generalized morbilliform or maculopapular eruptions. Their immunologic mechanism of action is probably related to type IV delayed hypersensitivity.

Moderate reactions may present as generalized urticaria with associated angioedema of the face and tongue, which may occur within minutes of sclerosant injection. Mild stridor may be an associated finding. This symptom complex is related to type I immediate hypersensitivity.

Severe reactions also occur almost immediately after sclerosant injection. A typical sequence of events often ensues, beginning with itching, anxiety, and tachycardia, then progressing to generalized urticaria, angioedema, and bronchospasm, and often eventuating in cardiovascular collapse secondary to generalized vascular dilatation. This complex of anaphylaxis may occur after initial exposure to sclerosant antigen; however, more commonly, it occurs following reexposure to the sensitizing antigen. A distinguishing factor of anaphylaxis that helps to differentiate it from a syncopal episode is the development of tachycardia in the former clinical setting while bradycardia is more commonly found in the vasovagal or syncopal setting.

Hypersensitivity Potential of Commonly Employed Sclerosants

Only hypertonic saline (HS) presents with no antigenic allergenicity potential. However, the utilization of additives such as benzoate, lidocaine, or heparin can negate this and lead to the development of hypersensitivity reactions in susceptible individuals.

Sodium tetradecyl sulfate (STS), which is in common use in this country, has a surprisingly low allergenic potential (approximately 0.3%). These reactions are most commonly nonfatal delayed hypersensitivity maculopapular eruptions developing 30 to 90 minutes after injection.

Polidocanol (POL) reactions also occur with minimal incidence (approximately 0.01%). Both urticarial and generalized morbilliform reactions have been reported. A rare death due to anaphylaxis has been reported.

In perspective, the extensive worldwide usage of both STS and POL is associated with a minimal incidence of adverse allergenic events.

Chromated glycerin (CG) has been associated with rare systemic hypersensitivity reactions, although contact sensitivity to chromium occurs in approximately 5% of treated individuals.

Sodium morrhuate (SM) has a more significant allergenic potential. A spectrum of reactions varying from urticaria to severe anaphylactic reactions has been reported in up to 3% of treated individuals.

Ethanolamine oleate (EO) has been associated with rare urticarial and fatal anaphylactic reactions which may be related to either the ethanolamine or oleic acid moieties.

Polyiodide iodine (PII) has been associated with local cutaneous allergic reactions (approximately 0.01%) but no systemic hypersensitivity. Because it is a mixture of iodide ions, sodium iodine and benzyl alcohol, this agent should be utilized with caution in patients with hyperthyroidism and known hypersensitivity to iodine or benzyl alcohol.

Prevention

Of greatest importance, patients should be counseled about the allergic potential of sclerosant agents during the initial consultation, and, this should be reemphasized when informed consent is obtained. If the patient is not willing to undertake this risk then a nonallergenic agent such as HS should be employed as a sclerosing agent.

Other helpful hints that may be helpful in prevention (Table 13-18) include scheduling an initial test treatment session. Finally, it is prudent to have the patient sit in the waiting room for 15 to 30 minutes, particularly following the first treatment session, when using agents other than HS.

Treatment

Mild reactions such as urticaria or morbilliform eruptions may be treated (Table 13-19) with diphenhydramine (Benadryl, 25 to 50 mg t.i.d. to q.i.d.

TABLE 13-18. PREVENTION OF ALLERGIC REACTIONS

Informed consent with explanation of incidence of hypersensitivity reactions associated with each sclerosing agent to be employed during the initial presclerotherapy consultation
Obtain history of lidocaine or preservative hypersensitivity
Small initial treatment session
Have patient sit in waiting room for 15–30 minutes following treatment sessions (particularly first) when using agents other than hypertonic saline

TABLE 13-19. TREATMENT OF ALLERGIC REACTIONS

Type of Reaction	Clinical Presentation	Treatment
Mild	Pruritus	Diphenhydramine (Benadryl, Warner–Wellcome, Morris Plains, NJ, U.S.A.) 50 mg t.i.d.–q.i.d.
	Urticaria	or
	Maculopapular eruptions Morbilliform eruptions	Epinephrine 1:1000, 0.2–0.5 mL s.c. (may repeat q3 min)
		Prednisone 40–60 mg/day × 7–10 days
Moderate	Generalized urticaria Angioedema	Epinephrine 1:1000, 0.2–0.5 mL s.c. (may repeat q3 min)
	Stridor Wheezing	Diphenhydramine (Benadryl) 50–80 mg i.m. or i.v. with theophylline i.v. 4–6 mg/kg infused over 15 min
		Methylprednisolone sodium succinate (Medrol, Upjohn, Kalamazoo, MI, U.S.A.) 60 mg i.v. (repeated q6h for 4–5 dosages)
Severe	Anaphylactic shock Cardiovascular collapse	Epinephrine 5–10 mL at 1:10,000 i.v. (0.5–1 mL of epinephrine 1:1000 diluted to 5–10 mL with saline (may repeat q5 min)
		Diphenhydramine (Benadryl) 50 mg i.v. with cimetidine (Tagamet, SmithKline Beecham, Philadelphia, PA, U.S.A.) 300 mg i.v.
		Methylprednisolone sodium succinate 60 mg i.v. repeated q6h for 4–5 dosages
		Theophylline (Roxane, Columbus, OH, U.S.A.) 4–6 mg/kg i.v.
		Oxygen (nasal cannula) 4–6 L/min
		Consider endotracheal intubation Tracheostomy Hospitalization

(Warner–Wellcome, Morris Plains, NJ, U.S.A.). Alternatively, a loading dose of diphenhydramine (Benadryl) 50 mg i.n. may be administered. More severe urticarial responses and those associated with mild bronchospasm may be controlled with subcutaneous administration of 0.2 to 0.5 mL of 1:1000 epinephrine with repeated dosages as required at 3-minute intervals. Type IV maculopapular eruptions may be treated with prednisone 40 to 60 mg/day for 7 to 10 days.

Moderate reactions such as urticaria associated with angioedema may be treated with diphenhydramine 50 to 75 mg given i.m. or i.v. administered in conjunction with cimetidine 300 mg i.v. (Tagamet, SmithKline Beecham, Philadelphia, PA, U.S.A.) in addition to epinephrine in the previously stated dosage. Wheezing associated with bronchospasm may be treated additionally with bronchodilators such as intravenous theophylline 4 to 6 mg/kg (Roxane, Columbus, OH, U.S.A.) infused over 15 minutes. Corticosteroids such as methylprednisolone sodium succinate (Medrol) (Upjohn, Kalamazoo, MI, U.S.A.) 60 mg given intravenously every 6 hours for 4 to 5 doses may help to prevent delayed recurrence of symptoms.

In the most severe anaphylactic reactions, such as those associated with impending cardiovascular collapse, oxygen is administered via a nasal cannula, and an intravenous line should be started with fluid replacement utilizing Ringer's lactate. Epinephrine is administered 0.5 to 1 mL (1:1000 diluted with 5 to 10 mL normal saline) yielding 5 to 10 mL of a 1:1000 dilution to be given intravenously and repeated every 5 minutes until vital signs and clinical symptoms are stabilized. Diphenhydramine, intravenous aminophylline, and methylprednisolone sodium succinate are administered in the previously stated dosage regimens. If respiratory compromise continues despite these measures, then transfer to a hospital critical care unit, endotracheal intubation, or tracheostomy must be considered.

Of greatest importance, all of the previously stated emergency treatment protocols must be readily available in the sclerotherapist's office for immediate activation. All of the above medications must be available on the cardiopulmonary resuscitation cart in association with intravenous lines and fluids. A designated member of the office staff should be responsible for carrying out these protocols and for ensuring that all medications are periodically reviewed. Protocols should be typed out and available to all office personnel for appropriate reference.

Thrombophlebitis

Superficial thrombophlebitis most commonly occurs as a rare isolated phenomenon. It most commonly occurs 1 to 3 weeks following sclerotherapy and presents as a tender, erythematous, nodular plaque over a treated vessel (Fig. 13-17). Large reticular veins 3 to 4 mm in diameter are the most susceptible vessels. The incidence of thrombophlebitis has varied from 0.1% to 5% in various series, although the former incidence is more consistent with the author's experience. The most common sequela of thrombi is hyperpigmentation, although in rare cases clot migration may involve perforating veins and the deep venous system, leading to valvular damage and a subsequent potential for the development of pulmonary emboli.

Prevention

Thrombophlebitis may be related to inadequate compression resulting in excessive intravascular thrombus. The use of adequate local spot compression and graduated hosiery at sufficient pressures (see Chapter 12) will help to minimize the development of postsclerotherapy thrombosis (Table 13-20).

Evaluation of postsclerotherapy thrombi with clot evacuation utilizing a number 11 Bard Parker blade may help eliminate tenderness and minimize the risk of hyperpigmentation (Fig. 13-18).

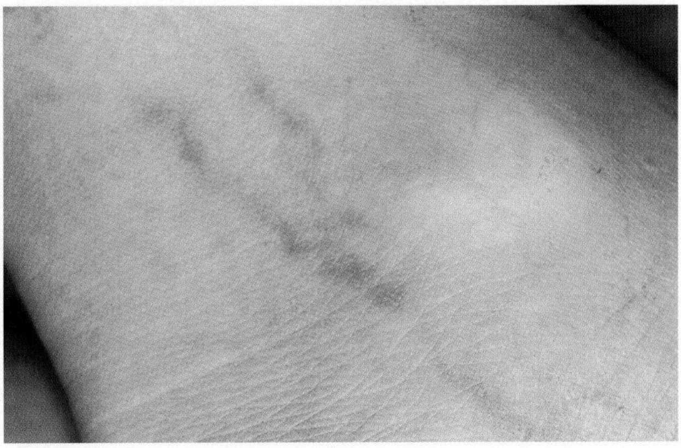

Figure 13-17

A tender erythematous, indurated plaque representing a focus of superficial thrombophlebitis appeared 2 weeks after sclerotherapy of a reticular vein 4 mm in diameter. Sodium tetradecylsulfate 0.25% was used as sclerosant, along with class II 20-mm Hg graduated compression.

TABLE 13-20. PREVENTION OF THROMBOPHLEBITIS

- ▶ Adequate local compression pads
- ▶ Adequate graduated compression hosiery
- ▶ Evacuation of postsclerotherapy thrombi (clot evacuation)
- ▶ Consideration of ambulatory phlebectomy rather than sclerotherapy for treatment of large (>4 mm in diameter) reticular veins

Because of the higher incidence of thrombi and thrombophlebitis in large reticular veins, these may, alternatively, be treated by ambulatory phlebectomy rather than sclerotherapy.

Treatment

Treatment of superficial thrombophlebitis (Table 13-21) is usually conservative. The cornerstones of therapy include evacuation of clot with adequate compression and frequent ambulation, which should be maintained until pain and inflammation have resolved. Tepid compresses, aspirin (325 to 1000 mg q.i.d.), and other nonsteroidal antiinflammatory drugs such as ibuprofen 300 to 800 mg t.i.d. (Motrin, Upjohn, Kalamazoo, MI, U.S.A.) may be helpful in limiting both inflammation and pain. These symptoms usually respond rapidly within 7 to 10 days.

Deep Venous Thrombosis/Pulmonary Embolus

Deep venous thrombosis and the subsequent development of pulmonary embolus is extremely rare after sclerotherapy of the superficial venous system. This is of

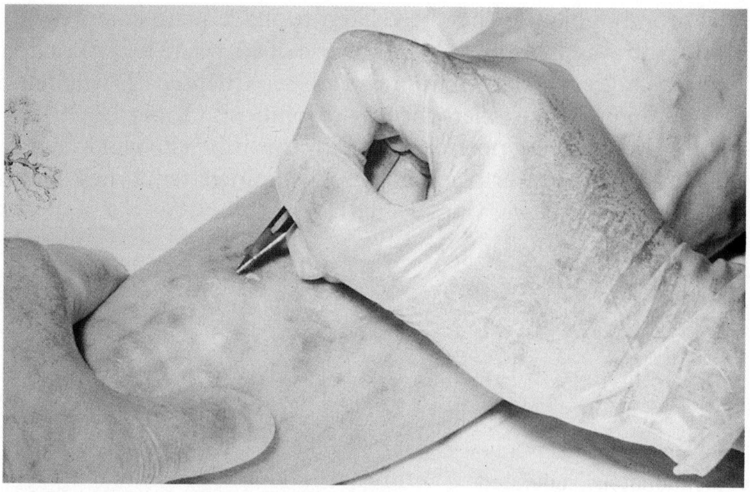

Figure 13-18

Area of superficial clot formation with associated thrombophlebitis. The clot was evacuated following stab incision utilizing a number 11 Bard Parker blade.

TABLE 13-21. TREATMENT OPTIONS FOR SUPERFICIAL THROMBOPHLEBITIS

Clot evacuation (Bard Parker number 11 blade)
Adequate graduated compression
Frequent ambulation
Tepid compresses
Aspirin (325 mg–1000 mg q.i.d.)
Nonsteroidal antiinflammatory drugs (i.e., ibuprofen 300–800 mg t.i.d.)

interest, considering the following three factors:

1. It is well known that the superficial venous system communicates with the deep venous system via communicating perforators.
2. Sclerosant action induces endothelial damage.
3. Sclerotherapy produces a microenvironment of vascular stasis.

These are all factors that, theoretically, predispose individuals to thrombophlebitis.

Despite these factors, the incidence of deep venous thrombosis and pulmonary embolus formation is so rare that it is reportable. The incidence is more frequent in the setting of hypercoagulable states with deficiencies of inhibitors of coagulation such as antithrombin III, protein C or protein S or in secondary hypercoagulable states such as pregnancy and related elevated estrogen states—i.e., hormonal ingestion, malignancy, and obesity.

Although rare, the risks of deep venous thrombosis and possible pulmonary embolic sequelae must be discussed with the patient during the initial consultation.

Presenting signs include deep, tender nodules, fever, dyspnea, and tachycardia. These symptoms usually ensue 9 to 12 hours after a given sclerotherapy treatment.

Prevention

There are a number of maneuvers that may help to minimize the incidence of thromboembolic phenomena (Table 13-22). These include:

- Limiting the amount of sclerosant to 0.5 to 1 mL per injection site in order to prevent retrograde movement of sclerosant into the deep venous system.
- Adequate compression utilizing class I support hose (20 to 30 mmHg) for smaller-diameter vessels (below 4 mm in diameter) and class II support hose (30 to 40 mm Hg) for larger-diameter vessels (above 4 mm in diameter) in association with rapid, frequent ambulation will help to prevent sludging stasis phenomena and ensure adequate emptying of deep leg veins. Pumping of the calf immediately posttreatment may also act as an adjuvant maneuver to ensure patency of the deep venous system. Because the incidence of thromboembolic phenomena is greatest within 9 to 12 hours after a given treatment session, consideration must be

TABLE 13-22. PREVENTION OF DEEP VENOUS THROMBOSIS/PULMONARY EMBOLUS

Limit the amount of sclerosant to 0.5–1 mL per injection site
Rapid, adequate, graduated compression
Calf massage and dorsiflexion of the ankle immediately postsclerotherapy treatment
Recognition of hypercoagulable states
- Antithrombin III deficiency
- Protein C deficiency
- Protein S deficiency
- Pregnancy
- Estrogen/progestin replacement
- Malignancy
- Obesity
- Elderly

given to wearing support hose throughout the night, particularly during the first evening postinjection, as indicated.

- Finally recognition of hypercoagulable states, as previously stated, will identify those patients at greatest risk for developing these untoward sequelae. Consideration for discontinuing all oral contraceptive therapy, as well as instituting weight reduction when indicated, must be individualized and discussed between the patient and physician.

Treatment

Deep venous thrombosis is a medical emergency and must be recognized by the practicing sclerotherapist. This will prevent valvular damage and the potential for subsequent pulmonary embolus. Goals of therapy are (Table 13-23):

- To prevent growth of the thrombus
- To avoid development of new thrombi
- To prevent pulmonary embolization

Anticoagulation is carried out with intravenous heparin loading dose of

TABLE 13-23. TREATMENT OF DEEP VEIN THROMBOSIS/PULMONARY EMBOLISM

Acute
- Immediate intravenous heparinization
  - Loading dose 100 U/kg
- Fibrinolytic therapy options (consider for fresh thrombosis present <72 h)
  - Streptokinase
  - Urokinase

Chronic
- Coumarin derivatives (Coumadin)
- Keep prothrombin time 2–2.5 times normal value
- Continue therapy 3 months for deep venous thrombosis
- Continue therapy 6 months for pulmonary emboli

Prophylaxis
- Aspirin
- Dipyramidole

100 U/kg body weight, with subsequent dosages determined by laboratory coagulation parameters. Most patients require 1000 to 2000 U/hour to achieve adequate anticoagulation.

Low-molecular-weight heparins are associated with fewer bleeding complications.

Oral anticoagulation is usually continued with a coumarin derivative. The commonly recommended dose is that which increases the prothrombin time to 2 to 2.5 times the normal value. In every case (thrombus present for less than 72 hours), fibrinolytic activators such as streptokinase or urokinase may help accelerate thrombolysis.

After a deep venous thrombosis, oral anticoagulation is continued for at least 3 months, as this is the time required for the development of venous collaterals and is also the period during which most recurrence is seen. After pulmonary embolism, 6 months of anticoagulation is indicated.

Other antiplatelet agents, such as aspirin and dipyramidole may be utilized for long-term prophylaxis in selected areas.

Arterial Injection

Perhaps arterial injection is the most significant side effect of sclerotherapy. As more injections are being carried out in an attempt to sclerose the proximal greater and lesser saphenous veins at the groin or popliteal regions, the incidence of complications due to arterial injection is increasing. These problems have continued despite, paradoxically, the present state-of-the-art ultrasound-guided injections, image magnification, and reliance upon a two-dimensional duplex ultrasound display.

The classic sign of intraarterial injection following sclerotherapy is burning pain propagating rapidly and distally in the injected limb. This sign is valuable but not immediately present in all instances, especially when the sclerosant is STS. The development of erythematous or cyanotic color changes is a useful diagnostic sign. An even more precise clinical clue than color changes themselves is recognition of a sharply demarcated color change in an area adjacent to a given injection site.

At times there may not be clearly reliable clinical signs; thus the sclerotherapist must be constantly on guard for subtle signs of arterial injection and institute immediate therapy when the index of suspicion seems sufficiently high.

Arterial injection produces a "sludge embolus," which leads to subsequent thrombosis and necrosis. Although necrotic damage to skin and subcutaneous tissues is the most common sequela, damage to muscles, nerves, and major vessels may lead to the need for limb amputation and, in severe cases, damage to internal organs as well.

Common predisposing high-risk locations for arterial injection are:

- ▶ The junction of the femoral and greater saphenous veins (greater saphenous vein injection)
- ▶ The junction of the greater and lesser saphenous veins (short saphenous vein injection)
- ▶ The posterior or medial malleolar regions (injection of internal ankle perforator veins)

TABLE 13-24. PREVENTION OF INTRAARTERIAL INJECTION

Blood aspiration technique
Open-needle technique (Sigg)
Injection of saphenofemoral junction by the sequestration technique 4–5 cm below the saphenofemoral junction (low risk anatomic zone)
Injection of a small test bolus looking for pain propagation (only helpful when hypertonic sclerosants are employed)
Utilization of Doppler needle devices

Prevention

As the treatment options for intraarterial injection are limited in terms of their efficacy, prevention (Table 13-24) in this case is definitely the best approach.

Aspiration of blood to ensure avoidance of intraarterial injection may suggest cannulation of an artery. However, varicose veins may contain highly oxygenated blood, and this maneuver although often helpful, is not always reliable.

The open-needle technique (Sigg technique), where vessels are cannulated under ultrasonic guidance with an open 18-gauge needle without a syringe, produces pulsatile blood flow as an artery is cannulated.

Injection of the saphenofemoral junction utilizing the sequestration technique with injection of the greater saphenous vein 4 to 5 cm below the saphenofemoral junction (a low-risk anatomic zone) may diminish the incidence of inadvertent intraarterial injection in this location.

Rapid distal propagation of pain, as previously stated, may be a useful clinical clue. The initiation of an injection with a small test bolus followed by a period of waiting before completing the injection can be effective in some circumstances. However, any strong hypertonic solution will produce this effect. Agents such as STS and sodium morrhuate cannot be relied upon to produce pain.

Finally, specialized needles containing Doppler devices (Smart Needle, Titronics Medical Instruments, Iowa City, IA, U.S.A.) or colorimetric visualization devices such as those employing piezoelectric crystals (Color Mark System, EchoCath, South Brunswick, NJ, U.S.A.) may help to minimize intraarterial events (see Chapter 14).

Treatment

This acute sclerotherapy emergency, like acute anaphylactic reactions, requires rapid and directed intervention (Table 13-25). A protocol should be in place so that if inadvertent arterial injection does ensue, rapid, efficient intervention will occur. One individual in the office should be designated as team leader and should be responsible for the rapid institution of the following therapeutic measures:

First, if arterial injection is suspected, aspiration of blood and sclerosing solution should be attempted in order to empty the artery as completely and rapidly as possible.

If possible, instillation of 10,000 U of heparin should be instituted through the same needle by means of a change of syringe.

If STS is employed, inactivation may occur by injecting 1% to 3% procaine periarterially.

TABLE 13-25. TREATMENT OF ARTERIAL ULCERATION

- Immediate
  - Aspiration of sclerosant
  - Cooling of limb
  - Arterial and periarterial infiltration with procaine 1% (inactivates sodium tetradecylsulfate)
  - Immediate heparinization, continue for 7–14 days
  - Intravenous dextran, 10%, 500 mg/day × 3 days
  - Hospital access
  - Thrombolytic therapy
    - Streptokinase 250,000–750,000 IU
  - Vasodilators
    - Prazosin
    - Hydralazine
    - Nifedipine
- Subacute
  - Subcutaneous heparin 10,000 U q.a.m.
    15,000 U q.h.s.

Ice immersion of the involved limb may decrease arterial perfusion.

The cornerstone of therapy is felt to be heparinization. The patient should be rapidly transported to a hospital setting where immediate intravenous heparinization should be instituted. This anticoagulation should be carried out for 7 to 14 days.

Intravenous infusion of dextran 10% (Medisan, Parsippany, NJ, U.S.A.) 500 mg/day for 3 days is recommended.

The role of thrombolytic agents such as streptokinase and/or vasodilators such as oral prazosin, hydralazine, or nifedipine may also be considered for 30 to 60 days.

Subcutaneous heparin following intravenous therapy has been suggested to decrease the incidence and severity of cutaneous necrosis.

Despite this long regimen of therapeutic interventions, their role in altering the course of arterial necrosis is questionable. Prevention, as previously stated, is the mainstay of therapy. Surgical debridement is often necessary to eradicate necrotic tissue and minimize the incidence of infection, which is a major source of morbidity in this setting.

Nerve Damage

Nerve damage may occur by one of two mechanisms. The nerve itself may be injected with sclerosant or, alternatively, perivascular inflammation may involve surrounding nerve sheaths.

Usually acute pain is the major presenting symptom. If continued, this pain may lead to hypesthesia and subsequent anesthesia.

TABLE 13-26. PREVENTION OF NERVE DAMAGE

- ► Recognition of anatomic landmarks and avoidance of the saphenous vein and sural nerve

TABLE 13-27. TREATMENT OF NERVE DAMAGE

▶ Nonsteroidal antiinflammatory agents such as ibuprofen (Motrin, Upjohn, Kalamazoo, MI, U.S.A.) 400–800 mg t.i.d.

The saphenous and sural nerves innervating the foot are the most common locations.

Permanent anesthesia, nerve palsy, and weakness have been reported; however, the majority of cases resolve in 6 to 12 weeks.

Prevention

Avoidance of the saphenous and sural nerves in high risk locations is the major mode of prevention (Table 13-26).

Treatment

As previously stated, most cases resolve spontaneously. Antiinflammatory approaches utilizing NSAIDs such as ibuprofen (Table 13-27) may help in shortening the course of inflammation and thus reduce the duration of symptoms.

▶ Conclusion

An astute recognition and understanding of appropriate management alternatives as related to postsclerotherapy complications is of utmost importance to the practicing phlebologist. It must be emphasized in closing this chapter that the prevention of complications by the use of fastidious technique, choice appropriate choice of sclerosant and MSC, and the utilization of adequate compression practices will optimize results and minimize complication profiles in the phlebologist's daily sclerotherapy practice.

BIBLIOGRAPHY

Biegeleisen K, Neilsen RD, O'Shaughnessy A. Inadvertent intra-arterial injection complicating ordinary and ultrasound guided sclerotherapy. *J Dermatol Surg Oncol* 1993;19:953–958.

Davis LT, Duffy DM. Determination of incidence and risk factors for post-sclerotherapy telangiectatic matting of the lower extremities: a retrospective analysis. *J Dermatol Surg Oncol* 1990;16:327–330.

Georgiev M. Post-sclerotherapy hyperpigmentation: a one year follow-up. *J Dermatol Surg Oncol* 1990;16:608–610.

Georgiev M. Post-sclerotherapy hyperpigmentation chromated glycerin as a screen for patients at risk (a retrospective study). *J Dermatol Surg Oncol* 1993;19:649–652.

Goldman MP. Post-sclerotherapy hyperpigmentation: treatment with a flashlamp-excited pulsed dye laser. *J Dermatol Surg Oncol* 1992;18:417–422.

Goldman PM, Kaplan RA, Duffy DM. Post Sclerotherapy hyperpigmentation: a histologic evaluation. *J Dermatol Surg Oncol* 1987;13:547–550.

Goldman MP, Sadick NS, Weiss RA. Cutaneous necrosis, telangiectatic matting and hyperpigmentation following sclerotherapy *Dermatol Surg* 1995;21:19–29.

Leibaschoff G, Brizzio E, Ferreira J, Banf J. Prevention of iatrogenic complications in the treatment of varicosities. *Am J Cosmet Surg* 1994;11:51–53.

Scott C, Selger E. Postsclerotherapy pigmentation: is serum ferritin level an accurate indicator? *Dermatol Surg* 1997;23:281–283.

Thibault P, Wlodarczyk J. Post sclerotherapy hyperpigmentation: the role of serum ferritin levels and the effectiveness of treatment with the copper vapor laser. *J Dermatol Surg Oncol* 1991;18:47–52.

Thibault PK, Wlodarczyk J. Correlation of serum ferritin levels and post-sclerotherapy pigmentation: a prospective study. *J Dermatol Surg Oncol* 1994;20:684–686.

Weiss RA, Weiss MA. Incidence of side effects in the treatment of telangiectasias by compression sclerotherapy: hypertonic saline vs. polidocanol. *J Dermatol Surg Oncol* 1990;16:800–804.

Zimmet SE. The prevention of cutaneous necrosis following extravasation of hypertonic saline and sodium tetradecyl sulfate. *J Dermatol Surg Oncol* 1993;19:641–646.

Zimmet SE. Hyaluronidase in the prevention of sclerotherapy induced extravasation necrosis: a dose response study. *Plastic Surg* 1996;22:73–76.

CHAPTER 14

NEW TECHNIQUES IN THE TREATMENT OF VARICOSE VEINS

A number of new modalities have evolved over the last decade for treating varicose and telangiectatic leg veins.

Although a detailed discussion of these entities is beyond the scope of this book, a basic knowledge and understanding of these procedures is of importance so that the sclerotherapist may refer a patient to a physician skilled in these newer techniques when he or she is unable to treat a particular venous problem utilizing the technologies described in this text. The reader is referred to the bibliography at the end of this chapter for more detailed discussions of the therapeutic entities outlined below.

Lasers/Noncoherent Pulsed Light Sources

Lasers and noncoherent flash-lamp pulsed-light sources have exploded upon the scene for the treatment of lower extremity telangiectasis. To date they have relegated to treatment of small microtelangiectasis noncannulizable by standard microsclerotherapy techniques. Their utilization is based upon the principle of selective photothermolysis, whereby light is selectively absorbed by hemoglobin (577-nm maximal absorption causing theoretical selective penetration to the full depth of the target blood vessel in order to thermocoagulate the entire wall without damaging perivascular tissue or overlying skin). This is accomplished by heating the vessel based upon its selective thermal relaxation time (TRT—time necessary to cool the target in comparison to surrounding tissue—i.e., for a 0.1-mm diameter vessel it is 5 ms). Pulse durations are chosen in order to provide selective gentle heating (Fig. 14-1). It is felt that the optimal laser that would accomplish

TABLE 14-1. LASER/FLASH-LAMP DEVICES FOR TREATMENT OF TELANGIECTASIAS

Manufacturer	Product Name	Laser Type	Wavelength	Energy Output	Pulse Duration	Price	Accessories
Aesculap-Meditec	Pro-Yellow	Diode/copper	511/578 nm	8.5 w	Continuous	$66,900	None
Candela	GentleLase	Alexandrite	755 nm	100 joules	3 ms	$69,500	Dynamic cooling device (cryogen)
	ScleroPLUS	Pulsed dye	up to 600 nm	up to 20 joules	1500 µsec	$99,500	Dynamic cooling device (add $19,500)
	SkinPlus	YAG (KTP)	532 nm	10–15 mJ	Quasi-CW	$89,500	SkinScan
	(KTP Alone)					$79,000	no scanner
Coherent	VersaPulse C	Multiple	1,064 nm	400 mJ	5 ns, 30 ms	$199,000	VersaSpot QS handpiece
			755 nm	450 mJ	45 ns		VersaSpot QS handpiece
			532 nm	200 mJ	4 ns		VersaSpot QS handpiece
	VersaPulse V	Green	532 nm	4,000 mJ	2–50 ms	$125,000	VersaSpot Chilled Tip
Continuum Biomedical	CB Diode/532	DPSS Green	532 nm	2 joules	10–100 ms	$55,000	Optional Scanner
	Medlite IV	Q-SW YAG	1,064/532 nm	up to 8 joules	5–7 ns	$95,000	Handpieces 585 nm (yellow), 650 nm (red), 532 nm, 1,064 nm
	Medlite	Q-SW YAG	1,064/542 nm	up to 12 joules	5–7 ns	$60,000	Safety eyewear handpieces 2 mm 3 mm
Cynosure	LPIR	Alexandrite	755 nm	up to 40 joules	5–10–20 ms	$139,500	
	Illustra	DPSS Green	532 nm		0.2–CW	$45,000	4 watt output
	PhotoGenica V	Dye	585 nm	5–10 joules	300–500 µsec	$89,500	
	PhotoGenica VLS	Dye	585–600 nm	5–20 joules	340–1,500 µsec	$154,500	
Diomed	LaserLite	Diode	810 nm	up to 350 joules	50–250 ms	$77,500	Includes 20 × 24 mm scanner/hair removal also
E.S.C.	MultiLight	Pulsed light	515–1,200 nm	3–90 joules	0.5–25 ms	$139,000	Handpiece: 8 mm × 35 mm
	VascuLight	YAG and pulsed light	1,064 nm 515–1,200 nm	40–150 joules	1–16 ms	$169,000	PhotoDerm upgrade costs $37,500
HGM	Corium 200	DPY	532	up to 3,820 J/cm^2	0–150 ms	$19,950	Smartscan handpiece/hard shell carrying case
	Corium 400	DPY	532	up to 5,730 J/cm^2	0–150 ms	$32,450	Smartscan handpiece/hard shell carrying case
	Spectrum K1	Krypton	520–567 568–575	Green 2W Yellow 1W	Continuous	$51,950	Digital autoscan Concour remote/Smartscan handpiece
	VeinLase	YAG	1,064/532 nm	5kW peak power in capt pulse	0.008–0.05 ms in captured pulse	$89,950	Spot size (collimated): 2 mm and 4 mm Concour remote/Smartscan handpiece
Iriderm	Diolite 532	DPSS Green	532 nm	up to 3W	1–100 ms	$44,500	Scanlite: optional, comes with 5 spot size handpieces, seymour light head set, carry-all case, safety glasses, patient goggles
Laserscope	Aura	KTP	532 nm	1–999 joules	1–50 ms	$49,000	StarPulse; DermaStats 1- ,2- , and 4 mm; SmartScan
Nidek	Prima KTP 532	YAG	532 nm	up to 990 joules	3 to 700 ms & CW	$42,500	PrimaScan pattern generator/optional

Note: Energy is expressed as fluence which varies with spot size. All lasers are approved for sale.

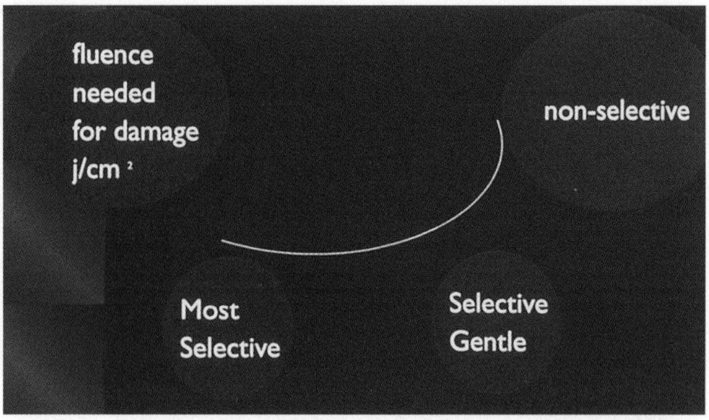

Figure 14-1

The effect of pulse duration is shown. Laser and flash-lamp approaches to lower extremity telangiectasias are based on the principle of selective endothelial heating of a target chromophore "hemoglobin." By treating the target (hemoglobin) selectively, based upon its thermal relaxation time, one may achieve gentle cavitation of the target tissue (blood vessel) while sparing the epidermis.

these goals is one with a wavelength spectrum of 800 to 1000 nm, a pulse duration of 50 to 100 ms and a spot size of 8 mm and up. These parameters will provide gentle cavitation, avoid hemorrhage, and allow epidermal temperature clamping in order to allow adequate thermal damage for vessels greater than 0.1 mm in diameter.

Lasers and flash-lamp sources of proven efficacy presently available to accomplish these goals are listed in Table 14-1.

As can be seen in Fig. 14-2A to D, each of these techniques can produce excellent results in selected cases. The problems associated with laser/flash-lamp treatment of lower extremity veins include the following:

1. *Multiple treatments.* Usually an average two to three of treatments will be necessary to produce complete clearing of a given treatment area utilizing all of the modalities mentioned above, which must be explained during the initial patient consultation.

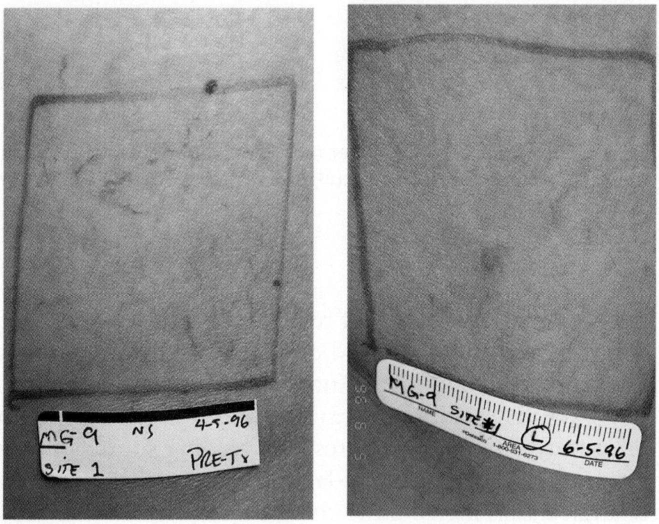

A

Figure 14-2

Pre/post treatment of lower extremity telangiectasias (1 to 2 mm in diameter) utilizing: A: Photoderm 500 to 1200 nm flash lamp (pre/posttreatment). (*Figure continues.*)

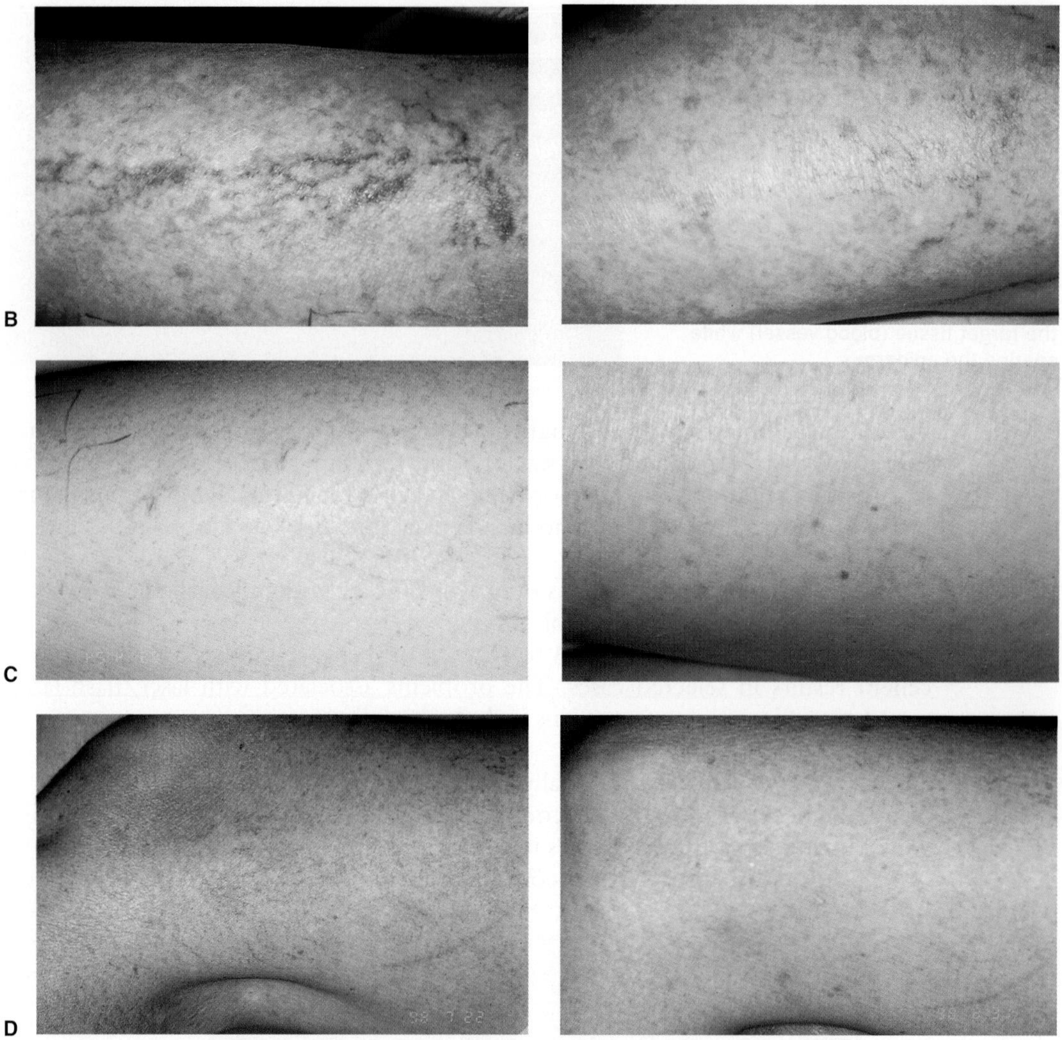

Figure 14-2 (continued)

B: Sclerolaser 595 to 600 nm pulsed dye laser (pre/posttreatment). **C:** Versapulse 532 green light laser (pre/posttreatment). **D:** Vasculight 1064-nm Nd:YAG infrared laser (pre/posttreatment).

2. *Inconsistent results.* Lack of reliable results may occur with each of the above modalities in selected cases due to the inherent characteristics of the various technologies. Another major cause of failure to achieve adequate results is failure to treat feeding sources of reflux by sclerotherapy prior to treating the small residual feeding source of telangiectasia.
3. *Cost factor.* Laser and flash-lamp sources utilized in the treatment of telangiectasias increase the cost of treatments. In general, when effective, sclerotherapy yield a greater and more reliable source of results form a cost effective point of view.

4. *Hyperpigmentation.* May occur in up to 10% of patients treated with laser and flash-lamp modalities. This is related to the increased hydrostatic pressure noted in the lower extremities and, as expected, is more common in Fitzpatrick skin types IV to VI.
5. *Epidermal surface changes.* Again, this may occur in 1% to 3% of patients treated with any of the above modalities and is related to factors discussed in the following section. Unfortunately, as compared with vascular therapy of the face, we have not been able to achieve the same degree of selective photothermolysis and epidermal bypass in treating the venous system of the lower extremity.
6. *Purpura.* Prolonged erythema is also noted in up to 33% of patients treated with the above modalities. True purpura is most commonly noted with pulsed dye laser modalities (i.e., ScleroLASER, Candela Corp., Wayland, MA, U.S.A.); however, it may be noted with other green light and intense pulsed light sources as well.
7. *Patient expectations.* Patients have come to expect medical miracles from laser technology. In the treatment of lower extremity vessels with laser and intense light source therapy, results have been less consistent and associated with more recurrences than with similar treatment of other cosmetic problems. Keeping patients properly informed as to what they may realistically expect will help to avoid later problems and disappointments.

There are four major reasons, in the author's opinion, why we have not been able to achieve consistent results with laser/pulsed light source treatment of leg veins, including the poorer results associated with treatment of larger diameter vessels (i.e., those greater than 3 to 4 mm in diameter). First, there is the deeper location of lower extremity vessels. As compared with the face, true total selective photothermolysis does not occur in the lower extremity as some energy is absorbed by the epidermis and superficial dermis, accounting for the higher-than-expected incidence of prolonged erythema, purpura, hyperpigmentation, and epidermal skin changes noted after laser/flash-lamp treatments.

Second, the increased hydrostatic pressure noted in the vasculature of the lower extremity also leads to more inconsistent total obliteration of the total vessel, frequent recurrences, and pigment dyschromia. Third, the vessels of the lower extremity have deeper basal lamina than those of the face, making it more difficult for laser/flashlamp light to get through and to obliterate the vessel. A fourth theoretic consideration is the altered cytokine pattern noted upon injury to lower extremity vessels.

In spite of these above issues, laser and flash-lamp light source treatment of lower extremity telangiectasia remains an exciting new area of phlebology research, as the alternatives for treating vessels that are noncannulizable with standard 30-gauge sclerotherapy needles are minimal. These include, as stated in Chapter 4, microsclerotherapy needles (i.e., insulin, tuberculosis, or disposable 31- to 33-gauge needles or microangiocaths (STD, Hereford, England; Kawasumi Lab, Tampa, FL, U.S.A.). In the setting of these small linear, noncannulizable vessels, lasers and flash lamps will play an increasing role in the future. Prospects for improving the technology of laser/flash-lamp treatment of the lower extremity include the delivery of high energies via dynamic cooling devices, as established by Candela (Wayland, MA, U.S.A.) (extended pulse duration dye laser) and ESC (Photoderm,

Needham, MA, U.S.A.) utilizing a nonozone cryogen attachment mechanism and by the Coherent Versapulse System (Coherent, Santa Ana, CA, U.S.A.), where water-cooled tips are employed.

The establishment of improved laser/flash-lamp parameters will also improve results and perhaps eventually allow treatment of larger-diameter vessels. One such advancement is the extended 50-ms pulse duration achieved with the Coherent Versapulse 532 nm green light laser (Coherent, Santa Ana, CA, U.S.A.) and the 1064 Nd:YAG technology for treating larger-diameter vessels (i.e., reticular veins Vasulight E.S.C, Veinlase HGM, Salt Lake City, UT, U.S.A.). Finally, improved technology will hopefully allow the achievement of more consistent results with lower side-effect profiles and capabilities for treating larger-diameter vessels.

Ambulatory Phlebectomy

Ambulatory phlebectomy is a minor office procedure for the complete removal of primary or secondary varicose veins. It involves removal of diseased venous segments by hook avulsion. All superficial veins with the exception of the groin termination of the long saphenous vein (LSV) can be avulsed easily by this technique (Table 14-2). Large veins, particularly well-demarcated branches of the greater or lesser saphenous veins or perforators, can be avulsed through microstab incisions. The thigh (i.e., anteromedial or posterolateral branches of the greater saphenous vein) is a good place for the beginner to initially implement this technique.

Preoperative Considerations

Doppler/photoplesythmography (PPG) and duplex ultrasound studies are necessary in order to confirm the competency of the saphenofemoral and saphenopopliteal junctions as well as that of the deep venous system.

TABLE 14-2. INDICATIONS FOR AMBULATORY PHLEBECTOMY

1. Side branches of the long saphenous (vein medial and lateral accessory veins posterior and anterior arch veins)
2. Isolated varicose veins of the dorsal foot, ankle, or popliteal region
3. Pudendal and vulvar varicosities
4. Insufficient perforating veins (e.g., popliteal)
5. Complementary procedure after crossectomy with or without stripping of the long or short saphenous vein
6. Varicosities draining leg ulcers
7. Reticular veins
8. Reticular veins feeding nets of telangiectasia
9. Telangiectasias in difficult-to-treat anatomic areas
10. Vein biopsy (inflammatory venous disease)
11. Facial telangiectasia

Preoperative Mapping

The varicose veins to be excised are marked with an indelible pen with the patient in a standing position. This technique is augmented by palpation of the veins just prior to marking (Fig. 14-3). Marking of appropriate venous segments will lead to facilitation and success of the procedure. Because of potential shift of veins up to 3 to 4 cm from an upright vertical or a transverse horizontal position, confirmation of venous position either by Doppler or transepidermal illumination (venoscopy), as previously described (Venoscope, Applied Biotech Products, Inc., Lafayette, LA, U.S.A.) may be helpful in overcoming this positional shift (Fig. 14-4).

Technique

Tumescent anesthesia has several advantages in performing ambulatory phlebectomy because it

- Eliminates multiple needle sticks
- Allows rapid anesthesia of extensive segments of diseased veins
- Produces temporary swelling and firmness of soft tissue, thus aiding vein removal by pressing the vein against the skin, which makes it easier to locate and hook
- Reduces blood loss
- Diminishes bruising
- Allows greater patient comfort over a larger period of time

Preanesthesia may be accomplished by any of the following options:

Diazepam 5 to 10 mg p.o.
Hydroxyzine hydrochloride 50 mg i.m.
Meperidine hydrochloride 50 mg i.m.
Promethazine hydrochloride 25 mg i.m.
Triazolam 0.25 mg p.o.

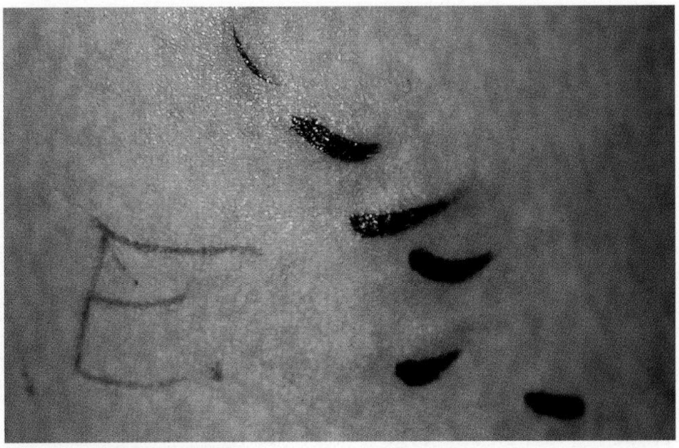

Figure 14-3
Marking of a proposed, potentially avulsed venous segment is performed with the patient in a standing position after appropriate palpation of diseased segments.

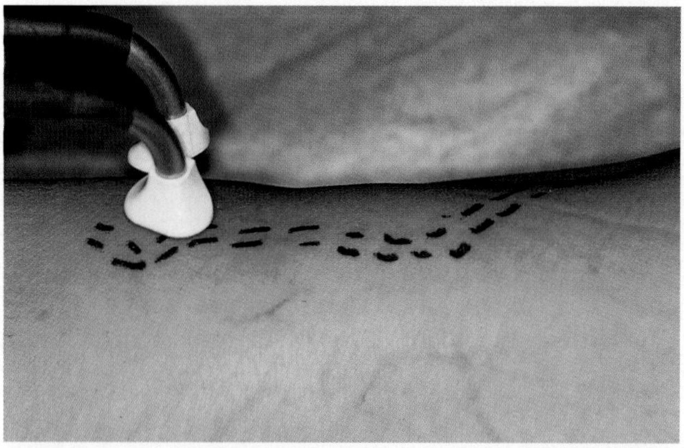
A

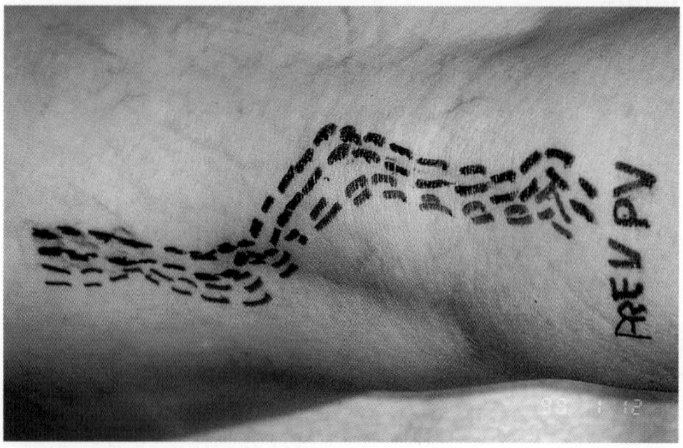
B

Figure 14-4

Transillumination (venoscopy) (Applied Biotech Products Inc., Lafayette, LA, U.S.A.) performed with the patient in a horizontal position (**A**) may reveal a shift of up to 3 to 4 mm of previously vertically marked venous segments. (**B**), which helps to facilitate the hooking of veins after infiltration with tumescent anesthesia.

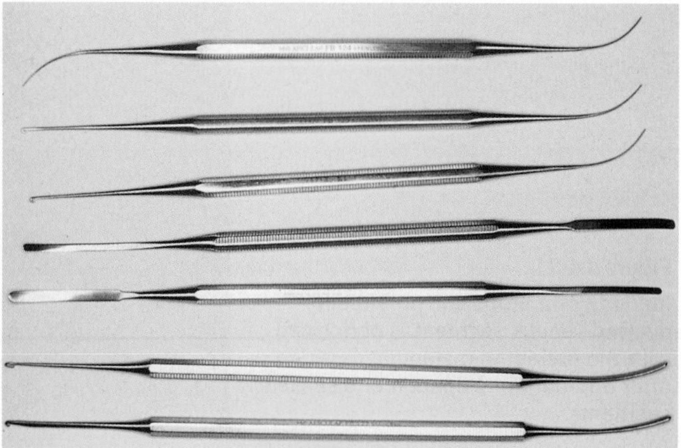

Figure 14-5

Assortment of phlebectomy hooks available for ambulatory phlebectomy procedure (available in small-, medium-, and large-diameters).

TABLE 14-3. INSTRUMENTATION FOR AMBULATORY PHLEBECTOMY

Sheet, 5 × 3 feet
Two fenestrated drapes
Sizes 2–4 phlebectomy hooks
Black-handled scissors
Bard Parker #11 blade (Becton Dickenson Acute Care, Franklin Lakes, NJ, U.S.A.)
Graefe iridectomy forceps (George Tiemann Inc., Hauppauge, NY, U.S.A.)
Mosquito clamp (hemostatic forceps)
Blunt-pointed probe
Gauze (4 × 4) (PSS, Plainview, NY, U.S.A.)
Kling mesh dressing (Johnson & Johnson, Piscataway, NJ, U.S.A.)
Betadine solution (PSS, Plainview, NY, U.S.A.)
Q-tips (PSS, Plainview, NY, U.S.A.)
10-mL syringes
20-mL syringes
18-gauge needles
16-gauge needles

The recipe for tumescent anesthesia for ambulatory phlebectomy (0.05%) is as follows:

Lidocaine 500 mg (50 mL of 1% lidocaine solution)
Epinephrine 1 mg (1 mL of 1:1000 solution)
Sodium bicarbonate 12.5 mEq (12.5 mL of an 8.4% $NaHCO_3$ solution)

Anesthesia is accomplished most easily by means of a peristaltic pump (i.e., the Klein pump), with pump settings at 2.0 to 7.0 and infusion rates 25 to 500 mL/min.

Instrumentation (Fig. 14-5) for the ambulatory phlebectomy procedure involves the use of a number of varied hook devices (small, medium, and large in di-

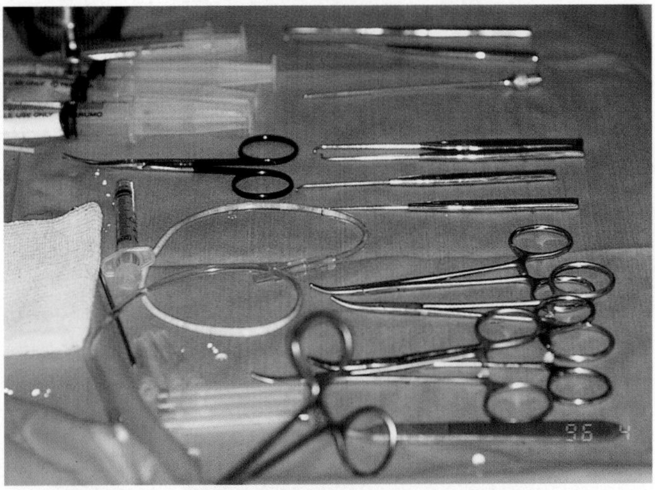

Figure 14-6
Pictorial view of the ambulatory phlebectomy setup tray.

ameter); sizes 2 to 4 are available from various manufacturers (Venosan, Houston, TX, U.S.A.; Bernsco, Seattle, WA, U.S.A.).

Phlebectomy hooks are manufactured by Müeller, Oesch, Ramlet, and Millet.

Several variants, including Varaday hooks, have tissue dissectors at one end which allow separation of vessels from underlying fascial attachments. Other instrumentation for the procedure is outlined in Table 14-3 and shown in Fig. 14-6.

"Micro" incisions measuring from 0.5 to 4 mm in length and parallel to the long axis of the extremity are made by an 18- or 16-gauge hypodermic needle. The vein is then delivered utilizing the phlebectomy hook. The exteriorized vein is then clamped proximally and distally and then either pushed or pulled, depending on operator preference, from each end until the vein is avulsed. A gentle rotation or rolling motion of the clamp in the same and/or opposite direction pulls and frees the vein from its secondary connective tissue sheath (Fig. 14-7A to D). The process is repeated every 3 to 5 mm along the length of the marked vein until the entire vein has been removed or adequate interruptions have been made. Bleeding is controlled with local pressure (Fig. 14-8A to C).

Postoperative Procedures

Postoperatively the area is cleansed. Antibiotic ointment and nonstick dressings are applied to the puncture sites and cotton padding is placed over the length of

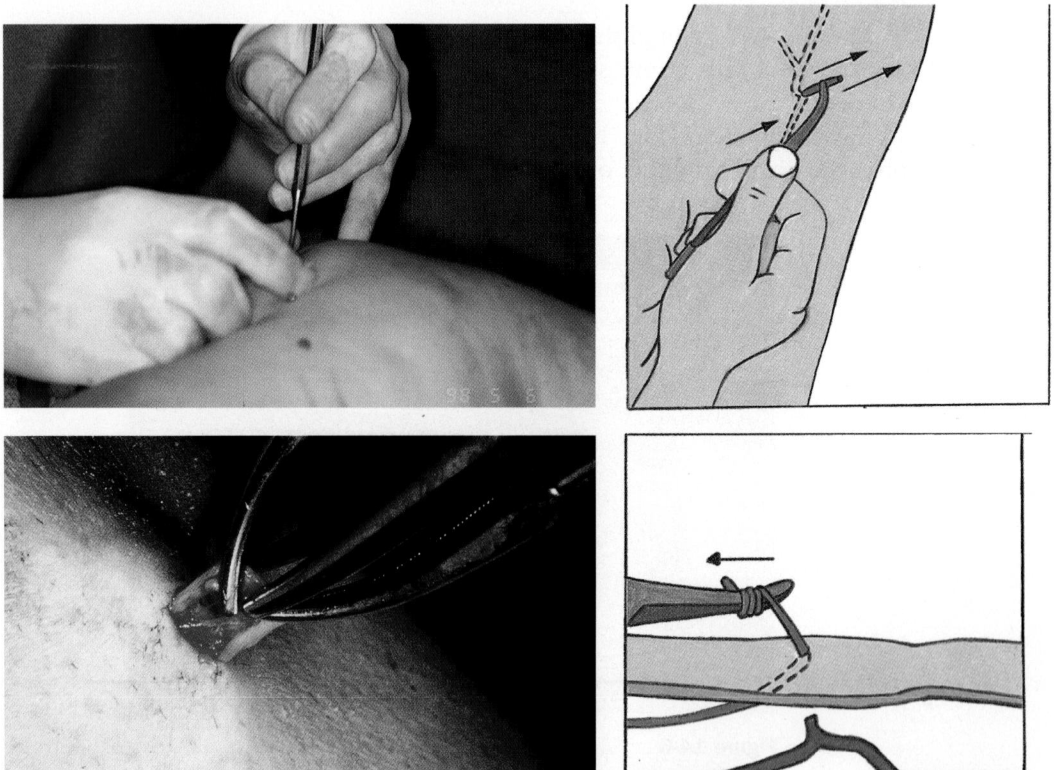

A

B

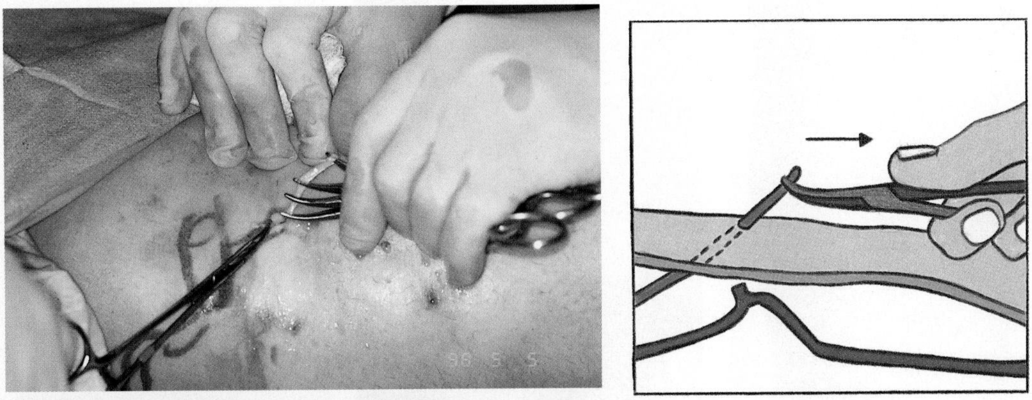

C

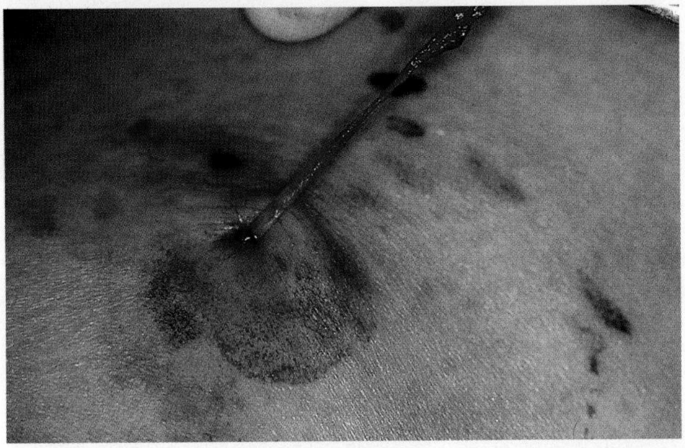

D

Figure 14-7

A: Hooking (venous segment with upward traction). **B:** Vein is then pulled and rolled to free it from surrounding connective tissue adventitial attachment. **C:** Successive clamping of the hooked vessel with a concomitant pushing or pulling motion allows avulsion of longer venous segments. **D:** Procedure continues until the diseased vein is broken free from the normal venous segment.

the surgical site (Fig. 14-9). The leg is then wrapped first with cotton gauze and then with an elastic compression dressing extending from the dorsum of the foot to the groin. This dressing helps to promote hemostasis, to reduce swelling of the foot and leg, and to speed wound healing (Fig. 14-10).

Walking is encouraged while the patient is still in the office to help mold the pressure wrap, so that the patient quickly returns to a fairly normal gait, thus generating normal function of the calf muscle pump. The week following surgery, the patient returns to the office for removal of the surgical dressing.

Major reported complications of the ambulatory phlebectomy procedure are less than 3%. These adverse sequelae are listed in Table 14-4.

Echosclerotherapy

Echo-guided sclerotherapy (EGS) is a treatment modality that increases the precision of sclerotherapy injection. It is beneficial in treating high-risk sites such as the saphenofemoral junction, saphenopopliteal junction, and retromalleolar area. It is also helpful for treating perforating veins, recurrent varicosities, and dilated veins associated with ulcerations. Finally, it can facilitate the treatment of obese patients and those with previous varicose vein surgical procedures, in whom administration of a sclerosant might otherwise be difficult.

A-C

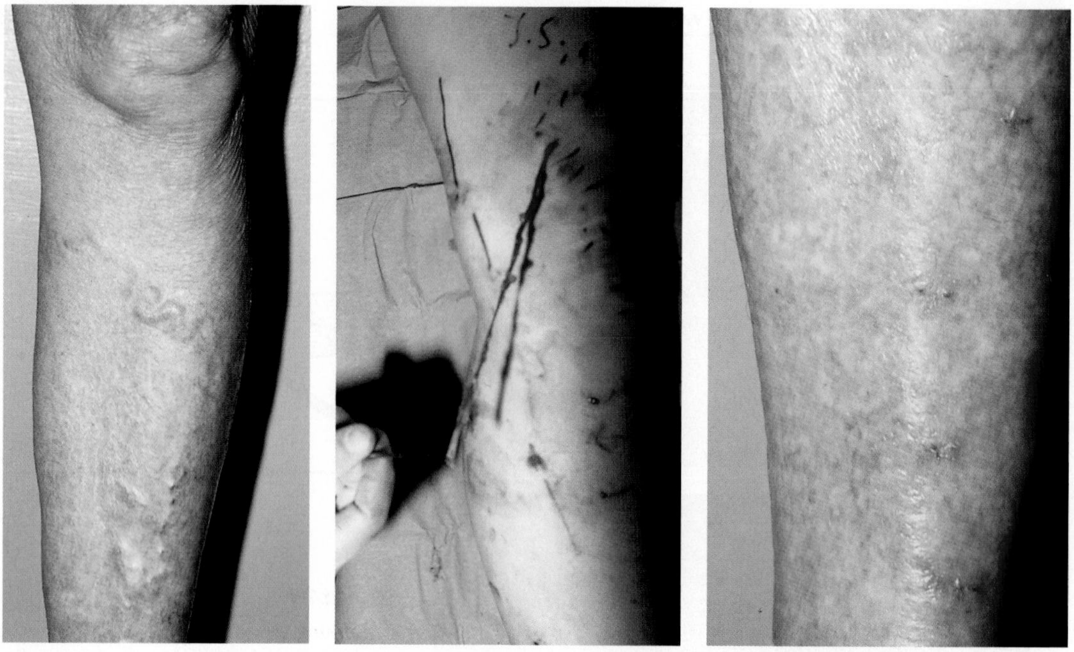

Figure 14-8

A: Preoperative ambulatory phlebectomy of a pretibial truncal varicosity. **B:** Interoperative avulsion of a long segment of diseased varicosity with a "pulling tension" maneuver. **C:** One week after ambulatory phlebectomy with total resolution of diseased segment of pretibial truncal varicosity.

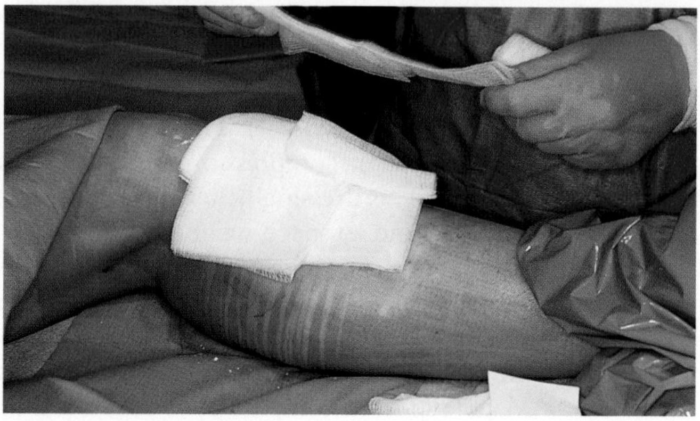

Figure 14-9

After ambulatory phlebectomy, antibiotic ointment and a nonstick dressing is applied to the puncture sites and cotton padding is placed over the length of the extremity.

TABLE 14-4. REPORTED COMPLICATIONS OF AMBULATORY PHLEBECTOMY

Blister formation
Infection
Bleeding
Temporary anesthesia
Lymphocoele
Localized superficial phlebitis
Telangiectatic matting
Pigmentation
Skin necrosis
Hematoma
Local anesthesia overdose

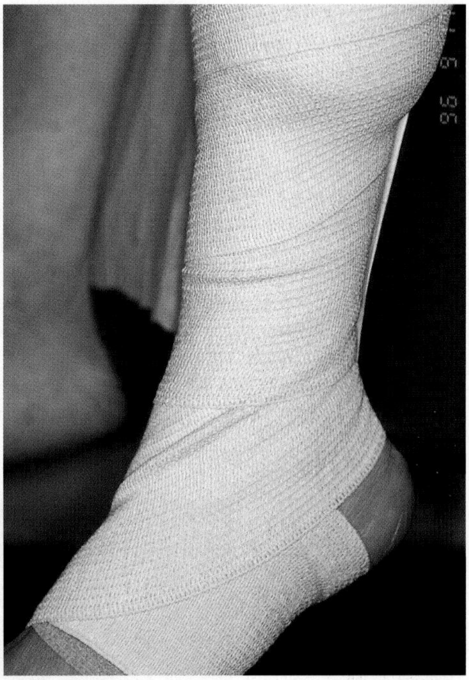

Figure 14-10
After placement of cotton gauze, Kling (Johnson & Johnson, Piscataway, NJ, U.S.A.) application the surgical limb is wrapped with an elastic compression dressing extending from the dorsum of the foot to the groin.

This procedure will ensure intravascular localization of sclerosant, particularly in difficult-to-treat anatomic locations (i.e., the saphenofemoral junction, veins that are impalpable when the patient is standing—even more so supine—and veins in obese individuals. By allowing direct visualization of the target vein, this approach prevents accidental extravascular, intraarterial, or deep venous injection and allows the minimal effective dose of sclerosants to be administered safely and accurately (Table 14-5).

Instrumentation

During sclerotherapy, echographic guidance may be obtained with instruments positioned either outside or inside the target vein.

Doppler-Guided Injections

This technique is utilized predominantly when vessels are present and palpable with the patient standing but impalpable in a supine position or impalpable but percussable in the standing position (Fig. 14-11). Injections are made with the Doppler transducer held adjacent to the injection target zone, directing the course of sclerosant instillation (Fig. 14-12).

Duplex Echography

The simplest means of duplex echographic guidance is gray-scale duplex echography, which targets sites of blood, localizes reflux, and clarifies the vessel's path-

TABLE 14-5. INDICATIONS FOR ECHOSCLEROTHERAPY

Varicose Vein	Clinical	Guide by Continuous-Wave Doppler	Duplex Ultrasound
Visiblé and palpable standing and supine	Yes	Unnecessary	Unnecessary
Palpable standing and impalpable supine	No	Yes	Unnecessary
Impalpable but percussable standing	No	Yes	Yes
Impalpable standing (even more so supine)	No	No	Yes

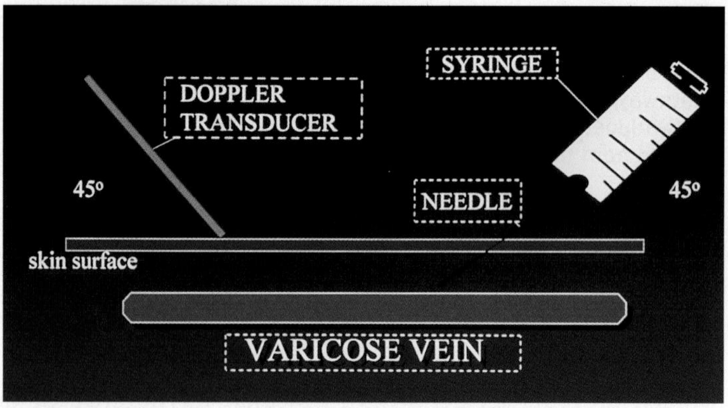

Figure 14-11

Schemata of Doppler transducer angled at 45 degrees with the needle pointed at an echogenically diagnosed varicosity.

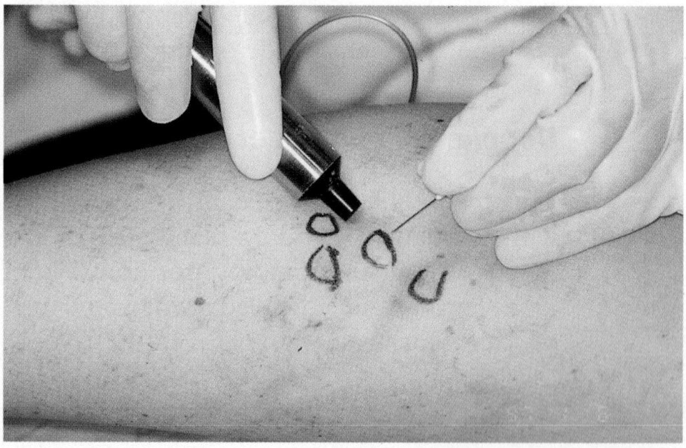

Figure 14-12

Clinical Doppler guidance of perforator vein injection. Note angulation of both continuous-wave Doppler and injecting needle of microcannula.

way. This approach combines (a) pulsed-wave Doppler ultrasonography and (b) real-time high-resolution gray-scale B-mode imaging (Fig. 14-13).

Color-Flow Doppler Imaging

This method adds colored imaging in the B-mode scan. The color changes from red to blue depending on whether blood is flowing toward or away from the transducer.

Intravenous echography

This technique yields two-dimensional cross-sectional images of intramural and extramural architecture. A disposable catheter containing a high-resolution 20- or 25-mHz ultrasound transducer allows a catheter to be introduced through either an 18-gauge needle or an introducer/dilator set with a side arm.

This technique allows immediate assessment of the vein's reaction to the instillation of sclerosant.

Improved Needle Visualization Techniques

Echosclerotherapy has been improved by the new adjuvant techniques. With the Smart Needle, visualization is enhanced by a Doppler probe incorporated into the needle's tip (Fig. 14-14). The probe is used to guide the needle toward the target vein or to confirm proper positioning within the vessel. In the other modification (the Color Mark System), the needle's location is indicated by a line of color generated by piezoelectrically induced flexural waves (Fig. 14-15).

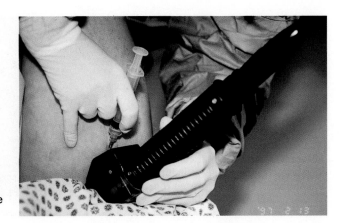

Figure 14-13

Duplex-guided injection of the saphenofemoral junction.

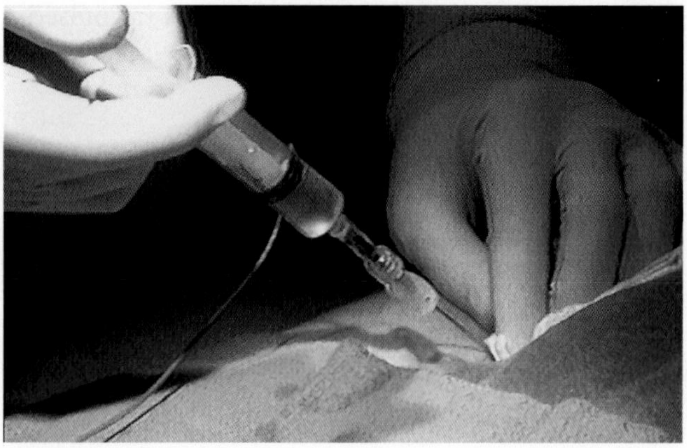

Figure 14-14
Smart Needle with Doppler probe in its tip. The operator differentiates audible sound produced by blood flow in arteries and veins. (Courtesy of Pauline Raymond Martimbeau.)

Technique of Echosclerotherapy

1. The length of the needle depends on the depth of the veins to be punctured.
2. Use of a catheter can increase the safety of the procedure.
3. Echosclerotherapy can be done with either duplex or B-mode scanning.
4. A 7- to 10-mHz probe should be used.

Venous Intravascular Coagulation

Venous obliteration utilizing intravascular monopolar electrocautery has been utilized to treat truncal varicosities in patients undergoing ligation of the saphenofemoral junction (Fig. 14-16).

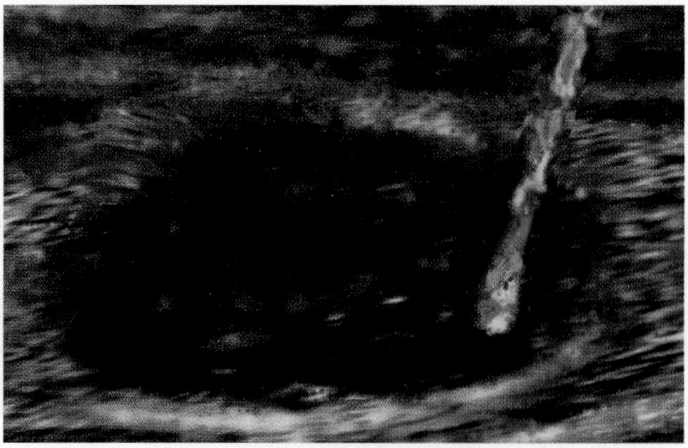

Figure 14-15
The Color Mark provides enhancement of needle visualization. It utilizes piezoelectric technology to induce micron-sized flexural waves in the needle. (Courtesy of Pauline Raymond Martimbeau.)

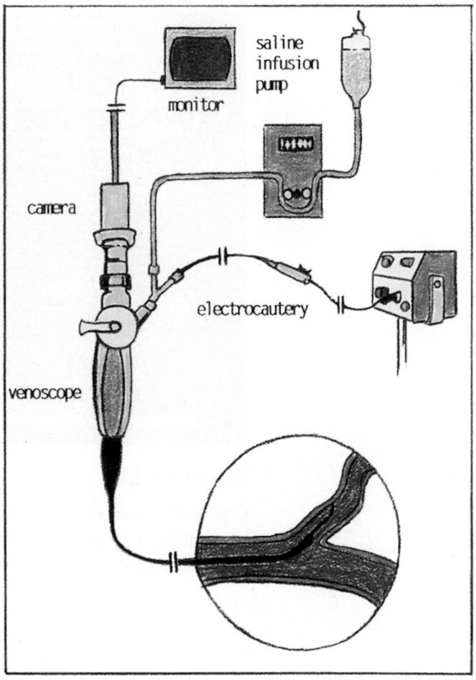

Figure 14-16
Diagrammatic representation of venoscopic electrocautery procedure for venous obliteration.

Some 55% of patients have significant improvement with this procedure.
33% of patients require no further sclerotherapy or ambulatory phlebectomy procedures.

Cryosurgery of Varicose Veins

An endovascular cryosurgical probe (−80°C) has been used to treat the long and short saphenous veins following classic ligation and interruption procedures.

A recurrence rate of 25% to 30% is felt to be compatible with classic surgery/stripping procedures.

The major sequela of this procedure is hyperpigmentation (55%) most cases of which clear within 6 months. Localized hematomas are noted in 10% of cases (Fig. 14-17).

Endovenous Shrinkage Utilizing Radiofrequency Heating

Known as the closure procedure, this incorporates bipolar electrodes to heat the vein wall by radiofrequency waves (Fig. 14-18). The electrodes collapse when the vein shrinks. Endothelial denudation with denaturation of the media and intramural collagen leads to a subsequent fibrotic seal of the vein lumen (Fig. 14-19A to C).

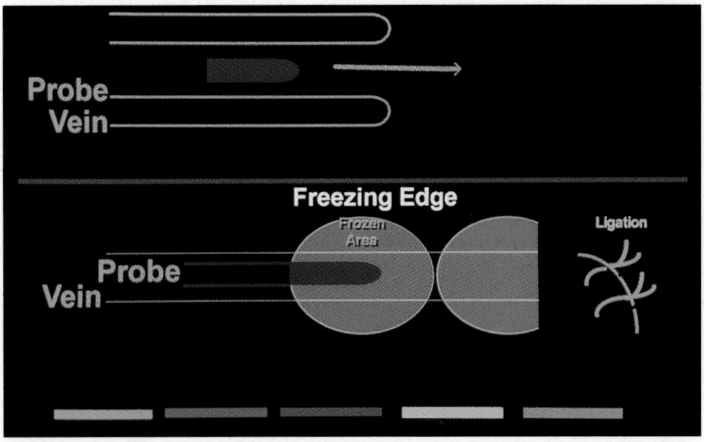

Figure 14-17

Cryosurgery of varicose veins utilizing an endovascular −80°C cryosurgical probe leads to permanent obliteration of truncal varicosities in approximately 75% of treated patients with truncal varicosities.

Conclusion

An array of new technologic advances has expanded the therapeutic armamentarium of the practicing phlebologist. Exciting new techniques will no doubt continue to evolve as we approach the millennium, leading to improved patient care in the treatment of venous disease.

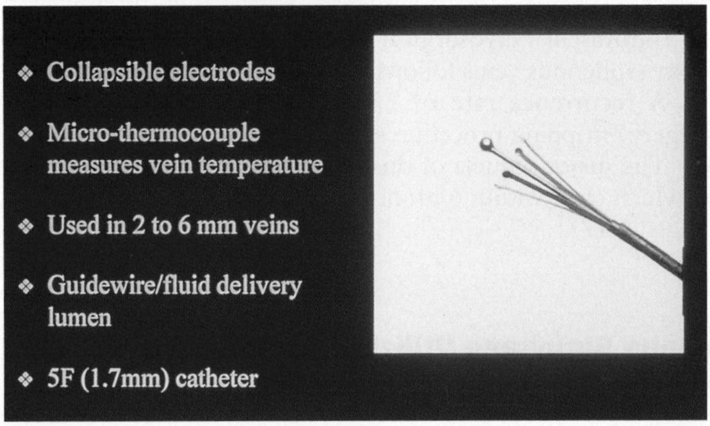

Figure 14-18

Radiofrequency bipolar electrode catheters (Closure catheter) can heat veins up to 70°C, producing collagen denaturation and subsequent endovascular fibrosis. (Courtesy of Robert Weiss, M.D.)

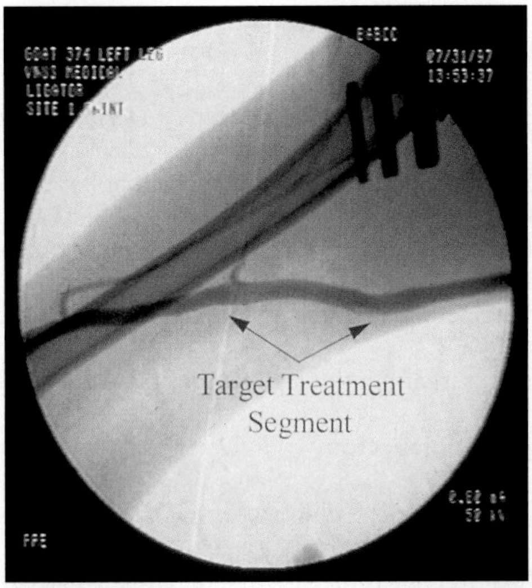

A

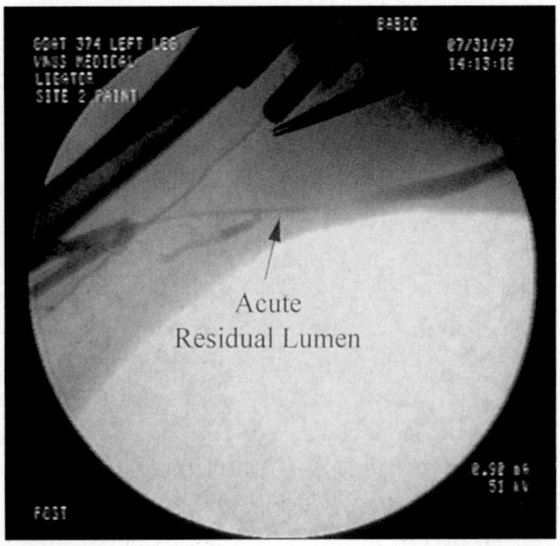

B

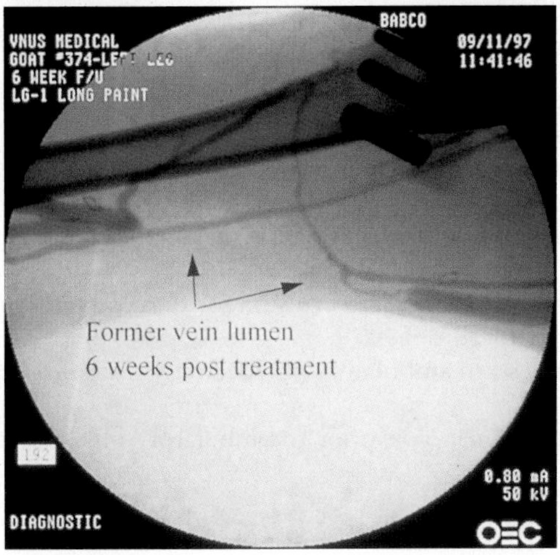

C

Figure 14-19

Animal study of endovenous vein shrinkage technique utilizing (closure) radiofrequency catheter. A: Pretreatment vein diameter, 8 mm. B: After treatment, vein is closed. C: Vein 6 weeks after treatment. (Courtesy Robert Weiss, M.D.)

BIBLIOGRAPHY

Adrian RM. Treatment of leg telangiectasias using a long pulse frequency *Dermatol Surg* 1998;24:19–23.

Bakst AA. Micro multi-vein incisions for the treatment of spider telangiectasia. *Am J Cosmet Surg* 1994;11:139–141.

Chess C, Chess Q. Cool laser optics treatment of large telangiectasia of lower extremities. *J Derm Surg Oncol* 1993;19:74–80.

Cornu-Thenard A, DeCottreau H, Weiss RA. Sclerotherapy continuous wave Doppler-guided injections. *Dermatol Surg* 1995;21:867–870.

Fratila A, Rabe E, Kreysel HW. Percutaneous minisurgical phlebectomy. *Semin Dermatol* 1993;12:117–122.

Garde C. Ambulatory phlebectomy. *Dermatol Surg* 1995;21:628–630.

Garde C. Cryosurgery of varicose veins. *J Dermatol Surg Oncol* 1994;20:56–58.

Georgiev M, Ricci S, Carbone D, Antignani P, Moliterno G. Stab avulsion of the short saphenous vein technique and Duplex evaluation. *J Dermatol Surg Oncol* 1993;19:456–468.
Goldman MP, Eckhimse S. Photothermal sclerosis of leg veins. *Dermatol Surg* 1996;22:323–330.
Gradman WS. Venoscopic obliteration of variceal tributaries using monopolar electrocautery. *J Dermatol Surg Oncol* 1994;20:482–485.
Hsia J, Lavery JA, Zelickson B. Treatment of leg telangiectasia using a long-pulse dye laser at 595 nm. *Lasers Surg Med* 1997;20:1–5.
Kanter A, Thibault P. Saphenofemoral incompetence treated by ultrasound-guided sclerotherapy. *Dermatol Surg* 1996;22:648–652.
Kienle A, Hibst R. Optimal parameters for laser treatment of leg telangiectasia. *Lasers Surg Med* 1997;20:346–353.
Neumann HAM. Ambulant minisurgical phlebectomy. *J Dermatol Surg Oncol* 1992;18:53–54.
Olivencia JA. Maneuver to facilitate ambulatory phlebectomy. *Dermatol Surg* 1996;22:654–655.
Olivencia JA. Complications of ambulatory phlebectomy: review of 1000 consecutive cases. *Dermatol Surg* 1997;23:51–54.
Ramelet AA. Complications of ambulatory phlebectomy. *Dermatol Surg* 1997;23:941–954.
Raymond-Martimbeau P. Advanced sclerotherapy treatment of varicose veins with duplex ultrasound guidance. *Semin Dermatol* 1993;12:123–128.
Ramelet AA. Muller phlebectomy—a new phlebectomy hook. *J Dermatol Surg Oncol* 1991;17:814–816.
Ricci S. Ambulatory phlebectomy—principles and evolution of the method. *Dermatol Surg* 1998;24:459–464.
Sadick NS, Schanzer H. Combined high ligation and stab avulsion for varicose veins in an out-patient setting. *Dermatol Surg* 1998;28:475–479.
Smith S, Goldman MP. Tumescent anesthesia in ambulatory phlebectomy. *Dermatol Surg* 1995;21:628–630.
Weiss RA, Goldman MP. Transillumination mapping prior to ambulatory phlebectomy. *Dermatol Surg* 1998;24:447–450.

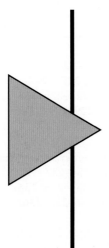

Subject Index

Page numbers followed by *f* refer to figures. Page numbers followed by *t* refer to tables.

R